TRANSLATIONS SERIES IN MATHEMATICS AND ENGINEERING

M.I. Yadrenko
Spectral Theory of Random Fields
1983, viii + 259 pp.
ISBN 0-911575-00-6 Optimization Software, Inc.
ISBN 0-387-90823-4 Springer-Verlag New York Berlin Heidelberg Tokyo
ISBN 3-540-90823-4 Springer-Verlag Berlin Heidelberg New York Tokyo

G.I. Marchuk
Mathematical Models In Immunology
1983, xxv + 353 pp.
ISBN 0-911575-01-4 Optimization Software, Inc.
ISBN 0-387-90901-X Springer-Verlag New York Berlin Heidelberg Tokyo
ISBN 3-540-90901-X Springer-Verlag Berlin Heidelberg New York Tokyo

A.A. Borovkov, Ed.
Advances In Probability Theory: Limit Theorems and Related Problems
1984, xiv + 378 pp.
ISBN 0-911575-03-0 Optimization Software, Inc.
ISBN 0-387-90945-1 Springer-Verlag New York Berlin Heidelberg Tokyo
ISBN 3-540-90945-1 Springer-Verlag Berlin Heidelberg New York Tokyo

V.A. Dubovitskij
The Ulam Problem of Optimal Motion of Line Segments
1985, xiv + 114 pp.
ISBN 0-911575-04-9 Optimization Software, Inc.
ISBN 0-387-90946-X Springer-Verlag New York Berlin Heidelberg Tokyo
ISBN 3-540-90946-X Springer-Verlag Berlin Heidelberg New York Tokyo

N.V. Krylov, R.S. Liptser, and A.A. Novikov, Eds.
Statistics and Control of Stochastic Processes
1985, xiv + 507 pp.
ISBN 0-911575-18-9 Optimization Software, Inc.
ISBN 0-387-96101-1 Springer-Verlag New York Berlin Heidelberg Tokyo
ISBN 0-540-96101-1 Springer-Verlag Berlin Heidelberg New York Tokyo

Yu. G. Evtushenko
Numerical Optimization Techniques
1985, xiv + 561 pp.
ISBN 0-911575-07-3 Optimization Software, Inc.
ISBN 0-387-90949-4 Springer-Verlag New York Berlin Heidelberg Tokyo
ISBN 3-540-90949-4 Springer-Verlag Berlin Heidelberg New York Tokyo

Continued on page 381

VISTAS IN APPLIED MATHEMATICS

Vistas in Applied Mathematics

Numerical Analysis
Atmospheric Sciences
Immunology

Edited by
A.V. Balakrishnan
A.A. Dorodnitsyn
J.L. Lions

Optimization Software, Inc.
Publications Division, New York

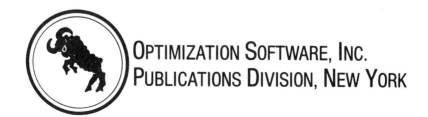

Editors

A.V. Balakrishnan
School of Engineering
University of California
Los Angeles, CA, U.S.A.

A.A. Dorodnitsyn
Director
Computing Center
The USSR Academy of Sciences
Moscow, U.S.S.R.

J.L. Lions
Collège de France
Paris, France

Library of Congress Cataloging-in-Publication Data

Vistas in applied mathematics.

"This volume is dedicated to Gurij Ivanovich Marchuk on the occasion of his 60th birthday."
Bibliography: p.
1. Numerical analysis. 2. Atmosphere—Mathematical models. 3. Immunology—Mathematical models.
I. Balakrishnan, A.V. II. Dorodnitsyn, Anatolii Alekseevich, 1910– . III. Lions, Jacques Louis.
IV. Marchuk, G. I. (Gurii Ivanovich), 1925–
QA297.V47 1986 519.4 86–8340
ISBN 0–911575–38–3

Published 1986. Printed in the United States of America.

Worldwide Distribution Rights by Springer–Verlag New York Inc., 175 Fifth Avenue, New York, New York 10010, U.S.A. and Springer–Verlag Berlin Heidelberg New York Tokyo, Heidelberg Platz 3, Berlin–Wilmersdorf–33, The Federal Republic of Germany.

ISBN 0–911575–38–3 Optimization Software, Inc., Publications Division
ISBN 0–387–96376–6 Springer–Verlag New York Berlin Heidelberg Tokyo
ISBN 3–540–96376–6 Springer–Verlag Berlin New York Heidelberg Tokyo

This volume is dedicated
to Gurij Ivanovich Marchuk
on the occasion of his
60th birthday

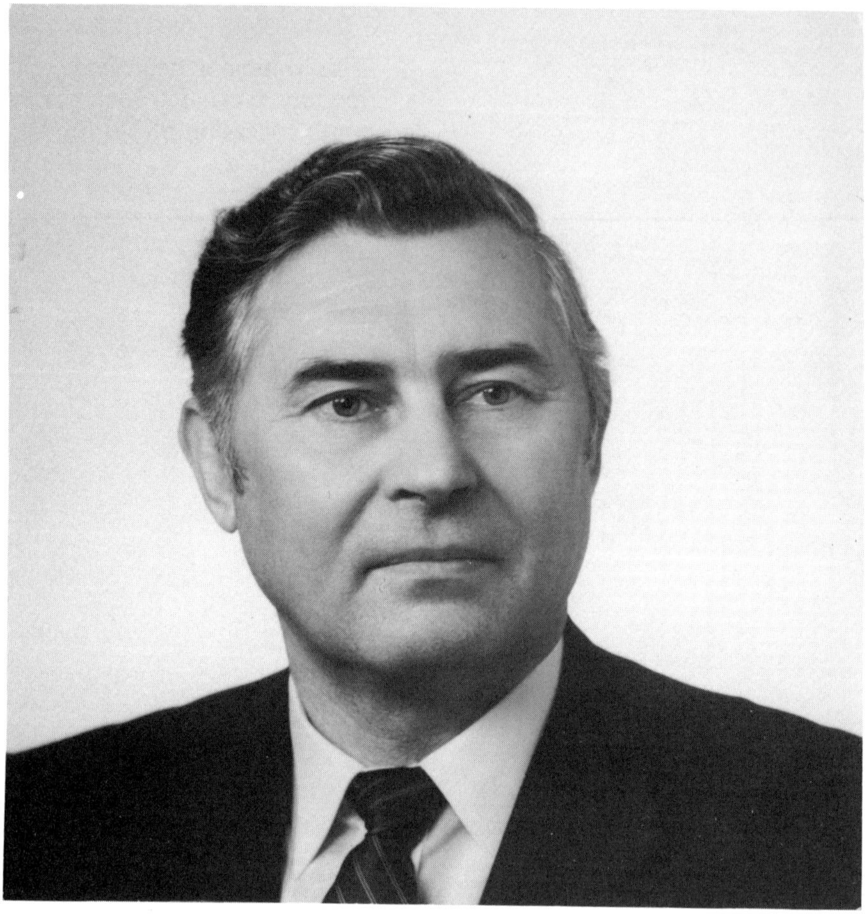

Gurij Ivanovich Marchuk

Gurij Ivanovich Marchuk began his scientific career at the Leningrad State University. In 1952 he wrote his Master's thesis, "The Dynamics of Large-scale Fields of Meteorological Elements in Baroclinic Atmosphere" and in 1956 his doctoral dissertation, "Numerical Methods for Calculating Nuclear Reactors." He was appointed professor in 1958, and in 1962 he was elected a Corresponding Member of the USSR Academy of Sciences, becoming a full Member in 1968. He is a three-time winner of the Order of Lenin—the highest Soviet award.

From 1953 to 1962 Gurij Ivanovich was the chief of a department of the Institute of Physics and Power in Obninsk, Siberia. In 1962 he became Deputy Director of the Novosibirsk Institute of Mathematics and in 1964 Director of the Novosibirsk Computing Center of the Siberian Branch of the USSR Academy of Sciences. In 1962 Gurij Ivanovich became professor and in 1966 Chairman of the Department of Numerical Methods in Dynamic Meteorology at the Novosibirsk State University.

Since 1980 Gurij Ivanovich has been Chairman of the Department of Mathematical Modelling of Physical Processes at the Moscow Physical-Technical Institute and Director of the Moscow Institute of Numerical Mathematics of the USSR Academy of Sciences.

In 1975 Gurij Ivanovich was elected the Chairman of the Presidium of the Siberian Branch of the USSR Academy of Sciences and Vice President of the USSR Academy of Sciences. In 1980 he was appointed Chairman of the USSR State Committee for Science and Technology and Deputy Chairman of the USSR Council of Ministers. He is a member of the Central Committee of the Communist Party of the USSR and deputy to the USSR Supreme Council (Verkhovnyj Sovet).

Gurij Ivanovich was instrumental in promoting extensive scientific cooperation between Soviet scientists and scientists of Bulgaria, Czechoslovakia, France, India, among other countries. He is the recipient of honorary doctorate degrees from France (Toulouse University), Czechoslovakia (Karlov University), the Technical University of Dresden and that of Budapest, and he is an Honorary member of the Academies of Science of the German Democratic Republic, Bulgaria, and Czechoslovakia. Gurij Ivanovich Marchuk received a medal 'For great service to mankind' from the Czechoslovakian Academy of Sciences and the 'Silver Core' from the International Federation for Information Processes (IFIP).

Gurij Ivanovich serves on the Editorial Boards of several Soviet and International journals: *Izvestiya Akademii Nauk SSR*, *Meteorologia i gidrologiya*, *Sibirskij matematicheskij zhurnal*, *Journal of Computational Physics*, *Numerische mathematik*, *Journal of Computer and System Sciences*, *Applied Mathematics and Optimization*, *Advances in Applied Mathematics*, *Calcolo*, among others.

Gurij Ivanovich has directed over ten doctoral candidates in physics and mathematics. He is the author of over 400 publications in Numerical Mathematics, Mathematical Modelling in Atmosphere and Ocean Physics, Immunology, and Environmental Protection.

CONTENTS

Atmospheric Sciences

Immunology

NUMERICAL ANALYSIS

SPLITTING–UP TECHNIQUES FOR COMPUTATIONS OF INDUSTRIAL FLOWS

J.P. Benque, O. Daubert, J. Goussebaile, and A. Hauguel
Laboratoire National d'Hydraulique, E.D.F.
Chatou, France

Summary

This article presents a wide range of applications of the splitting–up method, to the development of which G.I. Marchuk made a significant contribution, in industrial hydraulics computations involving extensive modelling (turbulence, head loss, etc.) in complex geometric patterns. These applications, from the earliest to the most recent ones, include space (co–ordination), operators (specific solvers), and geometric patterns (substruc–tures). Varied cases of industrial application as well as test cases provide a good illustration of the efficient use of the splitting–up method.

Introduction

Today, the use of similarity equations in numerical models in industrial hydraulics or in environmental science is commonplace. The classical approach to design such models is to start from the Navier–Stokes equation in which specific changes are made. The resulting equations have the following general form:

$$
\begin{array}{l|l|l|lll}
\dfrac{1}{C^2(p)}\dfrac{\partial p}{\partial t} & & + \nabla . u & & = 0 & (1) \\
\dfrac{\partial u}{\partial t} & + \nabla(u(U) \times u & + \nabla p & - \mathrm{Diff}(u) & = F(u,T) & (2) \\
\dfrac{\partial T}{\partial t} & + \nabla(u(U).T) & & - \mathrm{Diff}(T) & = S(u,T) & (3) \\
 & \text{advection} & \text{continuity} & \text{diffusion} & &
\end{array}
$$

Equation (1) defines mass conservation, equation (2) momentum conservation, and equation (3) the scalar conservation (temperature). Here the U is the flux associated with momentum, $u(U)$ is velocity, p is linked to the pressure, $C(p)$ is pressure–wave celerity (infinite for an incompressible fluid).

The change in u and T is given by equations (2) and (3) and corresponds to the advection due to the current, and to the diffusion, subject to the continuity condition (1) and the associated pressure gradient.

The mathematical operators associated with these mechanisms show the difference between them. Advection is hyperbolic and polarizes the behavior downstream; diffusion is parabolic, often nonlinear and expresses mostly turbulent effects; continuity is hyperbolic (elliptical for an incompressible fluid), always isotropic and couples the velocity components.

Nearly all numerical models developed at the "Laboratoire National d'Hydraulique" (LNH) of E.D.F. over the last decade are based on the simple idea that an algorithm is efficient when it has a single objective. These models are constructed using equations split into simpler parts, allowing a specific treatment of each. Hence the systems to be solved are of moderate size, symmetric and not too ill–conditioned. The precision of linking–up solutions has been improved. Initial simple fractional steps have led to transparent formulations. Furthermore, a greater computing capacity allows one to solve problems of growing complexity. At the beginning, only one–dimensional equations could be processed; today, it is possible to solve three–dimensional problems.

Solution of problems comprising 40^3 points in a cubic domain involves processing of the continuity step, uncoupling each velocity component as well as pressure. More sophisticated models of turbulence occurring near the walls have been designed for parallel computing, with a more accurate description of the boundaries by devising finite differences on curvilinear grids first and finite elements later. The general quality of the results has been enhanced through an increased computational load.

In industrial computations, it is convenient to take advantage of the regularity property of the grid (as in finite–difference method) while preserving the accurate desciption of the boundaries (as in the finite–element method); an attractive solution then emerges in the use of geometrical substructures with specific solutions. This notion is behind most recent codes being developed today and is useful for matching different equations.

General principles

As mentioned earlier, the use of realistic numerical simulation of industrial flows implies the treatment of complex equations with several variables, discretized over a large number of nodes. The splitting–up technique is the best remedy to offset the increasing computations and to ensure the most effective solvers: equations were initially split up in space (with co–ordination); later, the operators were split up (in relation to specific solvers); and today, equations are split up by domain. These methods are referred to as splitting–up techniques. G.I. Marchuk made a well–known, major contribution to the development of these techniques.

The finite–difference method and the time–marching method were used for initial numerical modelling of hydrodynamic problems, especially for nonlinear equations (calculations are made for transient equations, even in steady flows). For two–dimensional problems (only some years later did it become possible to solve three–dimensional problems) which require implicit solution, splitting–up techniques—such as the alternating–direction method of Peaceman and Rachford and later the fractional–step method of Marchuk and Yanenko—were used to reduce the size of the systems to be solved, since each direction in space was treated separately.

However, it soon turned out that in some applications the results obtained with an implicit centered discretization of spatial derivatives were least accurate when the advection terms were too high. It then became clear that a special effort had to be made to discretize these terms. Consequently, a one–dimensional equation expressing only transport was studied. It appeared that the method of integrating along the characteristic curves was the best to provide unconditionally stable results and minimize errors in phase and amplitude. But how can such a specific integration scheme be included in an aggregate problem involving continuity and diffusion phenomena? Simply by extending the notion of fractional steps and uncoupling both directions in space and the different operators in the partial differential equations.

Each fractional step could then be easily improved. In fact, among the various problems involving industrial or surface–free flows, the splitting–up of directions in space sometimes degrades the quality of results: for instance, in compressible or free–surface flows, the results were polarized along the grid lines. The "splitting–up technique with co–ordination," which can be used for the propagation (continuity) step (described below in more detail) was a decisive improvement. Furthermore, the advection step, which for a long period of time had been solved line by line on the finite–difference grid is now often replaced by a two– and even three–dimensional algorithm of characteristics, which allows a longer time step with the same degree of accuracy, especially when the velocity field is nonhomogeneous in intensity and duration.

The principle of a multidimensional routine in treating the advection step by the method of characteristic curves was so efficient in finite–difference codes that it was also applied to the Navier–Stokes equation in a finite–element code; it then became possible to overcome the difficulties in the cases where the Reynolds number was high and to include a turbulence model.

At the same time, finite–difference methods were developed for two–dimensional curvilinear grids; the method of fractional steps was generalized without any difficulty; the splitting–up of directions in space was, again, simply abandoned in the diffusion step because of the cross derivatives introduced by the transformation of coordinates.

As will be shown in the sequel, the transition of the fractional–step method from finite–differences to finite elements has led to a new "weak formulation" of the Navier–Stokes equations, which seems very attractive, accurate and enlightening since it can do away with some of the difficulties inherent in the classical splitting–up technique: the first–order approximation over time; nonsymmetric and time–varying matrices resulting from the discretization of advective terms are spontaneously placed on the right–hand side of the aggregate system to be solved without loss of accuracy; the conservation property can be nearly guaranteed.

The splitting–up of operators [10], [3]

The fractional–step method, designed by Yanenko and Marchuk [10], had an early use because of the initial choice of problems: transient equations for proper processing of nonlinearity and implicit methods, without any time–step limitation.

The principle is quite simple; for instance, to solve the classical transport–diffusion equation

$$\frac{\partial f}{\partial t} + \nabla(\underset{\sim}{u}f) - K\Delta f = 0 \tag{4}$$

of the type mentioned above, one introduces an intermediate variable $\tilde{f}$ between time steps n and $n+1$ such that

$$\frac{\tilde{f} - f^n}{\Delta t} + \nabla(\underset{\sim}{u}f^n) = 0\,, \tag{5a}$$

$$\frac{f^{n+1} - \tilde{f}}{\Delta t} = K\Delta f^{n+1}\,. \tag{5b}$$

The advantage of the fractional–step method is that special solvers can be fitted to the mathematical property of the operators. The disadvantage is that the method is a first–order approximation over time.

The method has been in wide use in nearly all numerical models (for example, see [3]). In the Navier–Stokes equation, initially the advective terms were solved, later the diffusion terms and finally the pressure and continuity constraint. Splitting–up in space (solving in the x direction with $\partial/\partial y$–type terms) was also used in the original models.

The solution of the advective terms and the mass–conservation condition are presented below in more detail.

Advection [4]

The basic idea is to make advective terms explicit by using an upwind scheme, as physically as possible, to construct a scheme of higher order of accuracy, to guarantee the unconditional stability with low numerical diffusion. This can be done by upwinding along the physical characteristics of equation (5a), using

$$\frac{dx}{dt} = \underset{\sim}{u}[t^n, t^{n+1}] ,$$

$$x^{n+1} = M , \text{ each node of the natural grid .}$$

The computation of these curves is a simple problem reversed in time, solved by means of the second–order Runge–Kutta method. In the finite–element approach, the idea of upwinding prompted RONAT to use test functions transported along the characteristic curves [4]:

$$\frac{\partial \psi}{\partial t} + \underset{\sim}{u} \nabla \psi = 0 \ [t^n, t^{n+1}] , \tag{6}$$

$$\psi(t{=}t^{n+1}, x) = \psi^{n+1}(x) = \varphi(x) \text{ (classical Galerkin shap function) .}$$

Then the $\{\psi\}$ defines two grids: the natural grid at time t^{n+1} and the upwind grid at time t^n, constructed at the foot of the characteristic curves. Before processing an advection equation, we note that this "weak" formulation of the advective terms leads to the projection of the velocity field onto the space associated with the upwind grid. An earlier application of characteristic curves in the finite–differences models (strong formulation) consists in integrating equation (5a) along the characteristic curves, according to the finite–difference approach:

$$\frac{df}{dt} = -f \nabla \underset{\sim}{u}. \tag{7}$$

This requires the value of f^n obtained by (parabolic and then cubic) interpolation at the foot of the characteristic curves.

Interpolation at the foot of the characteristic curves uses numerical diffusion with "strong" advection rather than the projection technique employed with "weak" formulation. Besides, "strong" advection implies the use of explicit splitting–up, with the first–order accuracy over time; the second–order accuracy over time (Crank–Nicholson scheme) can be obtained using "weak" advection, with still greater accuracy for processing advection alone (see figure 1). In both cases, at each time step, the use of advective terms leads to computing the right–hand term and then solving a linear–type problem, as shown below in the standard equation; see [4].

TEST OF THE ROTATING CONE

Weak Formulation   Finite–Elements Discretization

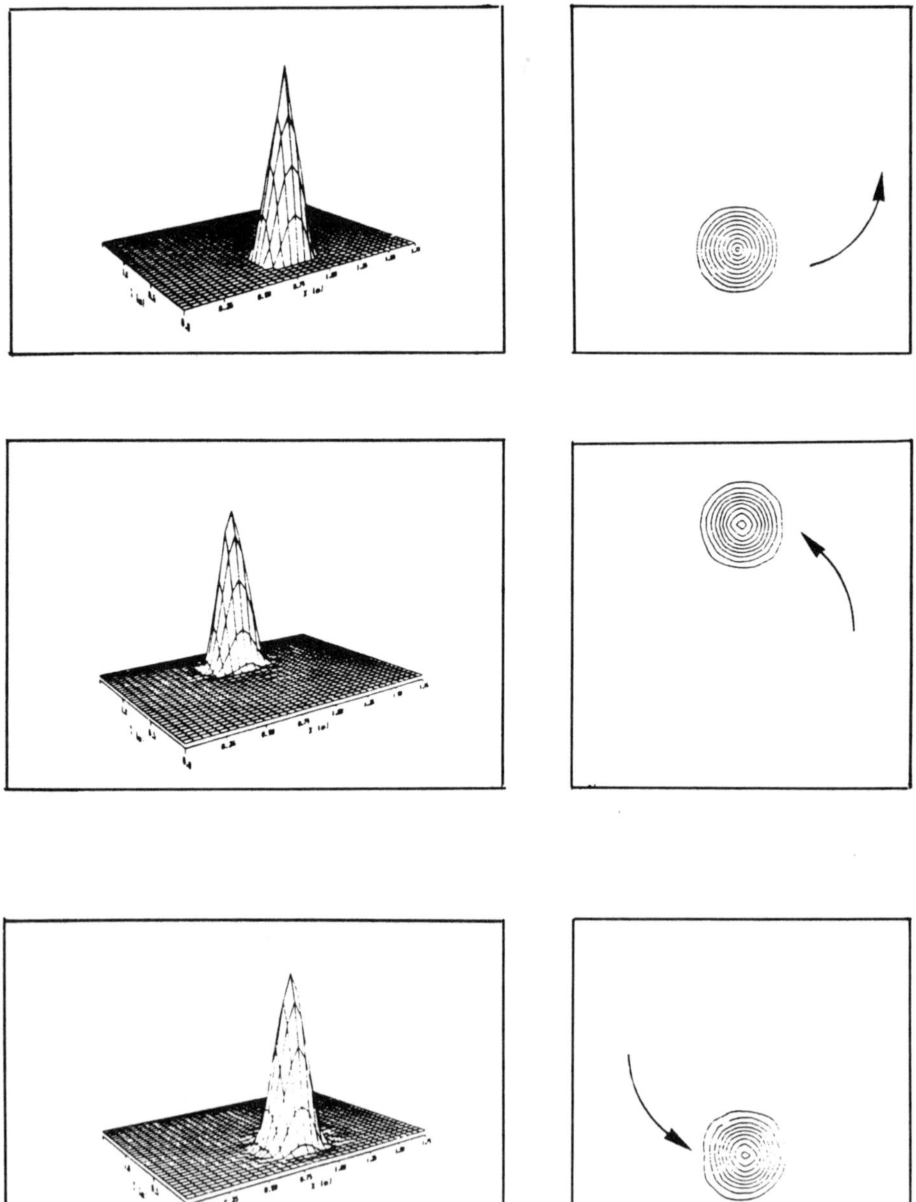

Fig. 1

TEST OF THE CONE ADVECTED IN A UNIFORM VELOCITY FIELD

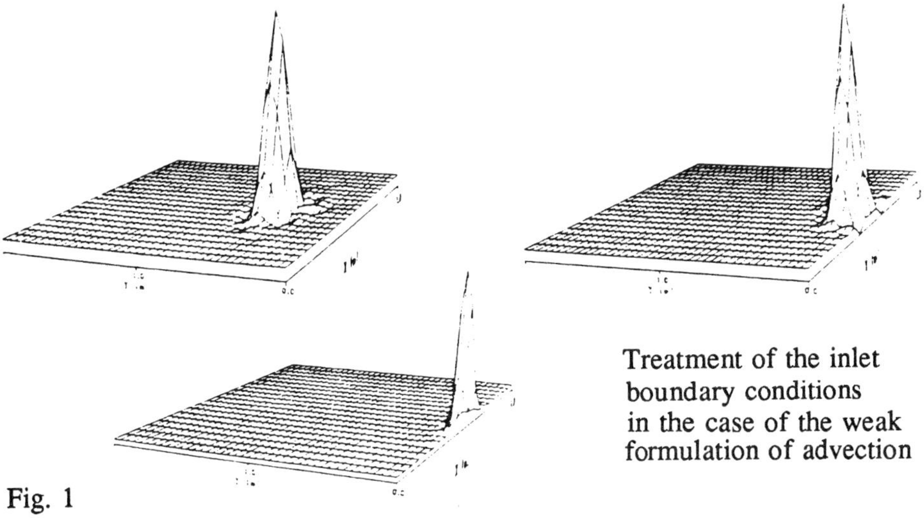

Treatment of the inlet boundary conditions in the case of the weak formulation of advection

Fig. 1

Integrating the weak formulation of equation (4) in space and over time between t^n and t^{n+1} and making some transformations taking equation (6) into account, we have

$$\int_\Omega f^{n+1}\,\psi^{n+1}\,d\Omega - \int_\Omega f^{n+1}\,\psi^n\,d\Omega + \int_{t^n}^{t^{n+1}} dt \int_\Omega K\,\nabla f\,\nabla\psi\,d\Omega$$
$$= \text{boundary terms.}$$

For the Crank–Nicholson discretization of the diffusion term, we have

$$\int_\Omega f^{n+1}\,\psi^{n+1}\,d\Omega + \frac{\Delta t}{2}\int_\Omega K\,\nabla f^{n+1}\,\nabla\psi^{n+1}\,d\Omega$$
$$= \int_\Omega f^n\,\psi^n\,d\Omega + \frac{\Delta t}{2}\int_\Omega K\,\nabla f^n\,\nabla\psi^n\,d\Omega + \text{boundary terms.} \tag{8}$$

The equation of diffusion and transport then takes the form of a simple diffusion equation. The whole advective effect has been done away with on the right-hand side in the upwind test functions ψ^n. This new formulation splits up the operators, but it is of second order over time.

It is possible to devise an exact integration rule for one-dimensional computations. The scheme obtained shows outstanding properties: negligible damping and phase shift for a wavelength which is greater than five space steps; see [4]. Numerical integration is easier for two-dimensional computations; however, it introduces a degree of damping. Nevertheless, performance remains very good. Figure 1 shows the results of a difficult test of the rotating cone with a P_2 discretization; the cone stands on only four elements; a damping ratio of 12% is observed after a revolution (48 time steps) and then stabilizes (12.2% after two revolutions). The last terms of equation (8) come from the boundary conditions. With respect to the inflow boundaries, a change of variable allows the boundary condition to be treated as a space integral in an extension of the computational domain; this extension is on the characteristic curves; see [4].

Treatment of the boundary condition provides excellent results in two–dimensional tests. The lower section of figure 1 shows the results obtained with this formulation in the case of a cone transported by a uniform velocity field.

Thus, much progress has been made in solving the aggregate problem, from the earlier strong advection with splitting–up in space to weak advection allowing for almost transparent splitting–up.

Diffusion – continuity [7], [2]

As was mentioned earlier, the treatment of the advective terms leads to computing the second member, possibly followed by computing the scalar diffusion and solving a general Stokes problem:

$$\frac{U^{n+1}}{\Delta t} - \text{Diff}\,(U^{n+1}) + \nabla\, p^{n+1} = S^n \,, \tag{9a}$$

$$\frac{1}{C^2\,(p)}\frac{p^{n+1}}{\Delta t} + \nabla . U^{n+1} = D^n \,. \tag{9b}$$

Algorithms (regardless equation (9b)) for efficient uncoupled computation of pressure and velocity components, were sought in accordance with the general principles described above. An equation for the pressure can be obtained by eliminating the velocity between (9a) and (9b). The Chorin–Temam projection method [5], which implies approximate boundary conditions for pressure and yields a good estimate of pressure for an incompressible fluid (C=0, D^n=0):

$$\begin{aligned} \Delta\, p^{n+1} &= \nabla . S^n \,, \\ \frac{\partial p^{n+1}}{\partial n} &= 0 \,. \end{aligned} \tag{10}$$

Consequently, the associated velocity field U^{n+1} is given by (9a), component by component. Initially, many finite–difference codes were developed at the L.N.H., using this approximate but effective method for estimating the pressure after a second fractional step solving implicit discretization of the Laplacian. A compatible discretization, i.e., the product of the divergence matrix by the gradient matrix, yields finer results regarding the continuity constraint. In the three–dimensional computations, the ESTET code then allows processing of 40,000 grid points in order to solve the Boussinesq equations with a k–ε eddy viscosity model. Figure 2 shows the rated flow in hot plenum of the fast reactor of Super Phenix 2; numerical results are confirmed by views of the salt–water scale model.

RATED FLOW IN THE HOT PLENUM OF A FAST BREEDER REACTOR

Three–dimensional computation with the ESTET finite–differences code

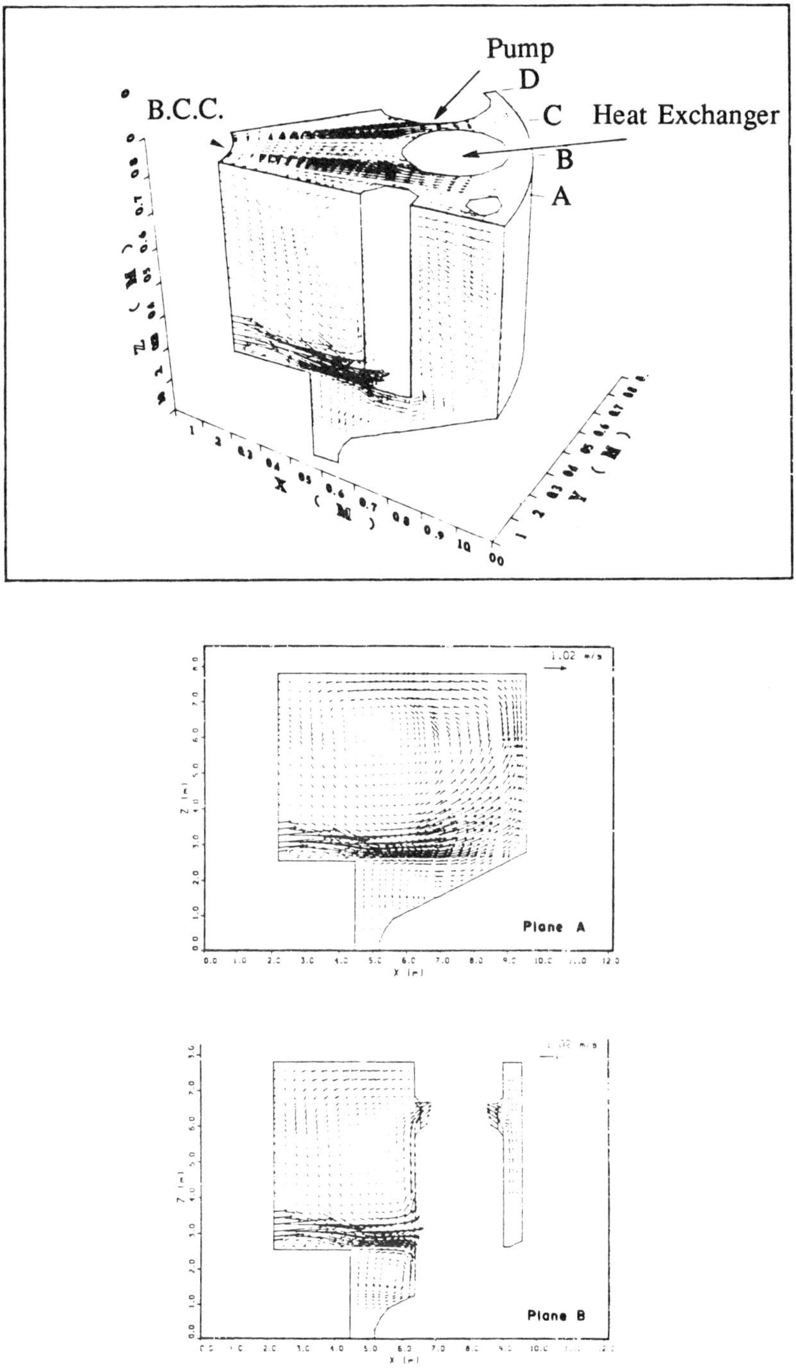

Fig. 2

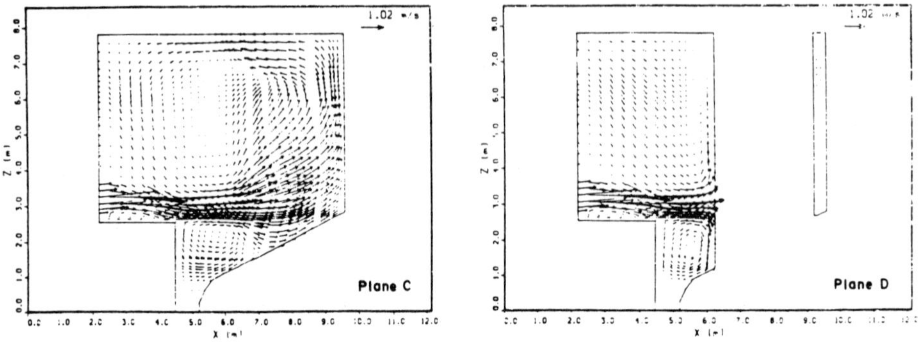

Fig. 2

SPACE SPLITTING WITH COORDINATION [8], [1]

In the finite–difference approach and in the compressible case, the solution of the pressure equation can also be split in space (see [8]). This has been done in the finite–difference code for the shallow–water model. In this case the pressure equation

$$\alpha p - \Delta p = S \tag{11}$$

can be split into two parts.

Find q, defining (p_1,p_2) by

$$\left\{ \begin{array}{ll} \frac{\alpha p_1}{2} - \frac{\partial^2 p_1}{\partial x^2} = \frac{S}{2} - q & \text{plus the Neumann boundary conditions} \\ \frac{\alpha p_2}{2} - \frac{\partial^2 p_2}{\partial y^2} = \frac{S}{2} + q & \end{array} \right. \tag{12}$$

satisfying the constraint

$$p_1 - p_2 = 0 \,.$$

The problem in q is endowed with all the appropriate properties (symmetric and positive definite) and can thus be solved by the conjugate–gradient method, which, too, requires only solving one–dimensional equations. This algorithm is very effective, but it cannot be transformed into the Poisson equation (α=0) due to the necessary existence of each splitted equation (12). A major feature of this algorithm is the fact that the number of iterations does not increase too fast with the size of the system.

Figure 5 shows the results obtained with this solver in the computations of tidal currents in the Canche estuary, in simulation of the uncovering tidal flows (see [1] for more detail).

PRECONDITIONED UZAWA ALGORITHM [2], [7]

In the finite–element approach, the construction of a compatible div–grad Laplacian discretization is cumbersome. Thus it is natural to solve the continuity and diffusion terms together. Hence, an iterative algorithm has been sought, using the efficient Chorin–Temam projection method as the first step to attain the proper level of mass conservation, without constructing the compatible matrix (for more detail, see [7]).

The classical finite–element discretization of equation (9) in the case of an incompressible fluid is given by

$$\begin{aligned} AU - BP &= S \,, \\ {}^{t}BU &= 0 \,. \end{aligned} \tag{13}$$

The standard Uzawa algorithm is a gradient algorithm solving the associated symmetric system:

$${}^{t}BA^{-1}BP = BA^{-1}S \,, \tag{14}$$

without constructing the ${}^{t}BA^{-1}B$ matrix.

The Chorin–Temam algorithm suggests that the solution of (14) should be preconditioned by the discretization of (10).

Equation (14) takes the form of the compatible discretization of a Poisson problem relating to pressure when diffusion is left out.

The preconditioned Uzawa algorithm then has two steps per iteration:

1. Find U^m, the solution of the momentum equation with a given pressure p^m:

$$AU^m = Bp^m + S \,.$$

2. Find p^{m+1}, the solution of

$$Cp^{m+1} = Cp^m - BU^m \,,$$

where the preconditioning matrix C is obtained by the discretization of (10). Note that the first iteration is equivalent to the Chorin–Temam algorithm and that preconditioning is more effective when the Reynolds number increases (matrix C comes closer to ${}^{t}BA^{-1}B$ because diffusion decreases); this fact, when verified by testing, is advantageous for solving industrial problems. This algorithm was implemented in one of the most recent three–dimensional codes N3S (for more detail, see [12]); the purpose of this finite–element code is to simulate industrial flows over roughly ten thousand nodes. In the near future, this code will combine the method of splitting–up of operators and geometry patterns. Figure 3 shows one of the first results obtained for the N3S code: the simulation of a cooling tower in a cross wind.

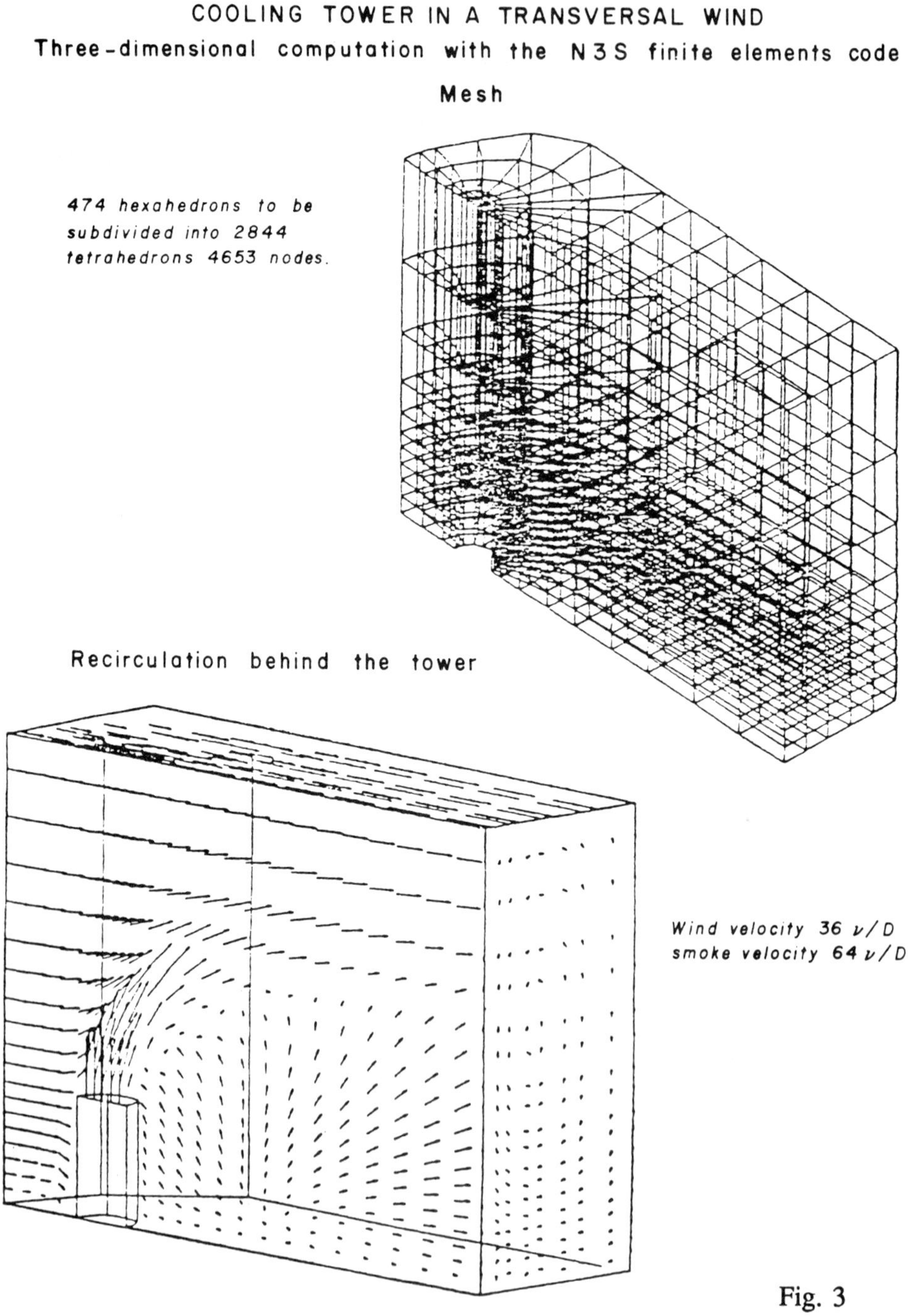

Fig. 3

Separation of variables

The chief advantage of these Stokes algorithms is that they uncouple pressure and velocity and dissociate the different velocity components when the boundary conditions are of the Dirichlet type. Approximate boundary conditions are used in the solvers mentioned above to calculate pressure or precondition its computation.

THE GLOWINSKI–PIRONNEAU ALGORITHM [7]

When physical boundary conditions are set for velocities, the boundary conditions relating to pressure can be computed so that divergence is cancelled in the weak sense (e.g., by solving a boundary operator). This principle, devised by Glowinski and Pironneau for the Stokes problem, has been generalized to shallow–water equations (compressible flow).

The original Glowinski–Pironneau algorithm has been implemented in an industrial code CEFALO, to solve the shallow–water equations. Figure 4 illustrates the prediction of the sea–surface level depending on the meteorological conditions in the northwest European continental shelf.

BOUNDARY CONDITIONS RELATING TO VELOCITY [6]

The role played by the boundary conditions has not been defined in the preceding discussion. Physical modelling may involve complex constraints on the boundary, which can couple the velocity components. In the case of flows with a high Reynolds number, the velocity gradient near a wall is very high and the use of zero Dirichlet conditions would make it possible that a superfine grid catches the boundary layer. Furthermore, the turbulence models with a high Reynolds number would not be applicable in this layer. In this regard, many researchers prefer to use a certain macroscopic physical law which simulates a logarithmic profile; this law meets the following two conditions:

– impermeability $\underset{\sim}{v} \cdot \underset{\sim}{v} = 0$ ($\underset{\sim}{n}$ is the normal to the boundary) (15a)

– mean velocity gradient near the wall linked to the tangential mean flow:

$$\frac{\partial(\underset{\sim}{v} \cdot \underset{\sim}{\tau})}{\partial n} + \alpha(\underset{\sim}{v} \cdot \underset{\sim}{\tau}) = \beta \tag{15b}$$

($\underset{\sim}{\tau}$ is tangent to the boundary, $\partial/\partial n$ is a normal derivative to the boundary).

The advantage of the preceding algorithms is that they allow processing of the new as well as the previous uncoupled conditions. For the Stokes

SURFACE / LEVEL AND CURRENTS
IN THE NORTH-WEST EUROPEAN CONTINENTAL SHELF

Shallow water equations computation with the CEFALO finite elements code

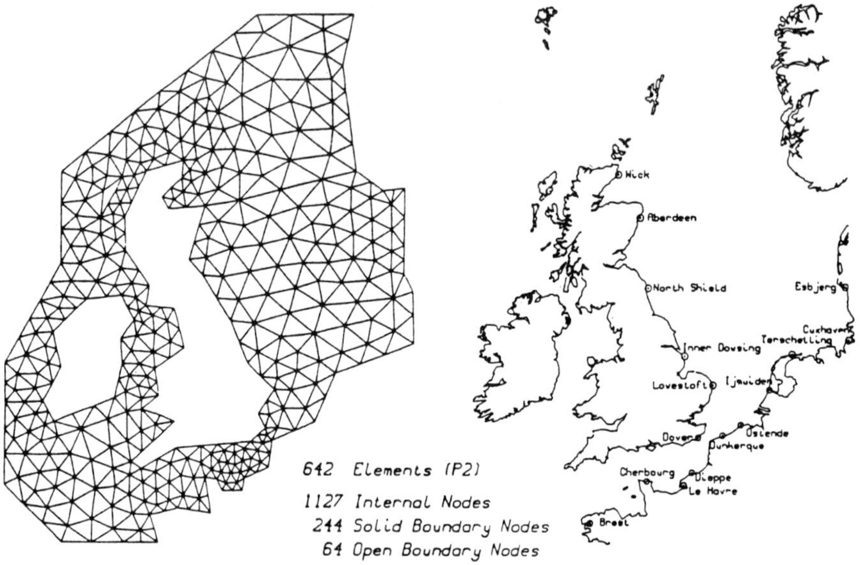

Finite Element Mesh of the North-West European continental shelf and position of ports

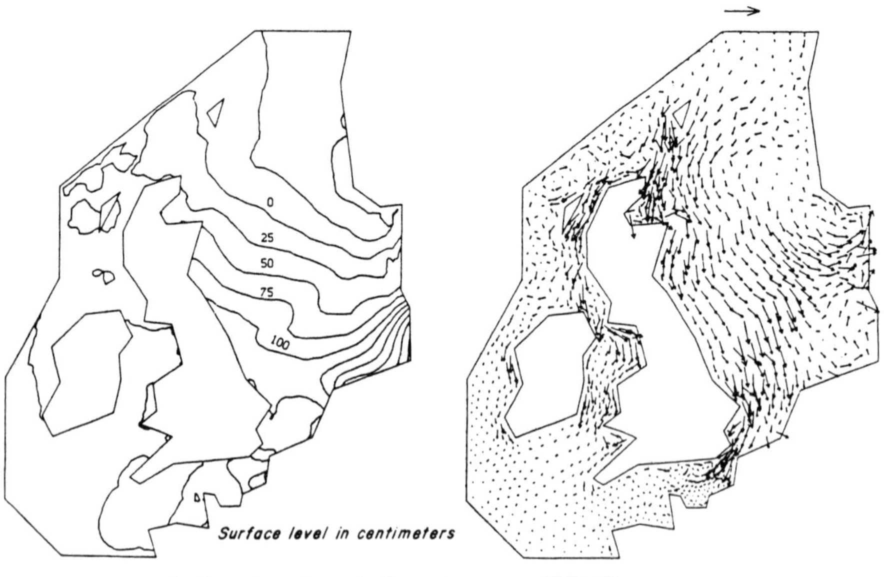

Surface Level and Currents - 19/11/73 at 13H

Fig. 4

problem, the use of boundary conditions (15) along a segment Γ_1 of the boundary Γ and of Dirichlet conditions $\underset{\sim}{u}_d$ along the remaining part $(\Gamma - \Gamma_1)$ yields the velocity field $\underset{\sim}{v}$ in subspace $\tilde{W}$:

$$W = \{\underset{\sim}{w} | w \in (H^1)^n,\ \underset{\sim}{w} = u_d/(\Gamma-\Gamma_1),\ \underset{\sim}{w}\cdot \underset{\sim}{n} = 0/\Gamma_1\},$$

which, for a given estimate of pressure $p \in L^2$, verifies:

$$\forall\ \underset{\sim}{\varphi} \in W_0 = \{\tilde{\varphi} | \underset{\sim}{\varphi} \in W,\ \underset{\sim}{\varphi} = 0/(\Gamma-\Gamma_1)\},$$

$$\int_\Omega \left(\frac{1}{\Delta t}\underset{\sim}{v}\cdot\underset{\sim}{\varphi} + \underset{\sim}{\nu}\nabla\underset{\sim}{v}\cdot \nabla\tilde{\varphi}\right) d\Omega + \int_{\Gamma_1} \alpha\underset{\sim}{v}\cdot \underset{\sim}{\varphi} d\Gamma \tag{16}$$

$$= \int_\Omega p\ \nabla\cdot\underset{\sim}{\varphi} d\Omega + \int_\Omega \underset{\sim}{S}\cdot \underset{\sim}{\varphi} d\Omega - \int_{\Gamma_1} \beta\underset{\sim}{\tau}\cdot \underset{\sim}{\varphi} d\Gamma .$$

A direct solution of equation (16)—the boundary conditions along Γ_1—would lead to coupling velocity components. Another approach is to determine the Dirichlet conditions relating to $\underset{\sim}{v}$ along Γ_1, which will yield an identical solution to that of the original problem.

Let γ_0 denote the trace operator of W in $(H^{1/2})^n$ $(\gamma_0(W) = W^{1/2})$ and let I denote the lifting operator of $W^{1/2}$ in W, such that

$$\forall\ \underset{\sim}{q} \in W^{1/2} = \{\underset{\sim}{q} | \underset{\sim}{q} \in (H^{1/2})^n,\ \underset{\sim}{q} = \underset{\sim}{u}_d/(\Gamma-\Gamma_1),\ \underset{\sim}{q}\cdot \underset{\sim}{n} = 0/\Gamma_1\},$$

$I(\underset{\sim}{q})$ is defined as the unique solution $\underset{\sim}{u}$ of:

$$\forall\ \underset{\sim}{\varphi}_0 \in (H_0^1)^n,$$

$$\left|\begin{array}{l} \displaystyle\int_\Omega \left(\frac{1}{\Delta t}\underset{\sim}{u}\cdot\underset{\sim}{\varphi}_0 + \underset{\sim}{\nu}\nabla\underset{\sim}{u}\cdot \nabla\underset{\sim}{\varphi}_0\right) d\Omega \\ \displaystyle\qquad = \int_\Omega p\ \nabla\cdot\underset{\sim}{\varphi}_0\ d\Omega + \int_\Omega \underset{\sim}{S}\cdot \underset{\sim}{\varphi}_0\ d\Omega , \\ \qquad\qquad \underset{\sim}{u} = \underset{\sim}{q}/\Gamma . \end{array}\right. \tag{17}$$

Due to (17) the problem (16) becomes essential for determining $\underset{\sim}{q} \in W^{1/2}$ such that the remaining equations in (16) hold, i.e.,

$$\forall\ \underset{\sim}{\varphi} \in W^{1/2},$$

$$\int_\Omega \left(\frac{1}{\Delta t}I(\underset{\sim}{q})\cdot\underset{\sim}{\varphi} + \underset{\sim}{\nu}\nabla I(\underset{\sim}{q})\cdot\nabla\underset{\sim}{\varphi}\right) d\Omega + \int_{\Gamma_1} \alpha\underset{\sim}{q}\cdot \underset{\sim}{\varphi} d\Gamma \tag{18}$$

$$= \int p\ \nabla\cdot\underset{\sim}{\varphi} d\Omega + \int_\Omega \underset{\sim}{S}\cdot \underset{\sim}{\varphi} d\Omega - \int_{\Gamma_1} \beta\underset{\sim}{\tau}\cdot \underset{\sim}{\varphi} d\Gamma .$$

The equivalence of (18) with the weak formulation of the logarithmic boundary condition (15b) can be observed in using the Green formula. Hence, the control problem is slightly more general: the pressure p and now the Dirichlet boundary conditions $\underset{\sim}{q}$ should be such that the associated state variable u, that is the solution of the Stokes problem (17), verify the continuity constraint (13b) and the logarithmic boundary condition (18). For instance, the Uzawa algorithm becomes, p^m and q^m being given ($p_0 = p^n$, $q_0 = \underset{\sim}{U}^n/\Gamma$):

- compute $\underset{\sim}{U}_m$, the solution of (17) (without coupling!);
- deduce the divergence error from (13.b) and then p_{m+1};
- deduce the error in the logarithmic profile from (18) and and then q_{m+1};
- iterate on p_m, q_m until the process converges.

In addition to making uncoupling impossible, another most interesting feature of this algorithm is fast convergence ensuring the correct Dirichlet boundary conditions. Three iterations are normally sufficient (see [6] for further details and examples).

Domain decomposition

The last but not the least point worth of interest is that the splitting–up technique is used for geometric patterns. The idea is to divide the computational domain into substructures without overlapping, to obtain independent problems in each subdomain, and next to use them and the appropriate solvers in each subdomain as operators. To be more specific, many industrial problems require an accurate description of the geometric pattern (i.e., irregular elements for the discretization); yet, a regular mesh is possible inside the subdomain, thus greatly reducing the computational cost, even in the finite–element discretization. Moreover, this method can be used in parallel computing.

For an easier implementation, one may match the finite elements and use compatible meshes (i.e., the same nodes on the junction between two subdomains).

The main difficulty in using the operator–splitting principle is to match the solution of the Stokes problem. Since characteristic curves have been used explicitly, advective terms are discarded on the right–hand side; near an inside junction of a subdomain where there is an inflow, the advective term is as easy to compute as in any other part of the subdomain. Indeed, the time–space transformation applied to the contribution of the boundary term allows its computation over the neighboring subdomain, using the characteristic curves.

For the Stokes problem, the adequate boundary conditions should be determined along the junction boundaries to uncouple the solving operation in each subdomain. The problem set out above is a matching problem which can be formulated as follows: find the Dirichlet conditions relating to velocity which yield equality of the stresses on each side of the junction (primal method) or vice-versa (dual method). The analysis of the continuous problem shows that this problem is linear, symmetric and V-elliptical, which ensures the success of the numerical method applied to the discretized problem (see [11] for further details).

The primal method is presented here in the framework of the Stokes equations (infinite celerity). As was mentioned earlier, once discretized, the Stokes equation can be written as

$$\begin{aligned} Au - {}^tBp &= S \text{ in } \Omega , \\ Bu &= 0 \text{ in } \Omega , \\ u &= u_D \text{ over } \Gamma . \end{aligned} \tag{19}$$

The domain Ω is partitioned, for simplicity, into two subdomains Ω^e, $e = 1, 2$. Let $\mathcal{T}h^e$, $e = 1, 2$ be the corresponding triangulations which are themselves a partition of $\mathcal{T}h$, triangulation of Ω.

Let Π^e, V^e, be the approximation spaces of pressure and velocities and let W^e be the space engendered by the basic functions associated with the nodes of $\partial\Omega^e$, boundary of Ω^e.

The subspace $\tilde{M}^e$ of W^e is thus defined by

$$\tilde{M}^e = \{\underset{\sim}{\lambda}^e \in W^e ; \underset{\sim}{\lambda} = \underset{\sim}{0} \text{ over } \Gamma^e \text{ and } \int_\varepsilon \underset{\sim}{\lambda}^e \cdot \underset{\sim}{n}^e = 0\} ,$$

where

$$\Gamma^e = \partial\Omega^e \cap \partial\Omega \quad \text{and} \quad \varepsilon = \partial\Omega_1 \cap \partial\Omega_2 .$$

We then write

$$\tilde{M} = \sum_{e=1}^{2} \tilde{M}^e .$$

If the bilinear form k over $\tilde{M} \times \tilde{M}$ is defined by

$$k(\underset{\sim}{\lambda}; \underset{\sim}{\mu}) = \sum_{e=1}^{2} \left(\int_{\Omega^e} \alpha \underset{\sim}{u}^e_{\lambda} \cdot \underset{\sim}{\mu}^e + \int_{\Omega^e} \nu \nabla \underset{\sim}{u}^e_{\lambda} \cdot \nabla \underset{\sim}{\mu}^e - \int_{\Omega^e} p^e_{\lambda} \cdot \nabla \underset{\sim}{\mu}^e \right)$$

and if the second member $\underset{\sim}{b}$ is defined by

$$(\underset{\sim}{b}, \underset{\sim}{\mu}) = \sum_{e=1}^{2} \left(\int_{\Omega^e} \alpha \underset{\sim}{u}^e_0 \cdot \underset{\sim}{\mu}^e + \int_{\Omega^e} \nu \nabla \underset{\sim}{u}^e_0 \cdot \nabla \underset{\sim}{\mu}^e - \int_{\Omega^e} p^e_0 \cdot \nabla \underset{\sim}{\mu}^e \right) ,$$

where $(\underset{\sim}{u}^e_\lambda, p^e_\lambda)$ and $(\underset{\sim}{u}^e_0, p^e_0)$ are solutions of

$$\begin{aligned} A^e u^e_\lambda - {}^tB^e p^e_\lambda &= 0 \text{ in } \Omega^e, \\ B^e u^e_\lambda &= 0 \text{ in } \Omega^e, \\ u^e_\lambda &= \lambda^e \text{ over } \varepsilon, \\ u^e_\lambda &= 0 \text{ over } \Gamma^e, \end{aligned} \tag{20a}$$

with $\lambda^e \in \tilde{M}^e$

$$\begin{aligned} A^e u^e_0 - {}^tB^e p^e_0 &= S^e \text{ in } \Omega^e, \\ B^e u^e_0 &= 0 \text{ in } \Omega^e, \\ u^e_0 &= W^e \text{ over } \varepsilon, \\ u^e_0 &= u^e_D \text{ over } \Gamma^e, \end{aligned} \tag{20b}$$

with $\underset{\sim}{w}^e$ such that

$$\int_{\partial\Omega^e} \underset{\sim}{u}^e_0 \cdot n = 0$$

(19) is then equivalent to

$$K\lambda^e = b, \tag{21.1}$$

$$A^e u^e_\lambda - {}^tB^e p^e_\lambda = S^e \quad \text{in } \Omega^e, \tag{21.2}$$

$$B^e u^e = 0 \quad \text{in } \Omega^e \tag{21.3}$$

for $e = 1,2$,

$$u^e = \lambda^e + w^e \quad \text{over } \varepsilon, \tag{21.4}$$

$$u^e = u^e_D \quad \text{over } \Gamma^e, \tag{21.5}$$

with the matching matrix K corresponding to the bilinear form k.

The primal algorithm of matching leads to

1. computing the matching matrix K: by (20a), for each junction node, compute the answer flowing from the the zero boundary condition except for the node considered;

2. at each time step:
   - computing the second number b: using (20b), compute the answer for an adequate boundary condition W on the junction and for the set boundary condition along the natural boundary;
   - solving the matching equation (21.1) to obtain the adequate Dirichlet boundary condition λ on the junction;
   - solving the system (21.2)–(21.5) in each subdomain.

The use of domain decomposition implies solving two problems of diffusion–continuity at each time step in every subdomain. Only when using the regularity of some subdomains, this method can be substantially efficient in non–parallel computing, notwithstanding the smaller size of the

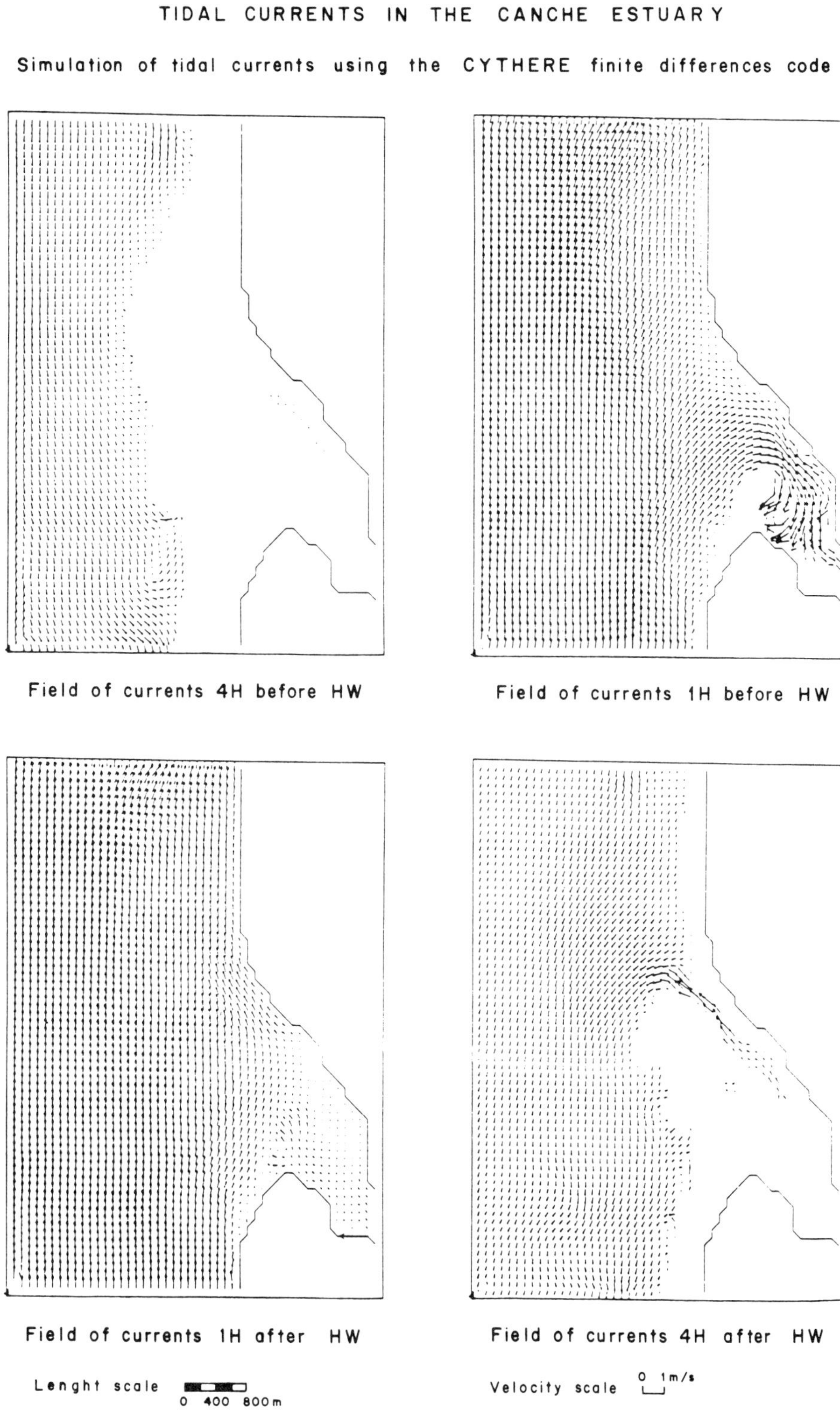
TIDAL CURRENTS IN THE CANCHE ESTUARY
Simulation of tidal currents using the CYTHERE finite differences code
Field of currents 4H before HW
Field of currents 1H before HW
Field of currents 1H after HW
Field of currents 4H after HW
Lenght scale
0 400 800m
Velocity scale
0 1m/s

Fig. 5

systems to be solved (see [11] for more details). It can also be noted that the method is independent of the solver used in each subdomain; this advantage is related to the fact that in this algorithm the pressure is not matched on the junction boundary: in fact, there are two pressures ensuring a divergence condition. This does not seem to be very important in test cases with the junction boundary in a region where the solution is "sufficiently" regular. Figure 6 gives the example presented earlier of the shallow–water equations relating to the northwest European shelf, processed with four substructures; matching of solutions is rather accurate, as observed in the aggregate solution which is very similar to the decomposed solution.

(a)

TEST RELATING TO DOMAIN SPLITTING

Test Case of the North–West European Continental Shelf

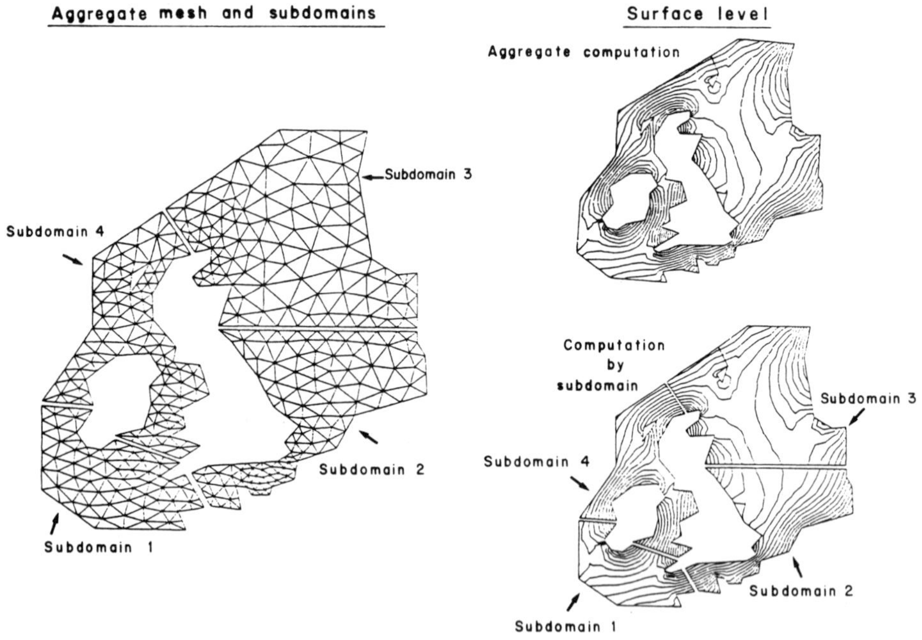

Fig. 6

(b)

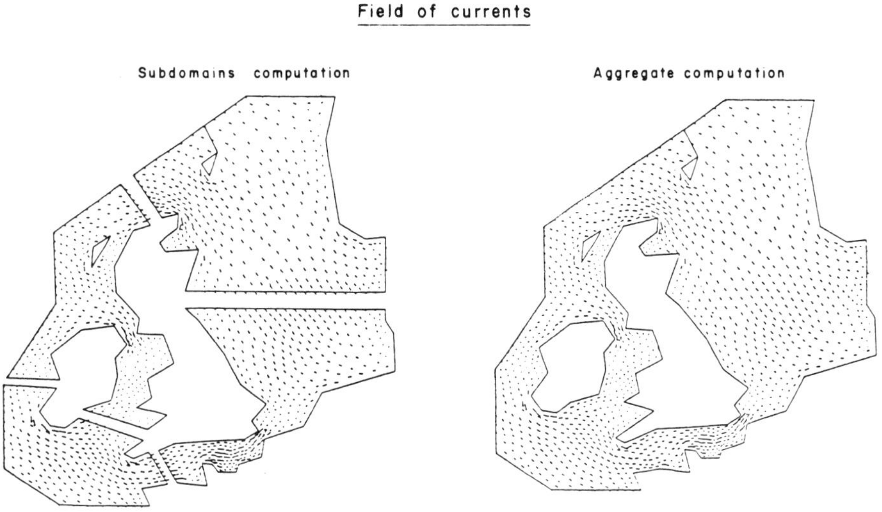

Fig. 6

Conclusion

As was stated earlier, the numerical simulation of industrial flows requires the consideration of a large number of variables in complex geo–metric patterns. Computational hydraulics covers several different fields: for instance, figure 2 is an illustration of the hot plenum of Super Phenix 2 and figure 4 indicates the sea–surface level depending on meteorological conditions in the northwest European continental shelf.

To treat different problems, one can use either the method of splitting operators, or uncoupling components, or domain decomposition. The splitting–up technique proved to be very efficient in modelling various phenomena—for example, turbulent viscosity, head loss terms, etc. On the one hand the "natural" splitting of large problems allows the broad application of the regular substructures and on the other hand this method makes the ap–plication of parallel computing quite promissing.

REFERENCES

[1] Benque, J.P., Cunge, J.A., Feuillet, J., Hauguel, A., and Holly, F.M., Jr. "New Method for Tidal Current Computation: Waterway Port, Coastal and Ocean Division." *The Proceedings of the ASCE* 108, no. WW3 (August 1982).

[2] Benque, J.P., Gregoire, J.P., Hauguel, A., and Maxant, M. "Application des méthodes de décomposition aux calculs numériques en hydraulique industrielle." *Proceedings of the Sixth International Conference on Computing Methods in Applied Sciences and Engineering*, Versailles, France, December 1983.

[3] Benque, J.P., Hauguel, A., and Viollet, P.L. *Applications of Computational Hydraulics*, vol. 2. London: Pitman, 1982.

[4] Benque, J.P., Labadie, G., and Ronat, J. "A New Finite–element Method for the Navier–Stokes Equations Coupled with a Temperature Equation." *Intern. J. of Numerical Methods in Fluids*. Forthcoming.

[5] Chorin, A.J. "Numerical Solution of Incompressible Flow Problems." *Numeric. Ann.*, 1968, no. 4:64–71.

[6] Goussebaile, G., Hecht, F., Labadie, G., and Reinhart, L. "Finite–element Solution of the Shallow–water Equations by a Quasi–direct Decomposition Procedure." *Intern. J. of Numerical Methods in Fluids.* Forthcoming.

[7] Labadie, G., and Lasbleiz, P. Quelques méthodes de résolution du problème de Stokes en éléments finis. Rapport EDF HE/41/83.01 et HI/44/72.07.

[8] Lions, J.L., and Marchuk, G.I. *Sur les méthodes numériques en science physiques et économiques*. Paris: Dunod, 1975.

[9] Marchuk, G.I. *Methods of Numerical Mathematics*. New York Berlin Heidelberg Tokyo: Springer–Verlag, 1975.

[10] Marchuk, G.I., and Yanenko, N.N. The application of the splitting–up method (fractional steps) to problems of mathematical physics. In *Some Problems of Numerical and Applied Mathematics* (in Russian). Novosibirsk: Izdatel'stvo "Nauka," 1966.

[11] Martinaud, J.P. Approximation éléments finis d'équations aux dérivees partielles par une méthode de décomposition des domains. Thèse de 3ème cycle soutenue le 20–6–84 à l'Universitè Pierre et Marie Curie, Paris VI.

[12] Gregoire, J.P., and Goussebaile, J. Avancement du projet N3S de Mécanique des fluides (mise à jour Janvier 1984). Rapport EDF HE/41/84.02 et HI/47/00.07.

RECENT RESULTS ON MIXED FINITE ELEMENT METHODS FOR SECOND ORDER ELLIPTIC PROBLEMS

F. Brezzi†, J. Douglas, Jr.††, and L.D. Marini†††

1. Introduction

The aim of this paper is to summarize certain relevant features of some new families of mixed finite elements recently introduced in [8] and [9]. These elements are similar to the well–known Raviart–Thomas–Nedelec elements [21], [22]; however, they provide essentially the same accuracy at lower cost. In the next section we recall the definition of the Raviart–Thomas–Nedelec elements and well as the definition of the new elements introduced in [8]. Then, in section 3, we show how they apply to a simple model problem. In section 4 we summarize the results proved in [8] and show that nearly all the nice properties which make the classical mixed elements useful remain valid for the new ones. A comparison of asymptotic error estimates is presented. Finally, we show in section 5 that the new elements can be applied to problems of linear elasticity in the plane in the same fashion as the Raviart–Thomas–Nedelec elements [1], [2], [4], [5], [20].

2. Description of the elements

For the sake of simplicity, we shall describe first the behavior of the trial (and test) functions on a single element (triangle or rectangle). We shall present the assembled spaces at the end of this section and their applications to second–order elliptic problems in the next section.

† Dipartimento di Meccanica Strutturale and Istituto di Analisi Numerica del C.N.R., 27100 Pavia, Italy
†† Department of Mathematics, University of Chicago, Chicago IL 60637, USA
††† Istituto di Analisi Numerica del C.N.R., 27100 Pavia, Italy

Let us consider first a triangle T with edges e_1, e_2, and e_3. For $k \geq 0$ let

$$\mathcal{P}_k(T) = \{\text{polynomials of degree} \leq k \text{ on } T\} , \tag{2.1}$$

$$\vec{\mathcal{P}}_k(T) = \{\text{vectors } \vec{v} = (v_1, v_2) \text{ such that } v_i \in \mathcal{P}_k(T)\} , \tag{2.2}$$

$$\vec{\mathcal{R}}_k(T) = \vec{\mathcal{P}}_k(T) \oplus \vec{x}\,\mathcal{P}_k(T) , \tag{2.3}$$

where $\vec{x} = (x_1, x_2)$. Note that

$$\vec{\mathcal{P}}_k(T) \subset \vec{\mathcal{R}}_k(T) \subset \vec{\mathcal{P}}_{k+1}(T) . \tag{2.4}$$

While it is not important for our immediate purposes to specify a choice of degrees of freedom for $\mathcal{P}_k(T)$, it is convenient to use some ad hoc degrees of freedom for the spaces $\vec{\mathcal{P}}_k(T)$ and $\vec{\mathcal{R}}_k(T)$. Denote the outer normal to ∂T by $\vec{n}$. Let $\vec{\mathrm{rot}}\ \varphi = (-\partial\varphi/\partial x_2, \partial\varphi/\partial x_1)$; let the barycentric coordinates of T be indicated by $\lambda_i = \lambda_i(\vec{x})$, $i = 1,2,3$, and let $b_3(\vec{x}) = \lambda_1(\vec{x})\lambda_2(\vec{x})\lambda_3(\vec{x})$.

Proposition 2.1 [21]. *For $k \geq 0$, a vector $\vec{v}$ in $\vec{\mathcal{R}}_k$ is uniquely determined by the following degrees of freedom:*

$$\int_{e_i} \vec{v}\cdot\vec{n}\, p\, ds , \quad p \in \mathcal{P}_k(e_i) , \quad i = 1,2,3 ; \tag{2.5}$$

$$\int_T \vec{v}\cdot\vec{p}\, d\vec{x} , \quad \vec{p} \in \vec{\mathcal{P}}_{k-1}(T) , \quad \text{if } k \geq 1 . \tag{2.6}$$

Proposition 2.2 [8]. *For $k \geq 1$, a vector in $\vec{\mathcal{P}}_k(T)$ can be uniquely determined by the following degrees of freedom:*

$$\int_{e_i} \vec{v}\cdot\vec{n}\, p\, ds , \quad p \in \mathcal{P}_k(e_i) , \quad i = 1,2,3 ; \tag{2.7}$$

$$\int_T \vec{v}\cdot \vec{\mathrm{grad}}\, p\, d\vec{x} , \quad p \in \mathcal{P}_{k-1}(T), \text{ if } k \geq 2 ; \tag{2.8}$$

$$\int_T \vec{v}\cdot \vec{\mathrm{rot}}(p b_3(\vec{x}))d\vec{x} , \quad p \in \mathcal{P}_{k-2}(T), \text{ if } k \geq 2 . \tag{2.9}$$

Let us now consider a rectangle Q, with edges $e_1,\ldots,e_4$ parallel to the axes. For $k \geq 0$ we set

$$\mathcal{Q}_k(Q) = \{\text{polynomials on } Q \text{ of degree} \leq k \text{ in each variable}\} , \tag{2.10}$$

$$\mathcal{P}_k(Q) \text{ and } \vec{\mathcal{P}}_k(Q) \text{ as in (2.1) and (2.2)} , \tag{2.11}$$

$$\vec{\mathcal{R}}_k(Q) = (\mathcal{Q}_k(Q) + x_1\mathcal{Q}_k(Q)) \times (\mathcal{Q}_k(Q) + x_2\mathcal{Q}_k(Q)) \,, \tag{2.12}$$

$$\vec{\mathcal{N}}_k(Q) = \vec{\mathcal{P}}_k(Q) \oplus \{\vec{\mathrm{rot}}(x_1 x_2^{k+1})\} \oplus \{\vec{\mathrm{rot}}(x_2 x_1^{k+1})\} \,. \tag{2.13}$$

Again, the choice of the degrees of freedom for $\mathcal{Q}_k(Q)$ is not relevant at this stage. For $\vec{\mathcal{R}}_k(Q)$ and $\vec{\mathcal{N}}_k(Q)$ we have the following parametrizations.

Proposition 2.3 [21]. *For $k \geq 0$, a vector $\vec{v}$ in $\vec{\mathcal{R}}_k(Q)$ can be uniquely determined by the following degrees of freedom:*

$$\int_{e_i} \vec{v}\cdot\vec{n}\, p\, ds \,, \quad p \in \mathcal{P}_k(e_i) \,, \quad i = 1,2,3,4 \,; \tag{2.14}$$

$$\int_Q \vec{v}\cdot\vec{p}\, dx \,, \quad \vec{p} \in \{\mathcal{Q}_k(Q)^2 \mid \frac{\partial^k p_1}{\partial x_1^k} = \frac{\partial^k p_2}{\partial x_2^k} = 0\} \,, \text{ if } k \geq 1 \,. \tag{2.15}$$

Proposition 2.4 [8]. *For $k \geq 1$, a vector $\vec{v}$ in $\vec{\mathcal{N}}_k(Q)$ can be uniquely determined by the following degrees of freedom:*

$$\int_{e_i} \vec{v}\cdot\vec{n}\, p\, ds \,, \quad p \in \mathcal{P}_k(e_i) \,, \quad i = 1,2,3,4 \,; \tag{2.16}$$

$$\int_Q \vec{v}\cdot\vec{p}\, d\vec{x} \,, \quad \vec{p} \in \vec{\mathcal{P}}_{k-2}(Q) \,, \quad \text{if } k \geq 2 \,. \tag{2.17}$$

Now let $\mathcal{T}_h$ be a decomposition of a given domain D into triangles (with the usual assumptions, see, e.g., [12]). We want to consider pairs $(\varphi,\vec{v})$, where φ is a piecewise polynomial function and $\vec{v}$ is a piecewise polynomial vector on D, drawn from the two following choices. The Raviart–Thomas–Nedelec spaces for $k \geq 0$ are given by pairs $(\varphi,\vec{v})$ such that

$$\varphi \in M_k^{-1}(\mathcal{T}_h) := \{\varphi \mid \varphi \in L^2(D),\, \varphi|_T \in \mathcal{P}_k(T),\, T \in \mathcal{T}_h\} \,, \tag{2.18i}$$

$$\vec{v} \in \vec{\mathcal{R}}_k^0(\mathcal{T}_h) := \{\vec{v} \mid \vec{v} \in (L^2(D))^2,\; \operatorname{div}\vec{v} \in L^2(D),\, \vec{v}|_T \in \vec{\mathcal{R}}_k(T),\, T \in \mathcal{T}_h\} \,. \tag{2.18ii}$$

The spaces of [8] for $k \geq 1$ consist of pairs $(\varphi,\vec{v})$ such that

$$\varphi \in M_{k-1}^{-1}(\mathcal{T}_h) \,, \tag{2.19i}$$

$$\vec{v} \in \vec{\mathcal{N}}_k^0(\mathcal{T}_h) := \{\vec{v} \mid \vec{v} \in (L^2(D))^2,\; \operatorname{div}\vec{v} \in L^2(D),\, \vec{v}|_T \in \vec{\mathcal{P}}_k(T),\, T \in \mathcal{T}_h\} \,. \tag{2.19ii}$$

If, instead, we consider a decomposition $\mathcal{Q}_h$ of D into rectangles with edges parallel to the axes, then the Raviart–Thomas–Nedelec spaces for $k \geq 0$ are given by

$$\varphi \in \tilde{M}_k^{-1}(\mathcal{Q}_h) := \{\varphi \mid \varphi \in L^2(D),\ \varphi|_Q \in \mathcal{Q}_k(Q),\ Q \in \mathcal{Q}_h\}\ , \tag{2.20i}$$

$$\vec{v} \in \vec{\mathcal{R}}_k^0(\mathcal{Q}_h) := \{\vec{v} \mid \vec{v} \in (L^2(D))^2,\ \operatorname{div} \vec{v} \in L^2(D),\ \vec{v}|_Q \in \vec{\mathcal{R}}_k(Q),\ Q \in \mathcal{Q}_h\} \tag{2.20ii}$$

and the spaces of [8] for $k \geq 1$ by

$$\varphi \in M_{k-1}^{-1}(\mathcal{Q}_h) := \{\varphi \mid \varphi \in L^2(D),\ \varphi|_Q \in \mathcal{P}_{k-1}(Q),\ Q \in \mathcal{Q}_h\} \tag{2.21i}$$

$$\vec{v} \in \vec{\mathcal{N}}_k^0(\mathcal{Q}_h) := \{\vec{v} \mid \vec{v} \in (L^2(D))^2,\ \operatorname{div} \vec{v} \in L^2(D),\ \vec{v}|_Q \in \vec{\mathcal{N}}_k(Q),\ Q \in \mathcal{Q}_h\}\ . \tag{2.21ii}$$

In all cases, note that the condition $\operatorname{div} \vec{v} \in L^2(D)$ is satisfied if and only if $\vec{v} \cdot \vec{n}$ is continuous across each interelement boundary.

It is easy to check that, *for the same value of k*, (which, as we shall see, roughly means *the same accuracy*) the choices (2.19) and (2.21) imply a lower number of degrees of freedom than (2.18) and (2.20), respectively. Actually, if NS is the number of edges of the decomposition and NE is the number of elements, then

$$\dim(M_k^{-1}(\mathcal{T}_h) \times \vec{\mathcal{R}}_k^0(\mathcal{T}_h)) = (k+1)NS + \frac{1}{2}(3k^2 + 5k + 2)NE\ ,$$

$$\dim(M_{k-1}^{-1}(\mathcal{T}_h) \times \vec{\mathcal{N}}_k^0(\mathcal{T}_h)) = (k+1)NS + \frac{1}{2}(3k^2 + k - 2)NE\ ,$$

and

$$\dim(\tilde{M}_k^{-1}(\mathcal{Q}_h) \times \vec{\mathcal{R}}_k^0(\mathcal{Q}_h)) = (k+1)NS + (3k^2 + 4k + 1)NE\ ,$$

$$\dim(M_{k-1}^{-1}(\mathcal{Q}_h) \times \vec{\mathcal{R}}_k^0(\mathcal{Q}_h)) = (k+1)NS + \frac{1}{2}(3k^2 - k)NE\ .$$

3. Application to a simple model problem

In this section we use the spaces (2.18)–(2.21) to approximate the solution of the simple model problem

$$-\Delta\psi = f \quad \text{in } D\ , \tag{3.1}$$

$$\psi = 0 \quad \text{on } \partial D\ . \tag{3.2}$$

A more general model problem with variable coefficients and nonhomogeneous boundary conditions is considered in [8].

The basic idea in the mixed method is simply to write the system (3.1)–(3.2) in the factored form

$$\vec{u} = \overrightarrow{\text{grad}}\, \psi \quad \text{in } D , \tag{3.3}$$

$$\psi = 0 \quad \text{on } \partial D , \tag{3.4}$$

$$-\text{div}\, \vec{u} = f \quad \text{in } D . \tag{3.5}$$

In variational form, we seek $\vec{u} \in H(\text{div};D)$ and $\psi \in L^2(D)$ such that

$$\int_D \vec{u} \cdot \vec{v}\, d\vec{x} + \int_D \psi \,\text{div}\, \vec{v}\, d\vec{x} = 0 , \quad \vec{v} \in H(\text{div};D) , \tag{3.6}$$

$$\int_D \varphi \,\text{div}\, \vec{u}\, d\vec{x} = -\int_D f\varphi\, d\vec{x} , \quad \varphi \in L^2(D) . \tag{3.7}$$

Note that (3.6) is derived from (3.3) and (3.4). It is very easy to check that (3.6)–(3.7) is well posed for $f \in L^2(D)$ (use, for instance, [7]). The equivalence with (3.1)–(3.2) is straightforward. Now we discretize (3.6)–(3.7) by means of the spaces (2.18)–(2.21); i.e., we seek $\vec{u}_h \in \vec{U}_h$ and $\psi \in \Psi_h$ such that

$$\int_D \vec{u}_h \cdot \vec{v}\, d\vec{x} + \int_D \psi_h \,\text{div}\, \vec{v}\, d\vec{x} = 0 , \quad \vec{v} \in \vec{U}_h , \tag{3.8}$$

$$\int_D \varphi \,\text{div}\, \vec{u}_h\, d\vec{x} = -\int_D f\varphi\, d\vec{x} , \quad \varphi \in \Psi_h , \tag{3.9}$$

where, for the triangular case,

$$\text{(case (2.18))} \quad \vec{U}_h := \vec{\mathcal{R}}_k^0(\mathcal{T}_h) , \quad \Psi_h := M_k^{-1}(\mathcal{T}_h) \tag{3.10}$$

or

$$\text{(case (2.19))} \quad \vec{U}_h := \vec{\mathcal{N}}_k^0(\mathcal{T}_h) , \quad \Psi_h := M_{k-1}^{-1}(\mathcal{T}_h) \tag{3.11}$$

and, for the rectangular case,

$$\text{(case (2.20))} \quad \vec{U}_h := \vec{\mathcal{R}}_k^0(\mathcal{L}_h) , \quad \Psi_h := \tilde{M}_k^{-1}(\mathcal{L}_h) \tag{3.12}$$

or

$$\text{(case (2.21))} \quad \vec{U}_h := \vec{\mathcal{N}}_k^0(\mathcal{L}_h) , \quad \Psi_h := M_{k-1}^{-1}(\mathcal{L}_h) . \tag{3.13}$$

Again it can be shown that all cases (3.10)–(3.13) lead to a well–posed, uniformly stable problem. A drawback of the formulation, however, consists in the fact that in all cases the corresponding matrix has the form

$$\begin{bmatrix} A & B \\ B^{\mathrm{T}} & 0 \end{bmatrix}$$

and is not positive definite. A way of circumventing this difficulty is found in the early works of Fraeijs de Veubeke [17] (see also [10], [11] for applications of this idea in a context closer to the present one). For the sake of simplicity, we shall recall his idea just for the choice (3.11). The application to the other choices (3.10), (3.12), and (3.13) is substantially identical. Let us introduce the space Λ_k of functions μ which are defined on the union $\mathcal{E}_h$ of internal edges and whose restriction to each $e \in \mathcal{E}_h$ is a polynomial of degree not greater than k. The functions in Λ_k are required to vanish on boundary edges. Set

$$\vec{\mathcal{N}}_k^{-1} = \{\vec{v} \mid \vec{v} \in (L^2(D))^2,\ \vec{v}|_T \in \vec{\mathcal{P}}_k(T),\ T \in \mathcal{T}_h\} . \tag{3.14}$$

For $\vec{v} \in \vec{\mathcal{N}}_k^{-1}$ and $\mu \in \Lambda_k$, let

$$\langle \vec{v} \cdot \vec{n}, \mu \rangle = \sum_{T \in \mathcal{T}_h} \int_{\partial T} (\vec{v} \cdot \vec{n})\, \mu \, ds . \tag{3.15}$$

It is quite obvious that $\vec{\mathcal{N}}_k^0 \subset \vec{\mathcal{N}}_k^{-1}$ and that

$$\vec{v} \in \vec{\mathcal{N}}_k^0 \iff (\vec{v} \in \vec{\mathcal{N}}_k^{-1} \text{ and } \langle \vec{v} \cdot \vec{n}, \mu \rangle = 0, \mu \in \Lambda_k) . \tag{3.16}$$

Proposition 2.2 implies that the map $\vec{v} \to \langle \vec{v} \cdot \vec{n}, \cdot \rangle$ is surjective from $\vec{\mathcal{N}}_k^{-1}$ to $(\Lambda_k)'$. This, together with (3.8) and (3.16), implies the existence of a unique $\lambda_h \in \Lambda_k$ such that

$$\int_D \vec{u}_h \cdot \vec{v}\, d\vec{x} + \sum_{T \in \mathcal{T}_h} \int_D \psi_h \operatorname{div} \vec{v}\, d\vec{x} - \langle \vec{v} \cdot \vec{n}, \lambda_h \rangle = 0, \quad \vec{v} \in \vec{\mathcal{N}}_k^{-1} . \tag{3.17}$$

It follows that the problem of finding $\vec{\tilde{u}}_h \in \vec{\mathcal{N}}_k^{-1}$, $\tilde{\psi}_h \in M_{k-1}^{-1}$ and $\tilde{\lambda}_h \in \Lambda_k$ such that

$$\int_D \vec{\tilde{u}}_h \cdot \vec{v}\, d\vec{x} + \sum_{T \in \mathcal{T}_h} \int_D \tilde{\psi}_h \operatorname{div} \vec{v}\, d\vec{x} - \langle \vec{v} \cdot \vec{n}, \tilde{\lambda}_h \rangle = 0\ , \vec{v} \in \vec{\mathcal{N}}_k^{-1}\ , \tag{3.18}$$

$$\sum_{T \in \mathcal{T}_h} \int_D \varphi \operatorname{div} \vec{\tilde{u}}_h\, d\vec{x} = -\int_D f\varphi\, d\vec{x}\ , \quad \varphi \in M_{k-1}^{-1}\ , \tag{3.19}$$

$$\langle \vec{\tilde{u}}_h \cdot \vec{n}, \mu \rangle = 0\ , \quad \mu \in \Lambda_k\ , \tag{3.20}$$

has a unique solution $(\vec{\tilde{u}}_h, \tilde{\psi}_h, \tilde{\lambda}_h)$, where $(\vec{\tilde{u}}_h, \tilde{\psi}_h)$ is the solution of (3.8)–(3.9). In spite of its appearance, (3.18)–(3.20) is simpler to treat algebraically than (3.8)–(3.9). Actually, the corresponding matrix now has the form

$$\begin{bmatrix} \tilde{A} & \tilde{B} & \tilde{C} \\ \tilde{B}^{\mathsf{T}} & 0 & 0 \\ \tilde{C}^{\mathsf{T}} & 0 & 0 \end{bmatrix},$$

where $\tilde{A}$ is block diagonal with each block corresponding to the unknowns for $\vec{\tilde{u}}_h$ inside one element. An *a priori* inversion of $\tilde{A}$ element by element leads now to a matrix

$$\begin{bmatrix} \tilde{B}^{\mathsf{T}}\tilde{A}^{-1}\tilde{B} & \tilde{B}^{\mathsf{T}}\tilde{A}^{-1}\tilde{C} \\ \tilde{C}^{\mathsf{T}}\tilde{A}^{-1}\tilde{B} & \tilde{C}^{\mathsf{T}}\tilde{A}^{-1}\tilde{C} \end{bmatrix}$$

(which is symmetric and positive definite) in the remaining unknowns $\tilde{\psi}_h$ and $\tilde{\lambda}_h$. Actually, $\tilde{B}^{\mathsf{T}}\tilde{A}^{-1}\tilde{B}$ is also block diagonal, so that we can proceed further with elimination and be left with a symmetric and positive definite system for the unknown $\tilde{\lambda}_h$, which allows a much wider choice of effective direct and iterative methods to be applied to solve the system [19], [6].

We remark explicitly that the definition of Λ_k *does not change* from one of the choices (3.10)–(3.13) to another. As we shall show in the next section, the introduction of the Lagrange multiplier $\tilde{\lambda}_h$ is not just a computational trick, but it also provides, through its knowledge, information about the values of ψ on the interelement boundaries which can lead to higher order accuracy than that provided by ψ_h.

4. Asymptotic error estimates

All of the choices (3.10)–(3.13) enjoy a basic property that makes their analysis much easier than that for other non-standard finite-element methods. We denote by P_h the L^2 projection onto Ψ_h.

There exists a projection $\Pi_h \in \mathcal{L}(\vec{H}^1(\mathrm{div};D), \vec{U}_h)$ *such that*

$$\begin{array}{ccc} \vec{H}^1(\mathrm{div};D) & \xrightarrow{\ \mathrm{div}\ } & L^2(D) \\ \Pi_h \big\downarrow & & \big\downarrow P_h \\ \vec{U}_h & \xrightarrow{\ \mathrm{div}\ } & \Psi_h \to 0\,. \end{array} \tag{4.1}$$

Note that (4.1) means that div $\Pi_h \vec{v} = P_h$ div $\vec{v}$ for all $\vec{v}$ in $\vec{H}^1(\mathrm{div};D)$ and that $\mathrm{div}(\vec{U}_h) = \Psi_h$. With the usual nondegeneracy assumptions on the decomposition (i.e., minimum angle condition for the $\mathcal{T}_h$'s and nonflattening for the $\mathcal{E}_h$'s),

$$\|\Pi_h\| \leq c \text{ , independent of } h \text{ .} \tag{4.2}$$

The use of (4.1) and (4.2) gives immediately the following error estimates [8].

Theorem 4.1. *Let* $(\psi,\vec{u})$ *and* $(\psi_h,\vec{u}_h)$ *be the solutions of* (3.6)–(3.7) *and* (3.8)–(3.9), *respectively. Then,*

$$\|\vec{u}-\vec{u}_h\|_0 \leq c\|\vec{u}-\Pi_h\vec{u}\|_0 \text{ ,} \tag{4.3}$$

$$\|\psi-\psi_h\|_0 \leq c\{\|\psi-P_h\psi\|_0 + h\|\vec{u}-\Pi_h\vec{u}\|_0 + h^{\min(2,k)}\|\mathrm{div}(\vec{u}-\Pi_h\vec{u})\|_0\} \text{ .} \tag{4.4}$$

Here, and in the following, c is a constant independent of h, and $\|\cdot\|_0$ denotes the $L^2(D)$ norm (for scalars or vectors).

It can also be shown that

$$\|\vec{u}-\Pi_h\vec{u}\|_0 \leq ch^{q+1}\|\psi\|_{q+1} \text{ , } 0 \leq q \leq k \text{ ,} \tag{4.5}$$

(with obvious notations) for all cases (3.10)–(3.13). On the other hand, it is clear that

$$\|\psi-P_h\psi\|_0 \leq ch^{q+1}\|\psi\|_{q+1} \text{ with } \begin{cases} 0 \leq q \leq k \text{ for (3.10) \& (3.12),} \\ 0 \leq q \leq k-1 \text{ for (3.11) \& (3.13).} \end{cases} \tag{4.6}$$

Combining (4.3)–(4.6), we end up with error estimates (for $\psi \in H^{k+2}(D)$) of the type:

$$\|\vec{u}-\vec{u}_h\|_0 \leq ch^{k+1} \tag{4.7}$$

for all the choices (3.10)–(3.13) and

$$\|\psi-\psi_h\|_0 \leq \begin{cases} ch^{k+1} & \text{for (3.10) \& (3.12) ,} \\ ch^k & \text{for (3.11) \& (3.13) .} \end{cases} \tag{4.8}$$

Hence it seems, at first sight, that the Raviart–Thomas–Nedelec spaces (3.10) and (3.12) provide better accuracy for the scalar field ψ than our choices (3.11) and (3.13). However, it must be pointed out that one generally uses the mixed approach (3.6)–(3.7) only if the main interest is in the approximation of the vector field $\vec{u}$. Also we shall see in what follows that we can obtain from the χ_h variable (introduced at the end of the previous section) a better approximation for ψ by a simple postprocessing. But first let us recall the negative norm estimates that can be obtained for (3.8)–(3.9). Here $\|\cdot\|_{-s}$ for $s \geq 0$ is the $(H^s(D))'$ norm (for scalars and vectors). We shall also assume that D has the following $(s+2)$–regularity property:

$$\begin{cases} \text{for any given } g \in H^s(D), \text{ the unique solution} \\ \varphi \in H_0^1(D) \text{ of } -\Delta\varphi = g \text{ satisfies} \\ \qquad \|\varphi\|_{s+2} \leq c\|g\|_s . \end{cases} \tag{4.9}$$

Actually, (4.9) is "rather contradictory" with the previous (implicit) assumption that D is the union of a finite number of triangles (or rectangles). In fact, what is done in [15], [16] and [8] is to assume (4.9) and then to use in $\mathcal{T}_h$ or $\mathcal{Q}_h$ generalized triangles (respectively, rectangles) with at most one curved edge. This can be done without jeopardizing (4.1) and (4.2) or (4.5) and (4.6), so that the previous estimates (4.7) and (4.8) remain valid. We chose not to introduce here the use of curved boundaries for the sake of simplicity.

Theorem 4.2. *Let* $(\psi,\vec{u})$ *and* $(\psi_h,\vec{u}_h)$ *be the solutions of* (3.6)–(3.7) *and* (3.8)–(3.9), *respectively. Then, for* (3.10) *or* (3.12),

$$\|\psi_h - P_h\psi\|_{-s} \leq ch^{s+k+2} , \quad 0 \leq s \leq k , \tag{4.10}$$

$$\|\vec{u}_h - u\|_{-s} \leq ch^{s+k+1} , \quad 0 \leq s \leq k+1 . \tag{4.11}$$

For (3.11) *or* (3.13),

$$\|\psi_h - P_h\psi\|_{-s} \leq ch^{\min(s+k+2,2k)} , \tag{4.12}$$

$$\|\vec{u}_h - u\|_{-s} \leq ch^{\min(s+k+1,2k)} . \tag{4.13}$$

The proofs of the bounds (4.10) and (4.11) are given in [16] and the proofs of (4.12) and (4.13) in [8]. Note that (4.10) and (4.12) can be viewed as superconvergence results.

Assume now that we solve (3.8)–(3.9) on the computer in the form (3.18)–(3.20). It can be shown (see [3], [8]) that it is possible to construct, element by element, a piecewise polynomial function $\tilde{\psi}_h$ such that

$$\|\psi-\tilde{\psi}_h\|_0 \leq ch^{k+2} \text{ (for (3.10) or (3.12))} , \tag{4.14}$$

$$\|\psi-\tilde{\psi}_h\|_0 \leq ch^{\min(k+2,2k)} \text{ (for (3.11) or (3.13))} . \tag{4.15}$$

For instance, in the triangular case ((3.10) or (3.11)) and for k even, $\tilde{\psi}_h$ on a triangle T can be defined as the unique element of $\mathcal{P}_{k+1}(T)$ satisfying

$$\int_{e_i} (\tilde{\psi}_h - \tilde{\lambda}_h)\, p(s) ds = 0 \,, \quad p \in \mathcal{P}_k(e_i),\ i = 1,2,3 \,; \tag{4.16}$$

$$\int_T (\tilde{\psi}_h - \psi_h) p \, d\vec{x} = 0 \,, \quad p \in \mathcal{P}_{k-2}(T) \,. \tag{4.17}$$

The definition is slightly more complicated in other cases.

The estimates (4.14) and (4.15) show that, except for the case k=1, the simpler choices (3.11) and (3.13) provide the same accuracy as the usual ones (3.10) and (3.12) for the scalar variable.

Remark. In some cases, it may be interesting to use polynomials of different degree in different parts of the domain. This requires the use of "transition elements" since the normal component of the vector field $\vec{v}$ is the only quantity that has to be continuous from one element to another. It follows that on a transition element $\vec{v} \cdot \vec{n}$ will be, say, of degree k on one edge and of degree k–1 on one (or more) of the other edges. This can be done for our mixed elements (3.11) and (3.13) without losing the crucial property (4.1) (see [9] for the proof). On the other hand, the same cannot be done (or, at least, not as easily) for the classical Raviart–Thomas–Nedelec spaces. Roughly speaking, the elements (3.11) and (3.13) have one degree more than necessary (in $\vec{v} \cdot \vec{n}$) in order to enforce (4.1) (because the scalar space Ψ_h is of degree k–1), so that one can lower by one (when necessary) the degree of $\vec{v} \cdot \vec{n}$ on one or more edges without losing (4.1). In the case of triangular elements (3.11), if we lower the degree of $\vec{v} \cdot \vec{n}$ by one on all the three edges, we obtain elements that are similar to the classical ones (3.10). This is not true, however, for the rectangular elements (3.13). Composite elements can be used in order to shift from the degree k to the degree k–2 (or k–3) in a single step. We refer to [9] for the details.

5. An application to linear elasticity problems

The Raviart–Thomas–Nedelec elements have been used as a starting point for building other families of elements in various applications. We show here a simple example of a similar use for our triangular element in the case k=1.

Let D be a polygon in $\mathbf{R}^2$. For any $\vec{v} = (v_1, v_2)$ we define as usual the strain tensor $\varepsilon(\vec{v})$ by $\varepsilon_{ij} = 1/2\ (\partial v_i/\partial x_j + \partial v_j/\partial x_i)$. We write the linear plane elasticity strain–stress relationship (Hooke's law) $\sigma = 2\mu\varepsilon + \lambda\ \mathrm{tr}(\varepsilon)\delta$ ($\mu > 0$ and $\lambda \in [0,\infty]$ being the Lamé coefficients) in the form $\sigma = E(\varepsilon)$ and its inverse in the form $\varepsilon = C(\sigma)$. Our model elasticity problem when $\lambda < \infty$ can now be written as follows:

$$\left\{\begin{array}{l} \text{find } \vec{u} \in (H_0^1(D))^2 \text{ such that} \\ \int_D E(\varepsilon(\vec{u})) : \varepsilon(\vec{v}) d\vec{x} = \int_D \vec{f} \cdot \vec{v}\, d\vec{x} \,,\ \vec{v} \in (H_0^1(D))^2 \,, \end{array}\right. \tag{5.1}$$

where $\vec{f}$ is a given vector in, say, $(L^2(D))^2$.

The usual mixed formulation of (5.1) is given by the following:

$$\left|\begin{array}{l} \text{find } \sigma \in H_s(\vec{\mathrm{div}};D) \text{ and } \vec{u} \in (L^2(D))^2 \text{ such that} \\ \int_D C(\sigma) : \tau\, d\vec{x} + \int_D \vec{u} \cdot \vec{\mathrm{div}}\, \tau\, d\vec{x} = 0 \,,\ \tau \in H_s(\vec{\mathrm{div}};D) \,, \\ \int_D \vec{v} \cdot \vec{\mathrm{div}}\, \sigma\, d\vec{x} = \int_D \vec{f} \cdot \vec{v}\, d\vec{x} \,,\ \vec{v} \in (L^2(D))^2 \,, \end{array}\right. \tag{5.2}$$

where $H_s(\vec{\mathrm{div}};D)$ is the set of *symmetric* tensors τ in $(L^2(D))^4$ with $\vec{\mathrm{div}}\ \tau \in (L^2(D))^2$. One would like to discretize τ in the form

$$\tau = \begin{bmatrix} z_1 & z_2 \\ w_1 & w_2 \end{bmatrix} \tag{5.3}$$

with both $\vec{z}$ and $\vec{w}$ in a Raviart–Thomas–Nedelec vector space. This attempt clearly fails because, in general, $z_2 \neq w_1$. In some cases (such as our model problem (5.1)), this difficulty can be avoided by working with non-symmetric tensors, as in Arnold and Falk (see [2], [5]). Following them we set

$$\rho := \mu\ \mathrm{grad}(\vec{u}) + (\mu + \lambda)(\mathrm{div}\ \vec{u})\delta \,. \tag{5.4}$$

Relation (5.4) can be inverted; we write

$$\mathrm{grad}(\vec{u}) = B(\rho) \,, \tag{5.5}$$

and consider the following problem:

$$\left|\begin{array}{l} \text{find } \rho \in H(\vec{\mathrm{div}};D) \text{ and } \vec{u} \in (L^2(D))^2 \text{ such that} \\ \int_D \mathrm{B}(\rho) : \tau\, d\vec{x} + \int_D \vec{u} \cdot \vec{\mathrm{div}}\, \tau\, d\vec{x} = 0 \,,\ \tau \in H(\vec{\mathrm{div}};D) \,, \\ \int_D \vec{v} \cdot \vec{\mathrm{div}}\, \rho\, d\vec{x} = \int_D \vec{f} \cdot \vec{v}\, d\vec{x} \,,\ \vec{v} \in (L^2(D))^2 \,. \end{array}\right. \tag{5.6}$$

Problem (5.6) makes sense because we can easily derive the relation $\vec{\mathrm{div}}\ \rho = \vec{\mathrm{div}}\ \sigma = \vec{f}$ from (5.4). Now, the tensor space $H(\vec{\mathrm{div}};D)$ has no symmetry requirements, and the choice (5.3) is allowable for $\vec{z}$ and $\vec{w}$ to be in one of the vector spaces (2.18)–(2.21); the variable $\vec{v}$ will also be chosen as a pair of scalars (ζ,χ), so that both components belong to the corresponding scalar space in (2.18)–(2.21). For instance, we can choose

$$H(\vec{\mathrm{div}};D) \simeq \left\{ \begin{bmatrix} z_1 & z_2 \\ w_1 & w_2 \end{bmatrix} \mid \vec{z} \in \vec{N}_k^0(\mathcal{T}_h),\ \vec{w} \in \vec{N}_k^0(\mathcal{T}_h) \right\} =: \Sigma_h \,, \tag{5.7}$$

$$(L^2(D))^2 \simeq \{(\zeta,\chi) \mid \zeta \in M_{k-1}^{-1}(\mathcal{T}_h), \chi \in M_{k-1}^{-1}(\mathcal{T}_h)\} =: \vec{S}_h \,. \tag{5.8}$$

An easy combination of the arguments of [5] (for the formulation (5.6)) and [8] (for the choice (5.7)–(5.8)) shows that

$$\|\rho_h - \rho\| \le ch^{k+1} \,, \quad \|\vec{u}_h - \vec{u}\| \le ch^k \,. \tag{5.9}$$

An estimate of type (4.15) for a better approximation of the displacement field can also be derived. From ρ_h one finally deduces an approximation σ_h of σ through simple element–by–element algebraic computations.

If one chooses, instead, to stay with the physical variable σ, then a possibility is found in relaxing the symmetry requirements via a Lagrange multiplier. See [18], [1], [4], [20] for various results in this direction. We shall show here how this can be done in the context of our elements (2.19).

Note first that, for each $\tau \in H(\vec{\mathrm{div}};D)$,

$$\int_D C(\sigma) : \tau \, d\vec{x} + \int_D \vec{u} \cdot \vec{\mathrm{div}}\, \tau \, d\vec{x} = -\int_D \gamma \, \mathrm{as}(\tau) d\vec{x} \,, \tag{5.10}$$

where $\gamma := 1/2\,(\partial u_2/\partial x_1 - \partial u_1/\partial x_2)$ and $\mathrm{as}(\tau) := \tau_{21} - \tau_{12}$.

In order to discretize this problem, we first choose $\vec{S}_h$ as in (5.8) for k=1; i.e., $\vec{S}_h$ consists of piecewise constants to approximate the displacement field $\vec{u}$. An approximation of the stress field σ can then be obtained by augmenting the space Σ_h given in (5.7) of piecewise linear vectors for k=1 by means of two internal shape functions per triangle; namely, we take

$$\tilde{\Sigma}_h := \Sigma_h \oplus \begin{bmatrix} \partial b/\partial x_2 & -\partial b/\partial x_1 \\ 0 & 0 \end{bmatrix} \oplus \begin{bmatrix} 0 & 0 \\ \partial b/\partial x_2 & -\partial b/\partial x_1 \end{bmatrix} , \tag{5.11}$$

where $b(\vec{x}) := b_3(\vec{x}) = \lambda_1(\vec{x})\lambda_2(\vec{x})\lambda_3(\vec{x})$. Finally, we introduce the following space for the discretization of γ:

$$\Gamma_h := \{\beta | \beta \in H_0^1(\overline{D}), \beta|_T \in \mathcal{P}_1(T)\} \,. \tag{5.12}$$

The corresponding discrete problem is to

find $(\sigma_h, \vec{u}_h, \gamma_h) \in \tilde{\Sigma}_h \times \vec{S}_h \times \Gamma_h$ such that

$$\begin{cases} \int_D C(\sigma_h) : \tau \, d\vec{x} + \int_D \vec{u}_h \cdot \vec{\mathrm{div}}\, \tau \, d\vec{x} + \int_D \gamma_h \, \mathrm{as}(\tau) d\vec{x} = 0 \,, \tau \in \tilde{\Sigma}_h \,, \\ \int_D \vec{v} \cdot \vec{\mathrm{div}}\, \sigma_h \, d\vec{x} = \int_D \vec{f} \cdot \vec{v} \, d\vec{x} \,, \vec{v} \in \vec{S}_h \,, \\ \int_D \mathrm{as}(\sigma_h) \, \beta \, d\vec{x} = 0 \,, \beta \in \Gamma_h \,. \end{cases} \tag{5.13}$$

Lemma 5.1. Let τ be an element of $H_s(\vec{\mathrm{div}};D)$ such that

$$\int_D \mathrm{tr}(\tau) d\vec{x} = 0 \,. \tag{5.14}$$

Then, there exists an element $\Pi_h \tau \in \tilde{\Sigma}_h$ such that

$$\|\tau - \Pi_h \tau\|_0 \le ch^2 \|\tau\|_2 \text{ (whenever } \|\tau\|_2 \text{ is finite)} \,, \tag{5.15}$$

$$\int_D \vec{\mathrm{div}}\, (\tau - \Pi_h \tau) \cdot \vec{v} \, d\vec{x} = 0 \,, \vec{v} \in \vec{S}_h \,, \tag{5.16}$$

$$\int_D \mathrm{as}(\Pi_h \tau) \beta \, d\vec{x} = 0 \,, \beta \in \Gamma_h \,, \tag{5.17}$$

$$\int_D \mathrm{tr}(\Pi_h \tau) \, d\vec{x} = 0 \,. \tag{5.18}$$

Proof. We shall construct five tensors $\tau^{(1)},\dots,\tau^{(5)}$ in $\tilde{\Sigma}_h$ such that each of them satisfies

$$\| \tau - \tau^{(i)} \|_0 \le ch^2 \|\tau\|_2 \,, \tag{5.19}$$

$$\int_D \vec{\mathrm{div}} (\tau - \tau^{(i)}) \cdot \vec{v} \, d\vec{x} = 0 \,, \quad \vec{v} \in \vec{S}_h \,. \tag{5.20}$$

Moreover, $\tau^{(4)}$ and $\tau^{(5)}$ will satisfy

$$\int_D \mathrm{as}(\tau^{(i)}) \beta \, d\vec{x} = 0 \,, \quad \beta \in \Gamma_h \,, \tag{5.21}$$

and finally

$$\int_D \mathrm{tr}(\tau^{(5)}) \, d\vec{x} = 0 \,, \tag{5.22}$$

so that the choice $\Pi_h \tau := \tau^{(5)}$ will end the proof. We start by choosing $\tau^{(1)}$ in Σ_h such that for each edge e in $\mathcal{T}_h$ we have

$$\int_e (\tau - \tau^{(1)}) \vec{n} \cdot \vec{p} \, ds = 0 \,, \quad p \in \vec{\mathcal{P}}_1(e) \,. \tag{5.23}$$

This is possible from Proposition 2.2. An easy computation gives (5.20; i=1) and standard Bramble–Hilbert techniques give (5.19; i=1). Now set

$$\eta := \frac{1}{|D|}\int_D \mathrm{as}(\underline{\tau}^{(1)})\, d\vec{x}\,. \tag{5.24}$$

Since $\mathrm{as}(\underline{\tau}) = 0$ (5.19; i=1) implies that $|\eta| \le ch^2$. Thus, setting

$$\underline{\tau}^{(2)} := \underline{\tau}^{(1)} + \begin{pmatrix} 0 & \eta \\ 0 & 0 \end{pmatrix}, \tag{5.25}$$

we have (5.19) and (5.20) for i=2; moreover,

$$\int_D \mathrm{as}(\underline{\tau}^{(2)})\, d\vec{x} = 0\,. \tag{5.26}$$

It is well known that (5.26) implies the existence of $\vec{z} \in (H_0^1(D))^2$ such that

$$\mathrm{div}\, \vec{z} = \mathrm{as}(\underline{\tau}^{(2)})\,, \tag{5.27}$$

$$\|\vec{z}\|_1 \le \|\mathrm{as}(\underline{\tau}^{(2)})\|_0 \le ch^2 \|\underline{\tau}\|_2\,. \tag{5.28}$$

Following [13] or [14] (see also [4] for a related argument) we can construct $\vec{z}^h \in (H_0^1(D))^2$, piecewise linear and continuous, such that

$$\|\vec{z}-\vec{z}^h\|_{r,T} \le ch_T^{1-r}\|\vec{z}\|_{1,T}\,,\quad r = 0,1,\quad T \in \mathcal{T}_h\,. \tag{5.29}$$

We now set

$$\underline{\tau}^{(3)} := \underline{\tau}^{(2)} + \begin{bmatrix} -\partial z_1^h/\partial x_2 & \partial z_1^h/\partial x_1 \\ -\partial z_2^h/\partial x_2 & \partial z_2^h/\partial x_1 \end{bmatrix}. \tag{5.30}$$

Note that $\underline{\tau}^{(3)} \in \Sigma_h$. We have $\vec{\mathrm{div}}\, \underline{\tau}^{(3)} = \vec{\mathrm{div}}\, \underline{\tau}^{(2)}$, so that (5.20) holds for i=3. Moreover, (5.28) and (5.29) imply (5.19, i=3). For all $\beta \in H_0^1(D)$ we have now from (5.27) and (5.30)

$$\int_D \mathrm{as}(\underline{\tau}^{(3)})\, \beta\, d\vec{x} = \int_D \mathrm{div}(\vec{z} - \vec{z}^h)\, \beta\, d\vec{x}$$

$$= -\int_D (\vec{z} - \vec{z}^h)\cdot \vec{\mathrm{grad}}\, \beta\, d\vec{x}\,. \tag{5.31}$$

Now, for any $T \in \mathcal{T}_h$, we define $\vec{\alpha} = \vec{\alpha}(T) \in \mathbf{R}^2$ by

$$\vec{\alpha}\int_T b(\vec{x})\, d\vec{x} = \int_T (\vec{z} - \vec{z}^h)\, d\vec{x}\,; \tag{5.32}$$

a simple scaling argument shows that

$$|\vec{\alpha}(T)| \le c\|\vec{z} - \vec{z}^h\|_{0,T} / \|b\|_{0,T}\,. \tag{5.33}$$

Next we set, in each T,

$$\tau^{(4)} := \tau^{(3)} + \begin{bmatrix} -\alpha_1 \partial b/\partial x_2 & \alpha_1 \partial b/\partial x_1 \\ -\alpha_2 \partial b/\partial x_2 & \alpha_2 \partial b/\partial x_2 \end{bmatrix} . \tag{5.34}$$

Clearly, $\tau^{(4)} \in \tilde{\Sigma}_h$. For $\beta \in \Gamma_h$ (which implies that $\overrightarrow{\text{grad}}\, \beta \in \vec{\mathcal{P}}_0(T)$ for all T) we have now from (5.31), (5.32) and (5.34)

$$\int_D \text{as}(\tau^{(4)})\, \beta\, d\vec{x} = \int_D \text{as}(\tau^{(3)})\, \beta\, d\vec{x} + \int_D b(\vec{x})\, \vec{\alpha} \cdot \overrightarrow{\text{grad}}\, \beta\, d\vec{x} = 0 . \tag{5.35}$$

On the other hand, (5.20; i=4) holds, and from (5.33) and (5.34) we have

$$\|\tau^{(3)} - \tau^{(4)}\|_{0,T} \le |\alpha(T)|\ \|b\|_{1,T} \le ch_T^{-1}\ \|\vec{z} - \vec{z}^h\|_{0,T} \tag{5.36}$$

so that (5.36), (5.29) and (5.28) give

$$\|\tau^{(3)} - \tau^{(4)}\|_0 \le ch^2\, \|\tau\|_2 \ ; \tag{5.37}$$

hence, we have (5.19; i=4) from (5.19; i=3) and (5.37). Note that (5.19; i=4) and (5.14) imply that

$$\left|\int_D \text{tr}(\tau^{(4)})\, d\vec{x}\right| \le ch^2 \ . \tag{5.38}$$

Now we set

$$\tau^{(5)} = \tau^{(4)} - \frac{1}{|D|} \int_D \text{tr}(\tau^{(4)})\, d\vec{x}\, \delta \ , \tag{5.39}$$

and we clearly have (5.19)–(5.21) for i=5, as well as (5.22).

Lemma 5.2. *For any* $\tau \in \tilde{\Sigma}_h$ *such that* $\int_D \text{tr}(\tau) d\vec{x} = 0$ *and* $\overrightarrow{\text{div}}\, \tau = 0$,

$$\int_D C(\tau) : \tau\, d\vec{x} \ge c\|\tau\|_0^2 \ , \tag{5.40}$$

with c *independent of* τ, h, *and the Lamé coefficient* $\lambda \in [0,+\infty]$.

The proof is identical to that of [4; Lemma 4.3].

Theorem 5.3. *Let* $(\sigma,\vec{u})$ *be the solution of* (5.2), *let* $\gamma := 1/2(\partial u_2/\partial x_1 - \partial u_1/\partial x_2)$, *and let* $(\sigma_h, \vec{u}_h, \gamma_h)$ *be the solution of* (5.13). *Then,*

$$\|\sigma - \sigma_h\|_0 \le ch^2(\|\sigma\|_2 + \|\gamma\|_2) \ , \tag{5.41}$$

$$\|\gamma - \gamma_h\|_0 \le ch^2(\|\sigma\|_2 + \|\gamma\|_2) \ , \tag{5.42}$$

$$\|P_h\vec{u} - \vec{u}_h\|_0 \le ch^2(\|\sigma\|_2 + \|\gamma\|_2) , \tag{5.43}$$

where $P_h\vec{u}$ is the projection of $\vec{u}$ onto $\vec{S}_h$ (piecewise constants), with the constant c independent of h and λ.

Proof. Taking $\tau = \delta$ in the first equation of (5.2) and of (5.23) shows that $\int_D \operatorname{tr}(\sigma)d\vec{x} = \int_D \operatorname{tr}(\sigma_h)d\vec{x} = 0$ (see [4] for more details). Set

$$\xi = \Pi_h\sigma - \sigma_h , \tag{5.44}$$

with Π_h given by Lemma 5.1. From (5.18),

$$\int_D \operatorname{tr}(\xi)\, d\vec{x} = 0 . \tag{5.45}$$

It follows from (5.2), (5.13), and (5.16) that

$$\vec{\operatorname{div}}\, \xi = 0 \tag{5.46}$$

and from (5.17) that

$$\int_D \operatorname{as}(\xi)\, \beta\, d\vec{x} = 0 , \quad \beta \in \Gamma_h . \tag{5.47}$$

Finally, from (5.15),

$$\|\sigma - \Pi_h\sigma\|_0 \le ch^2 \|\sigma\|_2 . \tag{5.48}$$

Now apply (5.40) to see that

$$\|\xi\|_0^2 \le c\int_D C(\xi)\colon \xi\, d\vec{x} \le c\,\{\int_D C(\sigma_h - \sigma)\colon \xi\, d\vec{x} + \|\xi\|_0\, \|\sigma - \Pi_h\sigma\|_0\} . \tag{5.49}$$

From (5.10), (5.13) and then (5.46) we have

$$\begin{aligned}\int_D C(\sigma_h - \sigma)\colon \xi\, d\vec{x} &= \int_D (\vec{u} - \vec{u}_h) \cdot \vec{\operatorname{div}}\, \xi\, d\vec{x} \\ &\quad + \int_D (\gamma - \gamma_h)\, \operatorname{as}(\xi)\, d\vec{x} \\ &= \int_D (\gamma - \gamma_h)\, \operatorname{as}(\xi)\, d\vec{x} .\end{aligned} \tag{5.50}$$

If γ^I is the interpolant of γ in Γ_h, we can use (5.47) in (5.50) to obtain the bound

$$\int_D C(\sigma_h - \sigma)\colon \xi d\vec{x} = \int_D (\gamma - \gamma^I)\, \operatorname{as}(\xi)\, d\vec{x} \le ch^2 \|\gamma\|_2 \|\xi\|_0 ; \tag{5.51}$$

thus, (5.48), (5.49), and (5.51) imply (5.41). From [4; Lemma 4.4] we know that there exists a nontrivial $\tau \in \Sigma_h$ such that

$$\vec{\operatorname{div}}\, \tau = 0 , \tag{5.52}$$

$$\int_D (\gamma^I - \gamma_h)\, \operatorname{as}(\tau)\, d\vec{x} \geq c \|\tau\|_0 \, \|\gamma^I - \gamma_h\|_0 . \tag{5.53}$$

Hence,

$$c\, \|\gamma^I - \gamma_h\|_0 \|\tau\|_0 \leq \int_D (\gamma^I - \gamma_h)\, \operatorname{as}(\tau)\, d\vec{x}$$

$$\leq \int_D (\gamma - \gamma_h)\, \operatorname{as}(\tau)\, d\vec{x} + ch^2 \|\gamma\|_2 \|\tau\|_0 . \tag{5.54}$$

On the other hand, using (5.52) and proceeding as in (5.50), we have

$$\int_D (\gamma - \gamma_h)\, \operatorname{as}(\tau)\, d\vec{x} = \int_D C(\sigma_h - \sigma) : \tau \, d\vec{x} , \tag{5.55}$$

so that from (5.54), (5.55), and (5.41) we find that

$$\|\gamma^I - \gamma_h\|_0 \leq ch^2 (\|\sigma\|_2 + \|\gamma\|_2) , \tag{5.56}$$

which implies (5.42) via the triangle inequality. Finally, we can choose τ (again by [4; Lemma 4.4]) such that

$$\int_D (P_h\vec{u} - \vec{u}_h) \cdot \vec{\operatorname{div}}\, \tau \, d\vec{x} \geq c \|\tau\|_0 \, \|P_h\vec{u} - \vec{u}_h\|_0 . \tag{5.57}$$

Since P_h is the L^2–projection onto $\vec{S}_h$, it follows from (5.10) and (5.13) that

$$\int_D (P_h\vec{u} - \vec{u}_h) \cdot \vec{\operatorname{div}}\, \tau \, d\vec{x} = \int_D (\vec{u} - \vec{u}_h) \cdot \vec{\operatorname{div}}\, \tau \, d\vec{x}$$

$$= \int_D C(\sigma_h - \sigma) : \tau \, d\vec{x} - \int_D (\gamma - \gamma_h)\, \operatorname{as}(\tau)\, d\vec{x} , \tag{5.58}$$

and (5.43) follows from (5.57), (5.58), (5.41), and (5.42).

Remark. An error bound for $\vec{u} - \vec{u}_h$ is easily derived from (5.42) and the triangle inequality:

$$\|\vec{u} - \vec{u}_h\|_0 \leq \|\vec{u} - P_h\vec{u}\|_0 + \|P_h\vec{u} - \vec{u}\|_0 \leq ch . \tag{5.59}$$

However, in general, it is better to introduce an interelement Lagrange multiplier $\vec{\lambda}_h$ as in Section 3 and then to derive approximations for $\vec{u}$ from both $\vec{u}_h$ and $\vec{\lambda}_h$, as in section 4. See [4] for similar arguments.

Remark. Since the constant c which appears in (5.41)–(5.43) does not depend on the Lamé coefficient λ, the discretization (5.13) will be uniformly good for nearly incompressible materials. For $\lambda = \infty$ (completely incompressible material) we have the same results (since $\lambda = \infty$ is allowed in Lemma 5.2), but the condition $\int_D \operatorname{tr}(\sigma_h)\, d\vec{x} = 0$ must be added explicitly to (5.13) (and to (5.2)). See [4] for more details in a very similar case.

REFERENCES

[1] Amara, M., and Thomas, J.M. "Equilibrium finite elements for the linear elastic problem," *Numer. Math.* 33 (1979): 367–383.

[2] Arnold, D.N. A new mixed formulation for the numerical solution of elasticity problems. In *Advances in Computer Methods for Partial Differential Equations*, ed. R. Vichnevetsky and R.S. Stepleman. New Brunswick, NJ: IMACS, 1984.

[3] Arnold, D.N., and Brezzi, F. "Mixed and nonconforming finite element methods: implementation, postprocessing and error estimates," *Modélisation Mathématiques et Analyse Numérique* 19 (1985): 7-32.

[4] Arnold, D.N., Brezzi, F., and Douglas, J., Jr. "PEERS: A New Mixed Finite Element for Plane Elasticity," *Japan J. Appl. Math.* 1 (1984): 347-367.

[5] Arnold, D.N., and Falk, R.S. Mixed finite elements for elasticity. In preparation.

[6] Axelsson, A., and Barker, V.A. *Finite Element Solution of Boundary Value Problems: Theory and Computation.* New York: Academic Press, 1984.

[7] Brezzi, F. "On the existence, uniqueness, and approximation of saddle point problems arising from Lagrangian multipliers," *R.A.I.R.O., Anal. numér.* 2 (1974): 129–151.

[8] Brezzi, F., Douglas, J. Jr., and Marini, L.D. "Two families of mixed finite elements for second order elliptic problems," *Numer. Math.* 47 (1985): 217-235.

[9] ————. "Variable degree mixed methods for second order elliptic problems," *Matemática Aplicada e Computacional* 4 (1985): 19-34.

[10] Brezzi, F., Marini, L.D., Quarteroni, A., and Raviart, P.A. "On an equilibrium finite element method for plate bending problems," *Calcolo* 17 (1980): 272–291.

[11] Chinosi, C., Della Croce, L., Marini, L.D., Quarteroni, A., Sacchi, G., and Scapolla, T. Implementation of some finite element methods. Report 231 of IAN–CNR, Pavia (1979).

[12] Ciarlet, P.G. *The Finite Element Method for Elliptic Equations.* Amsterdam New York: North Holland, 1978.

[13] Clement, P. "Approximation by finite element functions using local regularization," *R.A.I.R.O., Anal. numér.* 9 (1975): 33–76.

[14] Douglas, J. Jr., Dupont T., and Wheeler, M.F. "H^1–Galerkin methods for the Laplace and heat equations." In *Mathematical Aspects of Finite Elements in Partial Differential Equations*, ed. Carl de Boor. New York: Academic Press, 1974.

[15] Douglas, J. Jr., and Roberts, J.E. "Mixed finite element methods for second order elliptic problems," *Matémática Aplicada e Computacional* 1 (1982): 91–103.

[16] ——————. "Global estimates for mixed methods for second order elliptic equations," *Math. of Comp.* 44 (1985): 39–52.

[17] Fraeijs de Veubeke, B.X. Displacement and equilibrium models in the finite element method. In *Stress Analysis*, ed. O.C. Zienkiewicz and G. Holister, New York: Wiley, 1965.

[18] ——————. 1975. Stress function approach. Paper presented at the International Congress on the Finite Element Method in Structural Mechanics, Bournemouth.

[19] Marchuk, G.I. *Methods of Numerical Mathematics*. New York Berlin Heidelberg Tokyo: Springer Verlag, 1975.

[20] Morley, M.E. Paper in preparation.

[21] Nedelec, J.C. "Mixed finite elements in $\mathbf{R}^3$," *Numer. Math.* 35 (1980): 315–341.

[22] Raviart, P.A., and Thomas, J.M. A mixed finite element method for second order elliptic problems. In *Mathematical Aspects of the Finite Element Method*, ed. I. Galligani and E. Magenes. Lecture Notes in Mathematics 606. Berlin New York Heidelberg Tokyo: Springer–Verlag, 1977.

ON THE MATHEMATICAL FOUNDATIONS OF THE k–ε TURBULENT MODEL

T. Chacon
INRIA
Paris, France

O. Pironneau
INRIA and Paris–Nord University
Paris, France

Abstract

The k–ε model is a heuristic model developed in engineering to take into account subgrid scale turbulence. It is used extensively in industry even though frequently the results are essentially inferior to the experimental data. In this paper we show how k–ε type models can be derived from the asymptotic expansion developed in earlier works [8], [9].

Introduction

Numerical simulation of turbulent flows at a high Reynolds number is a challenging problem. In principle, a direct simulation of the Navier–Stokes equations at the Reynolds number R is possible only if the grid size is smaller that $R^{-3/4}$. Therefore $R^{9/4}$ points are needed, more than the computer can handle!

The Reynolds equations

$$u_t + u\nabla u + \nabla p + \nabla\cdot\langle u'\otimes u'\rangle = 0\,, \quad \nabla\cdot u = 0$$

are obtained by averaging the Navier–Stokes equations where the total velocity v has been decomposed into

$$v = u + u' \quad \text{with } \langle u'\rangle = 0\,.$$

Here u is the mean flow and u' the turbulent part; $\langle u'\rangle$ denotes the ensemble average of u'.

In the k–ε model the Reynolds stress tensor is assumed to be a diffusion tensor:

$$\langle u'\otimes u'\rangle = -\frac{k^2}{\varepsilon}\mu(\nabla u+\nabla u^{\mathrm{T}}) , \tag{H1}$$

where the kinetic turbulent energy k and the rate of turbulent viscous energy ε

$$k = \frac{1}{2}\langle u'^2\rangle \qquad \varepsilon = \frac{1}{R}\langle u'_{i,j},u'_{i,j}\rangle$$

each satisfy a complex convection–diffusion equation.

To derive the equation for k, one subtracts the Navier–Stokes equations from the Reynolds equations:

$$u'_t + (u+u')\nabla u' + u'\nabla u + \nabla p' - \nabla\cdot\langle u'\otimes u'\rangle - R^{-1}\Delta u' = 0 ;$$

$$\nabla\cdot u' = 0 ,$$

then multiplying by u' and averaging yields

$$\langle\frac{u'^2}{2}\rangle_t + \langle(u+u')\nabla \frac{u'^2}{2}\rangle + \langle u'\otimes u'\rangle\colon\ \nabla u + \langle u'\nabla p'\rangle + \varepsilon = 0 .$$

As this looks like a convection equation for k by a flow field of velocity $u+u'$ and since it is known [10] that convection by random fields yields dissipation, it is conjectured that the above equation is of the form

$$k_t + u\nabla k - \nabla\cdot b\nabla k - \frac{k^2}{\varepsilon}\mu(\nabla u+\nabla u^{\mathrm{T}})\colon\ \nabla u + \varepsilon = 0 .$$

Here (H1) has been used in the fourth term and $\langle u'\nabla p'\rangle$ has been ignored because of the ergodicity and isotropy properties:

$$\langle u'\nabla p'\rangle \simeq \frac{1}{|B|}\int_B u'\nabla p'\,dx = \frac{1}{|B|}\int_{\partial B} p'u'\cdot d\partial B = 0 .$$

To derive an equation for ε one proceeds similarly:

(a) multiply by $u'_{i,j}$;

(b) make several assumptions to close the systems.

It has been suggested that a possible equation is

$$\varepsilon_t + u\nabla\varepsilon - \nabla\cdot c\nabla\varepsilon - s(\nabla u+\nabla u^{\mathrm{T}})\colon\ \nabla u + \frac{\varepsilon^2}{k} = 0 ,$$

where c,s (like b above) are unknown functions determined experimentally.

In this paper we wish to discuss the possibility of deriving the k–ε model more rigorously. On the basis of frame invariance of the Reynolds equations, it is possible to justify hypothesis (H1). Indeed, it will be shown in section 4 that under certain approximations $\langle u'\otimes u'\rangle$ and $\nabla u+\nabla u^{\mathrm{T}}$ generates the same subspace of the second–order tensors; hence in 2–D

$$\langle u'\otimes u'\rangle = \alpha I + \beta(\nabla u+\nabla u^{\mathrm{T}}),$$

where α,β are functions of the only nontrivial invariant of $\nabla u+\nabla u^{\mathrm{T}}$, and possibly (Kolmogorov [11]) of k and ε only. But $\nabla\cdot(\alpha I)$ is a pressure gradient, therefore (H1) corresponds to a linear approximation for β in terms of the only dimensionally correct quantity, k^2/ε:

$$\beta(k,\varepsilon,\det(\nabla u+\nabla u^{\mathrm{T}})) \simeq -\mu\frac{k^2}{\varepsilon}.$$

However in 3–D the same theory yields

$$\langle u'\otimes u'\rangle = \alpha I + \beta(\nabla u+\nabla u^{\mathrm{T}}) + \gamma(\nabla u+\nabla u^{\mathrm{T}})^2,$$

for which hypothesis (H1) appears be only a linear approximation.

To justify the equations for k and ε one has to work harder; we propose, in the sequel, an asymptotic expansion for the initial value Euler problem with random initial data yielding a two–equation turbulent model; but these involve the kinetic turbulent energy and the turbulent helicity

$$r = \langle u'\cdot\nabla\times u'\rangle.$$

The derivation assumes uniqueness and continuous dependence properties on the Euler equation.

Since these properties are not known, the derivation is only formal. However, it has two main advantages:

a. it gives a set of hypotheses under which k–ε models may be valid;
b. it gives modification to the traditional k–ε models which may improve them considerably; to this end some preliminary tests are included.

1. The model problem

Consider the problem of finding the velocity and pressure field $\{u^\varepsilon,p^\varepsilon\}$ by solving

$$u_t + u\nabla u + \nabla p = 0, \tag{1}$$

$$\nabla\cdot u = 0 \quad \text{in}\ \Omega\times(0,T)\subset\mathbf{R}^3\times\mathbf{R} \tag{2}$$

satisfying the initial conditions

$$u(x,0) = u^0(x) + w^0(\frac{x}{\varepsilon},x) \tag{3}$$

and the boundary conditions

$$u\cdot n = 0 \quad \text{on}\ \Gamma\times(0,T). \tag{4}$$

In (3) w^0 is a zero mean, stationary in $y = x/\varepsilon$, random process. To avoid problems with the boundary, we assume that the support of w^0 is strictly inside Ω.

We expect to find the limit $\{u,p\}$ of $\{u^\varepsilon, p^\varepsilon\}$ as ε tends to zero by writing

$$u^\varepsilon(x,t) = u(x,t) + w\left(\frac{a(x,t)}{\varepsilon},\frac{t}{\varepsilon},x,t\right) + \varepsilon u^1\left(\frac{a(x,t)}{\varepsilon},\frac{t}{\varepsilon},x,t\right) + \varepsilon^2 u^2\left(\frac{a(x,t)}{\varepsilon},\frac{t}{\varepsilon},x,t\right), \tag{5}$$

$$p^\varepsilon(x,t) = p(x,t) + \pi\left(\frac{a(x,t)}{\varepsilon},\frac{t}{\varepsilon},x,t\right) + \varepsilon p^1\left(\frac{a(x,t)}{\varepsilon},\frac{t}{\varepsilon},x,t\right) + \varepsilon^2 p^2\left(\frac{a(x,t)}{\varepsilon},\frac{t}{\varepsilon},x,t\right) \ldots, \tag{6}$$

where $w, u^1, u^2, \ldots, \pi, p^1, p^2 \ldots$ are random zero–mean stationary processes with respect to the variable

$$\{y,\tau\} = \left\{\frac{a(x,t)}{\varepsilon},\frac{t}{\varepsilon}\right\}.$$

In (5), (6), $a(x,t)$ will be the position at time t of the particle that was on x at time zero, i.e., $a(x,t)$ is the solution of

$$\begin{cases} a_t + u\cdot\nabla a = 0 & \text{in } \Omega \times (0,T), \\ a(x,0) = x & \text{in } \Omega. \end{cases} \tag{7}$$

We accept this Anzats [12] because we expect that the first effect of u^0 on w^0 is a convection, i.e., $w^0(x)$ is transformed into $w^0(a(x,t))$. There are also other arguments for such a choice; for instance, (7) appears in the cascade of equations if u^ε is expanded in powers of $\varepsilon^{1/3}$ (see [1], [2]).

2. Asymptotic expansion

From (5) we see that

$$\frac{\partial u_i}{\partial t} = \frac{\partial u_i}{\partial t} + \left[\frac{\partial}{\partial t} + \frac{1}{\varepsilon}\left(\frac{\partial}{\partial \tau} + \frac{\partial a_k}{\partial t}\frac{\partial}{\partial y_k}\right)\right](w_i + \varepsilon u_i^1 + \varepsilon^2 u_i^2 + \ldots), \tag{8}$$

$$\frac{\partial u_i}{\partial x_j} = \frac{\partial u_i}{\partial x_j} + \left[\frac{\partial}{\partial x_j} + \frac{1}{\varepsilon}\left(\frac{\partial a_k}{\partial x_j}\frac{\partial}{\partial y_k}\right)\right](w_i + \varepsilon u_i^1 + \varepsilon + 2u_i^2 + \ldots), \tag{9}$$

We shall use the following notation:

$$v_\tau = \frac{\partial v}{\partial \tau}, \quad \nabla_y v = \left(\frac{\partial v}{\partial y_1}, \frac{\partial v}{\partial y_2}, \frac{\partial v}{\partial y_3}\right)^{\mathrm{T}}, \tag{10}$$

$$v_t = \frac{\partial v}{\partial t}, \quad \nabla v = \left(\frac{\partial v}{\partial x_1}, \frac{\partial v}{\partial x_2}, \frac{\partial v}{\partial x_3}\right)^{\mathrm{T}}. \tag{11}$$

Then (9), for instance, is

$$\nabla u = \frac{1}{\varepsilon}\nabla a \nabla_y w + \nabla u + \nabla w + \nabla a \nabla_y u^1 + \varepsilon(\nabla u^1 + \nabla a \nabla_y u^2) + \ldots \tag{12}$$

and, together with (7), (1), becomes

$$\begin{aligned}
&\frac{1}{\varepsilon}[w_\tau + (\nabla a^{\mathrm{T}} w)\cdot\nabla_y w + \nabla a \nabla_y \pi] + u^1_\tau + (\nabla a^{\mathrm{T}} w)\cdot\nabla_y u^1 + (\nabla a^{\mathrm{T}} u^1)\cdot\nabla_y w \\
&\quad + \nabla a \nabla_y p^1 + u_t + w_t + (u+w)\cdot\nabla(u+w) + \nabla\pi + \nabla p \\
&\quad + \varepsilon[u^2_\tau + (\nabla a^{\mathrm{T}} w)\cdot\nabla_y u^2 + (\nabla a^{\mathrm{T}} u^2\cdot\nabla_y w + \nabla a \nabla_y p^2 + u^1_t \\
&\quad + (u+w)\nabla u^1 + u^1\nabla(u+w) + (\nabla a^{\mathrm{T}} u^1)\cdot\nabla_y u^1) + \nabla p^1] + \varepsilon^2(\ldots) = 0.
\end{aligned} \tag{13}$$

Similarly (2) becomes

$$\frac{1}{\varepsilon}\nabla_y\cdot(\nabla a^{\mathrm{T}} w) + \nabla\cdot(u+w) + \nabla_y\cdot(\nabla a^{\mathrm{T}} u^1) + \varepsilon[\nabla_y\cdot(\nabla a^{\mathrm{T}} u^2) + \nabla\cdot u^1] = 0. \tag{14}$$

Therefore (13), (14) yield a set of equations which we will use to define $w, u^1, \ldots$ Let us rewrite the first equations in terms of

$$\tilde{w} = (\nabla a)^{\mathrm{T}} w; \tag{15}$$

it is

$$\begin{cases} \tilde{w}_\tau + \tilde{w}\nabla_y \tilde{w} + C\nabla_y \pi = 0, \\ \nabla_y\cdot\tilde{w} = 0 \quad w \text{ stationary in } \{y,\tau\}, \end{cases} \tag{16}$$

where

$$C = C(x,t) = (\nabla a)^{\mathrm{T}}\nabla a. \tag{17}$$

The other equations are of the type

$$\begin{cases} \tilde{u}^i_\tau + \tilde{w}\nabla_y \tilde{u}^i + \tilde{u}^i\nabla_y \tilde{w} + C\nabla_y p^i = \tilde{f}^i, \\ \nabla_y\cdot\tilde{u}^i = g^i, \quad \tilde{u}^i \text{ stationary in } \{y,\tau\}, \end{cases} \tag{18–19}$$

where

$$\tilde{u}^i = (\nabla a)^{\mathrm{T}} u^i . \tag{20}$$

With $i = 1$, (19) will define $\tilde{u}^1$ only if $\{\tilde{f}^i, g^i\}$ belong to the image of the linear operator L, in y,τ, on the left–hand side. To get a corrector of order 1 on u, we define $\tilde{u}^1$ by

$$L\tilde{u}^1 = \mathbf{P}\{\tilde{f}^1, g^1\} \tag{21}$$

and $\tilde{u}^2$ by

$$L\tilde{u}^2 = \{\tilde{f}^2, g^2\} + \frac{1}{\varepsilon}[\{\tilde{f}^1, g^1\} - \mathbf{P}\{\tilde{f}^1, g^1\}] , \tag{22}$$

where $\mathbf{P}$ is the projection operator on the image of L. To characterize $\mathbf{P}$, one may study the null space $\mathcal{N}^*$ of the adjoint of L. Furthermore, from (22) we see that $\tilde{u}^2$ exists only if

$$\langle v, \{\tilde{f}^2, g^2\} + \frac{1}{\varepsilon}(I-\mathbf{P})\{\tilde{f}^1, g^1\}\rangle = 0 \quad \forall\, v \in \mathcal{N}^* . \tag{23}$$

So far we have identified five relations of the type (23): three of them are obtained by taking the expected value of (19) and the other two are derived by multiplying (19) by $C^{-1}\tilde{w}$ and $\nabla a^{-\mathrm{T}}(\nabla a \nabla_y) \times (\nabla a^{\mathrm{T}} \tilde{w})$ (see [1] or [3] for more details).

To expand (23), it is equivalent to average directly (13) multiplied by 1, w and $(\nabla a \nabla_y) \times w$. It yields

$$\left\{ \begin{aligned} & u_t + u\cdot\nabla u + \nabla p + \nabla\cdot\langle w\otimes w\rangle + \varepsilon\nabla\cdot\langle u^1\otimes w + w\otimes u^1\rangle = 0(\varepsilon) , \\ & \nabla\cdot u = 0 , \end{aligned} \right. \tag{24}$$

$$\begin{aligned} & \langle\frac{w^2}{2}\rangle_t + u\cdot\nabla\langle\frac{w^2}{2}\rangle + \langle w\otimes w\rangle : \nabla u + \nabla\cdot\langle(\frac{w^2}{2} + \pi)w\rangle \\ & + \varepsilon[\langle u^1\cdot w\rangle_t + u\nabla\langle u^1\cdot w\rangle + \langle w\otimes u^1 + u^1\otimes w\rangle : \nabla u \\ & + \nabla\cdot\langle(p^1 + u^1\cdot w)w + (\pi + \frac{1}{2}w^2)u^1\rangle] = 0(\varepsilon) , \end{aligned} \tag{25}$$

$$\begin{aligned} & \langle w\tilde{\nabla}\times w\rangle_t + u\cdot\nabla\langle w\tilde{\nabla}\times w\rangle + 2\langle w\otimes\tilde{\nabla}\times w\rangle : \nabla u + 2\nabla\cdot\langle w\times w_\tau + (\pi + \frac{1}{2}w^2)\tilde{\nabla}\times w\rangle \\ & + \frac{\varepsilon}{2}[\langle u^1\cdot\tilde{\nabla}\times w\rangle_t + 2u\cdot\nabla\langle u^1\cdot\tilde{\nabla}\times w\rangle \\ & + (\langle w\otimes\tilde{\nabla}\times u^1 + u^1\otimes\tilde{\nabla}\times w\rangle + \langle\tilde{\nabla}\times u^1\otimes w + \tilde{\nabla}\times w\otimes u^1\rangle) : \nabla u \\ & + \langle w\nabla\cdot w\rangle\nabla\times u + \nabla\cdot(\langle u^1\times w_\tau\rangle \\ & + \langle(p^1 + u^1\cdot w)\tilde{\nabla}\times w + (\pi + \frac{1}{2}w^2)\tilde{\nabla}\times u^1\rangle)] = 0(\varepsilon) , \end{aligned} \tag{26}$$

where $a \otimes b$, $A{:}B$, $\tilde{\nabla}$ stand respectively for $a_i b_j$, $A_{ij}B_{ij}$, $\nabla a \nabla_y$.

So we notice that the three local invariants of the Euler equation, namely the mean u, the kinetic energy $\langle w^2/2\rangle$, the helicity $\langle w\tilde{\nabla} \times w\rangle$, play a special role. Thus the situation is as follows:

Equation (16) does not define w uniquely; additional conditions are necessary. There are reasons to believe that one may add to (16) the following:

$$\langle \tilde{w}\rangle = 0, \quad \frac{1}{2}\langle \tilde{w}C^{-1}w\rangle = q, \quad \langle \nabla a^{-\mathrm{T}}\tilde{w}\cdot(\nabla a \nabla_y) \times (\nabla a^{-\mathrm{T}}\tilde{w})\rangle = r\,, \tag{27}$$

for instance $(b+ic)\exp iky + (b-ic)\exp iky$ is a solution of (16) when $b\cdot k = c\cdot k = 0$ and it is possible to choose b and c with (27). Thus, even (16)+(27) does not have a unique solution; however, since (27) are the only invariants of (16), it is reasonable to assume that (16)+(27) defines isolated solutions which depend continuously on C. This hypothesis will be investigated in a future work of this author, in connection with the results of Arnold [4], Serre [5], Olver [6].

3. The macroscopic equations

The above considerations imply that all of the statistics of w will depend upon the following macroscopic parameters:

$$C(x,t) = \nabla a^{\mathrm{T}} \nabla a \qquad \text{(deformation tensor)}\,,$$

$$q(x,t) = \frac{1}{2}\langle w^2\rangle \qquad \text{(kinetic “turbulent” energy)}\,,$$

$$r(x,t) = \langle w.\tilde{\nabla} \times w\rangle \qquad \text{(“turbulent” helicity)}\,,$$

Now $\tilde{u}^1$ is defined by (21):

$$\begin{cases} \tilde{u}^1_\tau + w\nabla_y \tilde{u}^1 + \tilde{u}^1 \nabla_y \tilde{w} + C\nabla_y p^1 \\ \qquad = -\nabla a^{\mathrm{T}}(f^1 - \langle f^1 + g^1 w\rangle + \beta w + \gamma\tilde{\nabla} \times w)\,, \\ \nabla_y \cdot \tilde{u}^1 = g^1\,, \end{cases} \tag{28}$$

where (see (13))

$$f^1 = w_t + u\nabla w + w\nabla u + w\nabla w + \nabla\pi + \text{terms independent of } y$$

and β and γ are such that

$$\begin{cases} \beta\langle w^2\rangle + \gamma\langle w\cdot\tilde{\nabla} \times w\rangle + \langle f^1\cdot w\rangle = 0\,, \\ \beta\langle w\cdot\tilde{\nabla} \times w\rangle + \gamma\langle|\nabla \times w|^2\rangle + \langle f^1\cdot\tilde{\nabla} \times w\rangle = 0\,. \end{cases} \tag{30}$$

Therefore, (28) being linear, $\tilde{u}^1$ is a linear function of u and ∇u and the statistics of $\tilde{u}^1$ will also depend linearly upon these additional parameters; thus (24)–(26) has the general form

$$u_t + u\nabla u + \nabla p + \nabla\cdot(R+\varepsilon(\mathscr{C}\!: \nabla u + \mathscr{A}u + \mathscr{B})) = 0(\varepsilon)\,, \tag{31}$$

$$\nabla\cdot u = 0\,, \tag{32}$$

$$q_t + u\nabla q + R : \nabla u + \nabla\cdot b + \varepsilon(\nabla\cdot(B\nabla q) + \ldots) = 0(\varepsilon)\,, \tag{33}$$

$$r_t + u\nabla r + S : \nabla u + \nabla\cdot c + \varepsilon(\nabla\cdot(D\nabla r) + \ldots) = 0(\varepsilon)\,, \tag{34}$$

where all new quantities are functions of ∇a, q, r and have the following definitions:

$$R = \langle w\otimes w\rangle = \nabla a^{-\mathrm{T}}\langle\tilde{w}\otimes\tilde{w}\rangle\nabla a^{-1}\,, \tag{35}$$

$$\mathscr{C}_{kl}^{ij} = \langle w_k\chi_l^{ij} + \chi_k^{ij}w_l\rangle\,, \tag{36}$$

$$b = \langle(\frac{w^2}{2} + \pi)w\rangle\,, \tag{37}$$

$$B_{ij} = \langle(p^i + \xi^i\cdot w)w_j + (\pi + \frac{1}{2}w^2)\xi_j^i\rangle\,, \tag{38}$$

$$c = \langle(\frac{w^2}{2} + \pi)\tilde{\nabla}\times w\rangle\,, \tag{39}$$

$$S_{ij} = \langle w_i\langle(\tilde{\nabla}\times w)_j\rangle\,, \tag{40}$$

$$D_{ij} = \langle(p^{i\prime} + \xi^{i\prime}\cdot w)\cdot(\tilde{\nabla}\times w)_j + (\pi + \frac{1}{2}w^2)(\tilde{\nabla}\times\xi^{i\prime})_j\rangle\,, \tag{41}$$

with

$$\chi^{ij} = a_{i\,m}^{-1}\,a_{j\,n}^{-1}\tilde{\chi}^{m\,n} \tag{42}$$

and $\tilde{\chi}^{m,n}$, $\{\tilde{\xi}^i, p^i\}$, $\{\tilde{\xi}^i, p'^i\}$ being solutions of (with L as defined in (21):

$$L(\tilde{\chi}^{m,n}) = -\mathbf{P}\{C_m\tilde{w}_n, 0\}\,, \tag{43a}$$

$$L(\tilde{\xi}^i) = -\mathbf{P}\{\nabla a^{\mathrm{T}}(w_i\frac{\partial w}{\partial q} + \frac{\partial\pi}{\partial q}e^i), \frac{\partial w_i}{\partial q}\}\,, \tag{43b}$$

$$L(\tilde{\xi}^{i\prime}) = -\mathbf{P}\{\nabla a^{\mathrm{T}}(w_i\frac{\partial w}{\partial r} + \frac{\partial\pi}{\partial r}e^i), \frac{\partial w_i}{\partial r}\} \tag{43c}$$

$$(e^i = i^{\text{th}} \text{ basis vector})\,.$$

The analogy with the k–ε model appears when one retains only the diffusion terms in the ε factors in (31)–(34); $\varepsilon\nabla\cdot\mathscr{A}u$ is neglected because it is small compared with $u\nabla u$; similarly, $\varepsilon\nabla\cdot\mathcal{B}$ is small compared to $\nabla\cdot R$... Note, however, that since (31)–(34) is a coupled system, one should really keep the second derivatives of q and r in (31), the second derivatives of u and r in (33)...

Now we proceed to analyze the quantities defined by (35)–(41).

4. Isotropic w^0, planar mean flow

When w^0 is invariant by rotation, a great simplification arises because the mean–flow equations must, in turn, be invariant under the changed coordinate systems.

Let M be a unitary matrix; if u, x, a denote the velocity and positions in a coordinate system and V, X, A the same after transformation by M, we have

$$X = Mx, \quad U = Mu, \quad A = Ma, \quad \nabla_x u = M^{\top}\nabla_X UM\,, \tag{44}$$

$$u_t + \nabla_x\cdot[u\otimes u + pI + R(\nabla a)]$$
$$= M^{\top}[U_t + \nabla_X\cdot[U\otimes U + pI + MR(M^{\top}\nabla_X AM)M^{\top}]]\,. \tag{45}$$

Thus the frame invariance of (24) requires that

$$MR(M^{\top}\nabla_X AM)M^{\top} = R(\nabla_X A) \quad \forall\, M \text{ such that } M^{-1} = M^{\top}\,. \tag{46}$$

From (35) and (44) we see that this property holds also for $\tilde{R} = \langle\tilde{w}\otimes\tilde{w}\rangle$

$$M\tilde{R}(M^{\top}CM)M^{\top} = \tilde{R}(C) \quad \forall\, M^{-1} = M^{\top}\,. \tag{47}$$

But (47) implies that R and C are diagonal in the same basis [7].

If the mean flow u is planar, then $\{I,C\}$ is a basis for the space of matrices diagonal in the same basis as C and we must have

$$R(C) = \alpha(\mathrm{tr}\, C,q,r)I + \beta(\mathrm{tr}\, C,q,r)C\,, \tag{48}$$

where α and β are two unknown functions of the only nontrivial unvariant of C, its trace (the determinant of C is 1 by (7)). Turning to R, by (35) we find that

$$R(\nabla a) = \alpha[\nabla a\nabla a^{\top}]^{-1} + \beta I$$
$$= \gamma(\mathrm{tr}\, C,q,r)\nabla a\nabla a^{\top} + \delta(\mathrm{tr}\, C,q,r)I \tag{49}$$

(Cayley–Hamilton theorem) .

A similar analysis applies to $\mathscr{C}$: ∇u if we neglect the dependence upon ∇a. First, one can see from (42)–(43) that $\mathscr{C}_{kl}^{ij}$ is equal to $\mathscr{C}_{lk}^{ij}$ and so $\mathscr{C}$: ∇u is really linear in $\nabla u+\nabla u^{\mathrm{T}}$. Also, as above, they are diagonal in the same basis; therefore

$$\mathscr{C}:\ \nabla u \ = \ \lambda I - \mu(\nabla u+\nabla u^{\mathrm{T}}) \ , \tag{50}$$

where λ, μ are functions of q, r and all the invariants that can be built from C and $\nabla u+\nabla u^{\mathrm{T}}$. But now, taking the trace of (50) and using (2), we can see that λ is linear in ∇u and that μ depends only on i, q, r.

Finally we note that q and r are homogeneous to a velocity square and to a velocity square over a length, respectively. In our Anzats there is no other length than the fixed macroscopic length related to Ω; therefore γ, δ, λ, μ are proportional to q or $\sqrt{q}$ and functions of q/r only. Hence in the end (24) reduces, in two dimensions, to

$$\begin{cases} u_t + u\nabla u + \nabla p + \nabla\cdot[q\gamma(i,\frac{q}{r})\nabla a\nabla a^{\mathrm{T}}] - \varepsilon\nabla\cdot[\sqrt{q}\mu(i,\frac{q}{r})(\nabla u+\nabla u^{\mathrm{T}})] \ = \ 0(\varepsilon) \ , \\ \nabla\cdot u \ = \ 0 \ . \end{cases} \tag{51}$$

The k–ε model corresponds to the case $\gamma = 0$, $\mu = q/r$.

Similarly frame invariance and dimensional analysis allow us to rewrite (33), (34):

$$q_t + u\nabla q + q\gamma\nabla a\nabla a^{\mathrm{T}} : \nabla u + \nabla\cdot(q^{3/2}b')$$
$$- \varepsilon\nabla(B'\nabla q^{1/2} + E'\nabla r^{1/2}) \ = \ 0(\varepsilon) \ , \tag{52}$$

$$r_t + u\nabla r + r\sigma\nabla a\nabla a^{\mathrm{T}} : \nabla u + \nabla\cdot(r^{3/2}c')$$
$$- \varepsilon\nabla(D'\nabla r^{1/2} + F'\nabla q^{1/2}) \ = \ 0(\varepsilon) \ , \tag{53}$$

where $\underline{b}'$, $\underline{B}'$, σ, $\underline{c}'$, $\underline{D}'$ are functions of i and q/r which can be determined, in principle, from w and (35)–(41). Note finally that it may be more convenient to work with q and $\ell = q/r$ (a length scale) for which an equation is easily obtained from (52)–(53).

Conclusion

Homogenization theory [12] appears to be an efficient tool to derive two–equation turbulent models from the Euler problem with random initial data. The derivation is subject to local uniqueness and smoothness properties, which are not known for the Euler problem. The k–ε model appears to be similar to a first–order approximation of the general model for two–dimensional mean flows only with two major modifications:

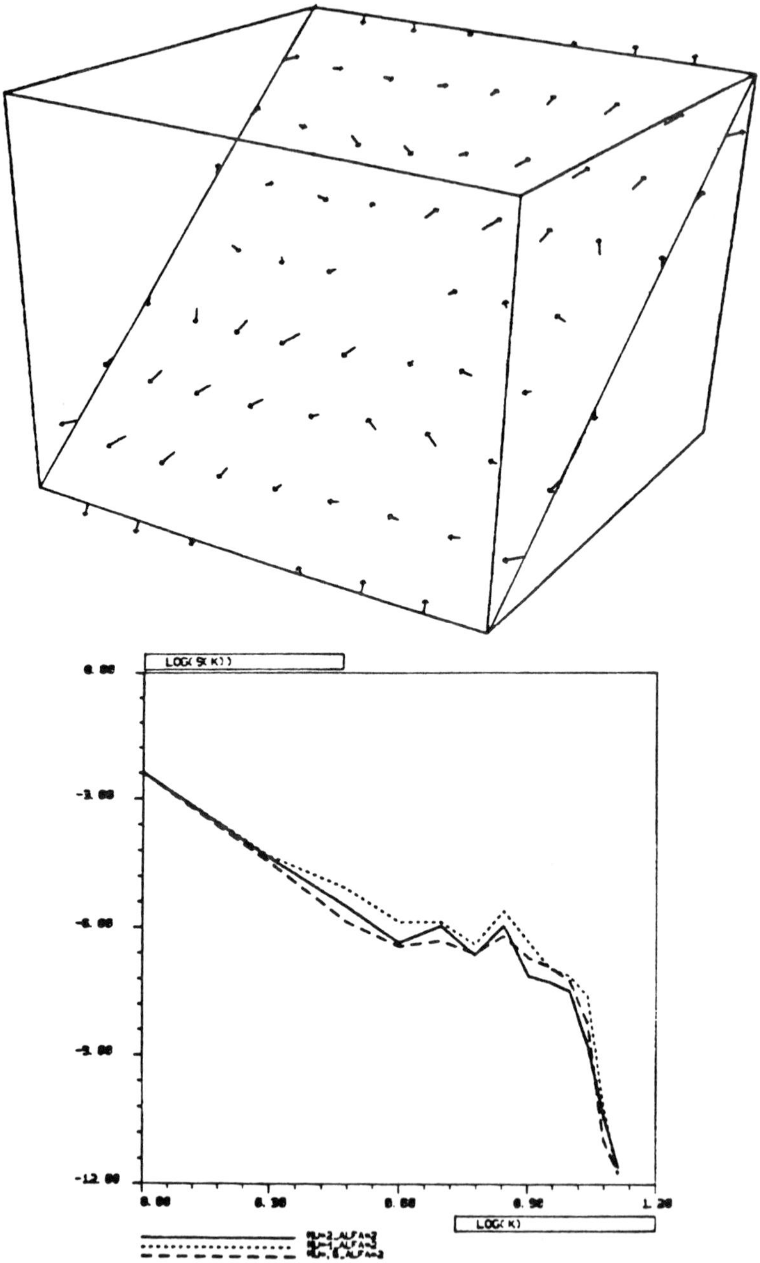

Fig. 1. Numerical solution of (16)

A typical stationary solution of (16) done by least squares method on the CRAY 1. Top: velocity field on the plane $y = 3$. Bottom: spectra of u^2. These computations are used to tabulate γ, in (51), in terms of i.

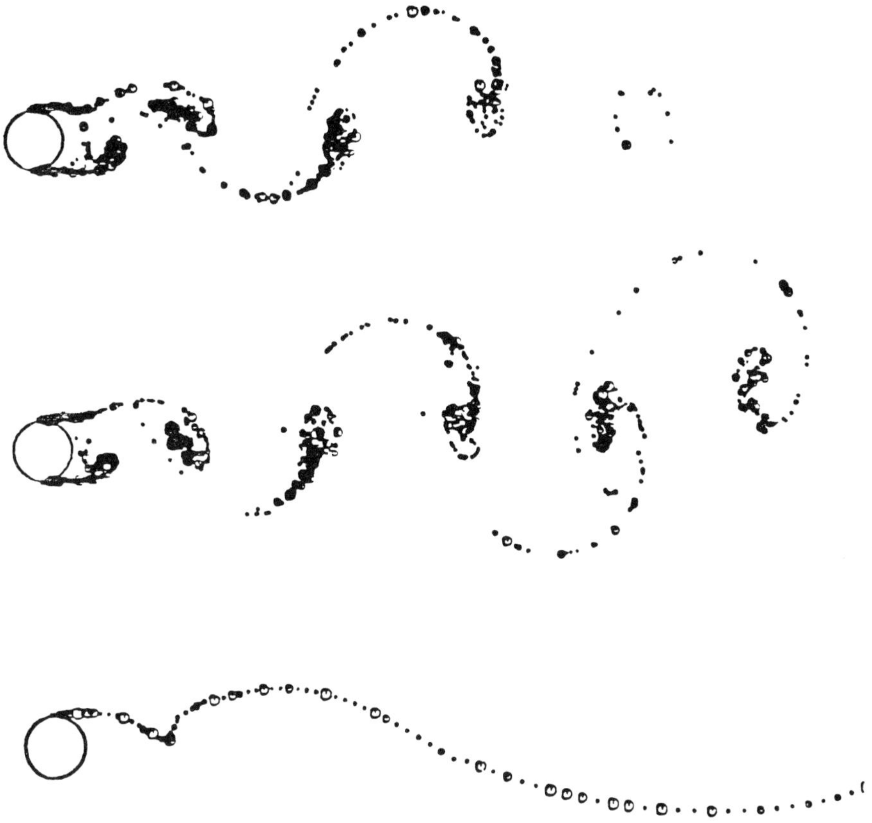

Fig. 2. Flow behind a cylinder (computed by C. Begue). Numerical solutions of (51)–(52) with $\mu = b' = B' = E' = 0$: effect of γ.

(a) the Reynolds stress tensor involves ∇a instead of ∇u;

(b) the rate of dissipated energy is replaced by the helicity r, or a length scale based on r.

Furthermore, the general derivation was done under the following hypothesis:

(a) existence of a spectral gap between the mean flow and the turbulent structures;

(b) local isotropy of the turbulence at places of production.

Now our investigation goes in two directions: (1) study of the local Euler problem (16)–(27) and tabulations of γ, μ, b',... and (2) numerical tests of the model on real flows. We have included some of the numerical tests already obtained.

Acknowledgement

This work has been done in collaboration with G. Papanicolaou, D. McLaughlin, and C. Begue (see the references).

This research was supported by contract DRET 81/683.

REFERENCES

[1] Leslie, D.C. Theoretical investigation of Schumann's model for subgrid Reynolds stress. QM TU Report 20/78 1978.

[2] McLaughlin, D., Papanicolaou, G., and Pironneau, O. "Convection of Microstructures." *Proc. INRIA Conf.*, Dec. 1981, ed. R. Glowinski. Amsterdam: North–Holland. Forthcoming.

[3] ————. "Convections of Microstructures and Related Problems." Submitted to *SIAM J. Appl. Math.*

[4] Arnold, V.I. *Mathematical Methods of Classical Mechanics*. New York Berlin Heidelberg Tokyo: Springer–Verlag, 1978. (English trans.)

[5] Serre, D. "Invariants et dégénérescence symplectique de l'équation d'Euler." *CRAS* 298, I, no. 14 (1984): 349–352.

[6] Olver, P.J. "A Nonlinear Hamiltonian System Structure for the Euler Equations." *J. Math. Anal. Appl.*, 89 (1982): 233–250.

[7] Ciarlet, P.G. *Lecture Notes on 3–D Elasticity*. Tata Notes. Bombay: Springer, 1983.

[8] Perrier, P., and Pironneau, O. "Subgrid turbulence modelling by homogenization." *Math. Modelling*, 2 (1981): 295–317.

[9] Papanicolaou, G., and Pironneau, O. On the asymptotic behavior of motion in random flow. In *Stochastic Nonlinear Systems*, ed. V.I. Arnold and J. Lefebvre. Berlin New York Heidelberg Tokyo: Springer–Verlag, 1981.

[10] Kester, H., and Papanicolaou, G. "A Limit Theorem for Turbulent Diffusion." *Commun. Math. Phys.* 65 (1979): 97–128.

[11] Monin, A.S., and Yaglom, A.M. *Statistical Fluid Mechanics of Turbulence*, vol. 2, 348. Cambridge, Mass.: MIT Press, 1985.

[12] Bensoussan, A., Lions, J.L., and Papanicolaou, G. *Asymptotic Analysis for Periodic Structures*. Amsterdam New York: North–Holland, 1978.

SPLITTING METHODS FOR THE NUMERICAL SOLUTION OF THE INCOMPRESSIBLE NAVIER–STOKES EQUATIONS

R. Glowinski†

Abstract

In this paper we discuss the solution by operator–splitting methods, of the time–dependent Navier–Stokes equations modelling incompressible, unsteady viscous flows. Using these methods, one can decouple the two main difficulties of the incompressible Navier–Stokes equations, namely the nonlinearity and the incompressibility, thus making the numerical solution of the global problem much easier.

1. Introduction. Synopsis

Solving the Navier–Stokes equations by numerical methods, in order to simulate unsteady flows of either *incompressible* or *compressible viscous fluids*, is still a challenging problem. This important problem has motivated the work of many scientists (see, e.g., Temam [1], Girault and Raviart [2], Rautmann [3], Thomasset [4], Glowinski [5] for references). Concentrating on the incompressible case, we would like to show in this paper that *operator–splitting methods*, like those advocated by Academician G.I. Marchuk in [6], provide quite efficient numerical schemes for solving the time–dependent Navier–Stokes equations. The content of the paper is the following.

In section 2 we describe and comment on the Navier–Stokes equations modelling unsteady flows for incompressible viscous fluids. In section 3 we discuss some general schemes using operator splitting and apply them to the

---

† University P. et M. Curie, Tour 55–65, place Jussieu 75230 Paris Cedex 05 and Institut National de Recherche en Informatique et Automatique, Domaine de Voluceau, Rocquencourt, 78153 Le Chesnay Cedex.

Navier–Stokes equations in order to *decouple the incompressibility and the nonlinearity* (in fact, we could not resist concluding that section by showing that the same principles also apply to *eigenvalue calculations*). In sections 4 and 5, we discuss the specific treatment of the nonlinearity and of the in–compressibility, respectively. *Finite–element approximations* are discussed in section 6, and finally in section 7 we show the results of several numerical experiments designed to test the methods previously discussed in the paper.

2. Formulation of the unsteady Navier–Stokes equations for incompressible viscous fluids

Let us consider a Newtonian viscous and incompressible fluid. If Ω and Γ denote the region of the flow and its boundary, respectively, then this flow is governed by the Navier–Stokes equations:

$$\frac{\partial \underset{\sim}{u}}{\partial t} - \nu \Delta \underset{\sim}{u} + (\underset{\sim}{u}.\underset{\sim}{\nabla})\underset{\sim}{u} + \underset{\sim}{\nabla} p = \underset{\sim}{f} \text{ in } \Omega , \tag{2.1}$$

$$\underset{\sim}{\nabla}.\underset{\sim}{u} = 0 \text{ in } \Omega \text{ (\textit{incompressibility condition})} . \tag{2.2}$$

In (2.1), (2.2):

(i) $\underset{\sim}{u} = \{u_i\}_{i=1}^N$ is the *flow velocity* ,

(ii) p is the *pressure*,

(iii) ν is the *viscosity* of the fluid (in normalized units we have $\nu = 1/\mathrm{Re}$, where Re is Reynold's number),

(iv) $\underset{\sim}{f}$ is a *density* of external forces.

In (2.1) $(\underset{\sim}{u}.\underset{\sim}{\nabla})\underset{\sim}{u}$ is a symbolic notation for the nonlinear vector term:

$$\left\{ \sum_{j=1}^{N} u_j \frac{\partial u_i}{\partial x_j} \right\}_{i=1}^{N} .$$

Boundary conditions have to be added; for example, in the case of the airfoil A of figure 2.1 below, we have (since the fluid is viscous) the following adherence condition:

$$\underset{\sim}{u} = \underset{\sim}{0} \quad \text{on } \partial A = \Gamma_A . \tag{2.3}$$

Typical conditions at infinity are

$$\underset{\sim}{u} = \underset{\sim}{u}_\infty , \tag{2.4}$$

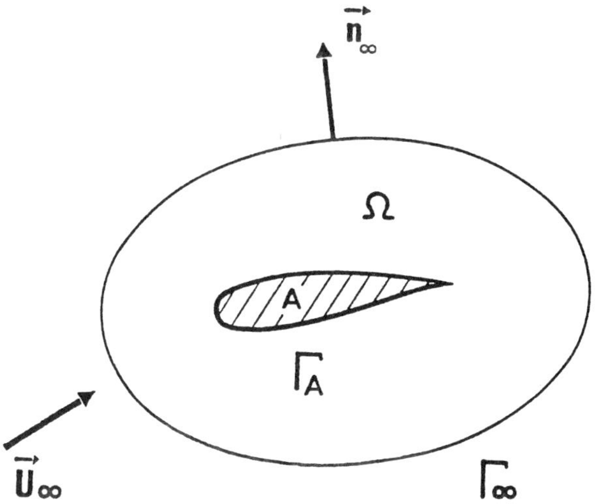

Fig. 2.1

where $\underset{\sim}{u}_\infty$ is a constant vector (with respect to the space variables, at least).

Finally, for the time–dependent problem (2.1), (2.2), an initial condition such as

$$\underset{\sim}{u}(x,0) = \underset{\sim}{u}_0(x) \quad \text{on } \Omega , \tag{2.5}$$

where $\underset{\sim}{u}_0$ is given (with $\underset{\sim}{\nabla}.\underset{\sim}{u}_0 = 0$), is usually prescribed.

With the methods described in this paper, we can also treat boundary con–ditions such as

$$\underset{\sim}{u} = \underset{\sim}{g}_0 \quad \text{on } \Gamma_0 , \quad \nu \frac{\partial \underset{\sim}{u}}{\partial n} - \underset{\sim}{n}p = \underset{\sim}{g}_1 \quad \text{on } \Gamma_1 , \tag{2.6}$$

where Γ_0, Γ_1 are subsets of Γ, such that $\Gamma_0 \cap \Gamma_1 = \emptyset$, $\Gamma_0 \cup \Gamma_1 = \Gamma$, and $\underset{\sim}{n}$ is the outward unit normal vector at Γ (see [5, appendix 3] for the numerical implementation of (2.6)).

In two dimensions, it may be convenient to formulate the Navier–Stokes equations using a *stream–function–vorticity* formulation (see, e.g., Fortin and Thomasset [7], Girault and Raviart [2], Glowinski and Pironneau [8], Reinhart [9], Keller and Schreiber [10], Glowinski, Keller, and Reinhart [11], Roache [12]).

Solving the above Navier–Stokes equations, even at moderate Reynold number (say Re $\simeq 10^3$), is a nontrivial task because of the following difficulties:

(i) it is a *nonlinear* system of partial differential equations;
(ii) we have the incompressibility condition (2.2).

In the next section we shall see how *time discretization* by operator–splitting methods can decouple the nonlinear and incompressibility difficulties.

To conclude this section, let us mention that a mathematical analysis of the Navier–Stokes equations for incompressible fluids can be found in Lions [13], Ladyzhenskaya [14], Temam [1] and Tartar [15], among others.

3. Time discretization by operator splitting methods. Applications

3.1. GENERALITIES. THE BASIC SCHEMES

Let us consider a real Hilbert space H; we consider in H the following initial–value problem:

$$\begin{cases} \dfrac{du}{dt} + A(u) = f, \\ u(0) = u_0, \end{cases} \tag{3.1}$$

where A is an operator from H to H, about which we are not very specific, f is a source term and u_0 the initial value, respectively. We suppose that A admits a nontrivial decomposition

$$A = A_1 + A_2 \tag{3.2}$$

(nontrivial means that A_1 and A_2 are individually simpler than A). With Δt (>0) a time–discretization step, let us define several schemes, taking advantage of the decomposition (3.2):

A. The Peaceman–Rachford time–discretization scheme.

The scheme is defined as follows:

$$u^0 = u_0 ; \tag{3.3}$$

then for $n \geq 0$, with u^n known, we compute successively $u^{n+1/2}$ and then u^{n+1} by

$$\frac{u^{n+1/2} - u^n}{\Delta t/2} + A_1(u^{n+1/2}) + A_2(u^n) = f^{n+1/2}, \tag{3.4}$$

$$\frac{u^{n+1} - u^{n+1/2}}{\Delta t/2} + A_1(u^{n+1/2}) + A_2(u^{n+1}) = f^{n+1}. \tag{3.5}$$

In (3.4), (3.5) $u^{n+\alpha}$ denotes an approximation of $u((n+\alpha)\Delta t)$, and $f^{n+\alpha} = f((n+\alpha)\Delta t)$.

B. The Douglas–Rachford time–discretization scheme.

It is a variant of the above scheme described by

$$u^0 = u_0 \; ; \tag{3.6}$$

then, for $n \geq 0$, define $\hat{u}^{n+1}$ and u^{n+1} from u^n by

$$\frac{\hat{u}^{n+1}-u^n}{\Delta t} + A_1(\hat{u}^{n+1}) + A_2(u^n) = f^{n+1} \; , \tag{3.7}$$

$$\frac{u^{n+1}-u^n}{\Delta t} + A_1(\hat{u}^{n+1}) + A_2(u^{n+1}) = f^{n+1} \; . \tag{3.8}$$

C. The three–stage operator–splitting scheme.

Let θ belong to the open interval (0,1/2). The idea behind this scheme is to split the time interval $[n\Delta t,(n+1)\Delta t]$ into three subintervals, as shown in figure 3.1, and integrate in time, using an implicit scheme for A_1 (respectively, an explicit scheme for A_2) on $[n\Delta t,(n+\theta)\Delta t]$. Next, one needs to switch

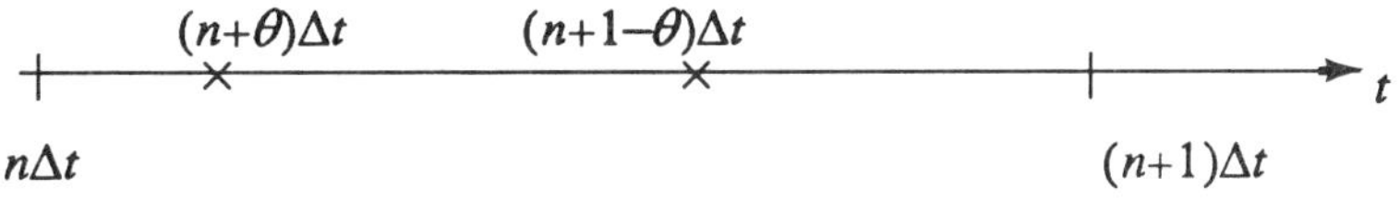

Figure 3.1

the role of A_1 and A_2 on $[(n+\theta)\Delta t,(n+1-\theta)\Delta t]$, and on $[(n+1-\theta)\Delta t,(n+1)\Delta t]$, $[n\Delta t,(n+\theta)\Delta t]$. Using these principles, we obtain the following scheme, some forms of which have been advocated by Strang [16], Beale and Majda [17], Leveque [18], Leveque and Oliger [19] (for $\theta = 1/4$):

$$u^0 = u_0; \tag{3.9}$$

then, for $n \geq 0$, we obtain $u^{n+\theta}$, $u^{n+1-\theta}$, u^{n+1} from u^n as follows:

$$\frac{u^{n+\theta}-u^n}{\theta\Delta t} + A_1(u^{n+\theta}) + A_2(u^n) = f^{n+\theta} \; , \tag{3.10}$$

$$\frac{u^{n+1-\theta}-u^{n+\theta}}{(1-2\theta)\Delta t} + A_1(u^{n+\theta}) + A_2(u^{n+1-\theta}) = f^{n+1-\theta} \; , \tag{3.11}$$

$$\frac{u^{n+1}-u^{n+1-\theta}}{\theta\Delta t} + A_1(u^{n+1}) + A_2(u^{n+1-\theta}) = f^{n+1} \; . \tag{3.12}$$

The convergence of (3.3)–(3.5) and (3.6)–(3.8) has been proved in Lions and Mercier [20] (see also Godlewsky [21]) under quite general monotonicity assumptions on A_1 and A_2; it is very likely that the methods used in [20] to prove the convergence of (3.3)–(3.5) and (3.6)–(3.8) still apply to (3.9)–(3.12).

3.2. CONVERGENCE AND STABILITY PROPERTIES OF THE BASIC SCHEMES

Following the approach used in [6], we shall consider for simplicity the case where $H = \mathbf{R}^N$, $f = 0$, $u_0 \in \mathbf{R}^N$, A is an $N \times N$ symmetric and positive definite matrix and

$$A_1 = \alpha A, \quad A_2 = \beta A, \quad \text{with } \alpha + \beta = 1, \quad 0 < \alpha, \beta < 1 . \tag{3.13}$$

In that case the solution of (3.1) is clearly given by

$$u(t) = e^{-tA} u_0 . \tag{3.14}$$

Analysis of the scheme (3.3)–(3.5) (see also [6]): We have from (3.4), (3.5), (3.13) that

$$u^{n+1} = (I + \beta\tfrac{\Delta t}{2}A)^{-1}(I - \alpha\tfrac{\Delta t}{2}A) \times (I + \alpha\tfrac{\Delta t}{2}A)^{-1}(I - \beta\tfrac{\Delta t}{2}A)u^n . \tag{3.15}$$

Using a vector basis consisting of eigenvectors of A, we have from (3.15), with obvious notation,

$$u_i^{n+1} = \frac{\left(1-\alpha\frac{\Delta t}{2}\lambda_i\right)\left(1-\beta\frac{\Delta t}{2}\lambda_i\right)}{\left(1+\alpha\frac{\Delta t}{2}\lambda_i\right)\left(1+\beta\frac{\Delta t}{2}\lambda_i\right)} u_i^n , \tag{3.16}$$

where λ_i (> 0, $\forall\, i=1,\ldots,N$) is the ith eigenvalue of A; we suppose that $\lambda_1 \le \lambda_2 \le \cdots \le \lambda_N$. Consider now the rational function R_1 defined by

$$R_1(x) = \frac{\left(1-\frac{\alpha}{2}x\right)\left(1-\frac{\beta}{2}x\right)}{\left(1+\frac{\alpha}{2}x\right)\left(1+\frac{\beta}{2}x\right)} ; \tag{3.17}$$

we observe that $|R_1(x)| < 1 \;\forall\, x > 0$, implying, in that simple case, the unconditional stability of the scheme (3.3)–(3.5). Since

$$\lim_{x \to +\infty} R_1(x) = 1 , \tag{3.18}$$

we see that for stiff problems, i.e., problems such that $\lambda_N/\lambda_1 >> 1$, the scheme (3.3)–(3.5) is not very good to damp, simultaneously, the components of u^n associated to the large and to the small eigenvalues of A; from this observation, we can expect that the scheme (3.3)–(3.5) is not well suited to capture the steady–state solutions of stiff problems (like those obtained from the discretization of partial differential equations); this has been confirmed by numerical experiments. Since

$$e^{-x} = 1 - x + \frac{x^2}{2} + x^2\varepsilon(x) \tag{3.19}$$

and, from (3.17),

$$R_1(x) = 1 - x + \frac{x^2}{2} + x^2\eta(x)\,, \tag{3.20}$$

with $\lim_{x\to 0} \varepsilon(x) = \lim_{x\to 0} \eta(x) = 0$, we have that the scheme (3.3)–(3.5) is *second–order accurate* in the simple case that we have considered. We see from (3.15) that if one takes $\alpha = \beta = 1/2$, then the two linear systems which have to be solved, at each full step, are in fact associated to the same matrix $I + (\Delta t/4)A$.

Analysis of the scheme (3.6)–(3.8): We have this time

$$u^{n+1} = (I+\alpha\Delta tA)^{-1}(I+\beta\Delta tA)^{-1}(I+\alpha\beta|\Delta t|^2A^2)u^n\,, \tag{3.21}$$

which implies

$$u_i^{n+1} = \frac{1+\alpha\beta|\Delta t|^2\lambda_i^2}{(1+\alpha\Delta t\lambda_i)(1+\beta\Delta t\lambda_i)}u_i^n\,. \tag{3.22}$$

If we now define R_2 by

$$R_2(x) = \frac{1+\alpha\beta x^2}{(1+\alpha x)(1+\beta x)}\,, \tag{3.23}$$

we see that $0 < R_2(x) < 1\ \forall\ x > 0$, implying in turn in this case under discussion, the unconditional stability of the scheme (3.6)–(3.8). Since we have again

$$\lim_{x\to+\infty} R_2(x) = 1\,, \tag{3.24}$$

the scheme (3.6)–(3.8) may behave poorly for stiff problems and not be too efficient for capturing steady–state solutions. With respect to the accuracy of the scheme (3.6)–(3.8), we easily prove that

$$R_2(x) = 1 - x + x^2 + x^2\eta(x)\,, \tag{3.25}$$

with $\lim_{x\to 0} \eta(x) = 0$, implying, if we compare to (3.19), that the scheme (3.6)–(3.8) is only first–order accurate.

The good choice for α and β is again $\alpha = \beta = 1/2$. Analysis of the scheme (3.9)–(3.12): We have (with $\theta' = 1-2\theta$)

$$u^{n+1} = (I+\alpha\theta\Delta tA)^{-1}(I-\beta\theta\Delta tA)(I+\beta\theta'\Delta tA)^{-1}$$

$$\times (I-\alpha\theta'\Delta tA)(I+\alpha\theta\Delta tA)^{-1}(I-\beta\theta\Delta tA)u^n\ , \tag{3.26}$$

which implies

$$u_i^{n+1} = \frac{(1-\beta\theta\Delta t\lambda_i)^2(1-\alpha\theta'\Delta t\lambda_i)}{(1+\alpha\theta\Delta t\lambda_i)^2(1+\beta\theta'\Delta t\lambda_i)}u_i^n\ . \tag{3.27}$$

Consider now the rational function R_3 defined by

$$R_3(x) = \frac{(1-\beta\theta x)^2(1-\alpha\theta' x)}{(1+\alpha\theta x)^2(1+\beta\theta' x)}. \tag{3.28}$$

Since

$$\lim_{x\to+\infty} |R_3(x)| = \beta/\alpha\ , \tag{3.29}$$

we should prescribe

$$\alpha \geq \beta \tag{3.30}$$

to obtain from (3.26), (3.27) the stability of the scheme (3.9)–(3.12) for large eigenvalues of A. Next, with respect to the accuracy of the scheme (3.9)–(3.12), we can show that

$$R_3(x) = 1 - x + \frac{x^2}{2}\{1 + (\beta^2-\alpha^2)(2\theta^2-4\theta+1)\} + x^2\eta(x)\ , \tag{3.31}$$

with $\lim_{x\to 0} \eta(x) = 0$. It follows from (3.31) that the scheme (3.9)–(3.12) is *second–order accurate* if either

$$\alpha = \beta \ \ (= 1/2 \text{ from } (3.13))\ , \tag{3.32}$$

or

$$\theta = 1 - \sqrt{2}/2 = .29289....\ ; \tag{3.33}$$

the scheme (3.9)–(3.12) is only *first–order accurate* if neither (3.32) nor (3.33) holds.

If one takes $\alpha = \beta = 1/2$, it follows from (3.27) that the scheme (3.9)–(3.12) is unconditionally stable $\forall\ \theta \in (0,1/2)$; however, since (from (3.29)) we have

$$\lim_{x\to+\infty} |R_3(x)| = 1\ , \tag{3.34}$$

the remark concerning the scheme (3.3)–(3.5), with regard to the integration of stiff systems, still holds. In general, we will choose α and β in order to have the same matrix for all the partial steps of the integration method, i.e., α, β, θ have to satisfy

$$\alpha\theta = \beta(1-2\theta) , \tag{3.35}$$

which implies

$$\alpha = (1-2\theta)/(1-\theta) , \quad \beta = \theta/(1-\theta) . \tag{3.36}$$

Combining (3.30), (3.36) yields

$$0 < \theta \leq 1/3 . \tag{3.37}$$

For $\theta = 1/3$, (3.36) implies $\alpha = \beta = 1/2$.

If $0 < \theta < 1/3$ and if α and β are given by (3.36), we have

$$\lim_{n \to +\infty} |R_3(x)| = \frac{\beta}{\alpha} = \frac{\theta}{1-2\theta} < 1 . \tag{3.38}$$

Indeed, we can prove that $\theta \in [\theta^*, 1/3]$ ($\theta^* = .087385580....$) and the α and β given by (3.36) imply the unconditional stability of the scheme (3.9)–(3.12); moreover, if $\theta \in (\theta^*, 1/3)$ (with α,β still given by (3.36)), property (3.38) endows the scheme (3.9)–(3.12) with good asymptotic properties as $n \to +\infty$ and, moreover, is well suited to compute steady–state solutions.

If $\theta = 1-\sqrt{2}/2$ (respectively, $\theta = .25$), we have $\alpha = 2-\sqrt{2}$, $\beta = \sqrt{2}-1$, $\beta/\alpha = 1/\sqrt{2}$ (respectively, $\alpha = 2/3$, $\beta = 1/3$, $\beta/\alpha = 1/2$).

3.3. THE APPLICATION TO THE SOLUTION OF THE TIME–DEPENDENT NAVIER–STOKES EQUATIONS

We discuss now the application of the schemes described in section 3.1 to the solution of the time–dependent Navier–Stokes equations (2.1), (2.2), with the initial–value condition (2.5); we suppose for simplicity that the boundary conditions are of the Dirichlet type, i.e.,

$$\underset{\sim}{u} = \underset{\sim}{g} \text{ on } \Gamma \text{ (with } \int_\Gamma \underset{\sim}{g} \cdot \underset{\sim}{n}\, d\Gamma = 0) . \tag{3.39}$$

3.3.1. The First Operator–Splitting Method

This method is directly derived from the *Peaceman–Rachford scheme* (3.3)–(3.5) and is the following:

$$\underset{\sim}{u}^0 = \underset{\sim}{u}_0 ; \tag{3.40}$$

then for $n \geq 0$ and starting from $\underset{\sim}{u}^n$, we compute $\{\underset{\sim}{u}^{n+1/2}, p^{n+1/2}\}$ and $\underset{\sim}{u}^{n+1}$ by solving

$$\left\{\begin{aligned} &\frac{\underset{\sim}{u}^{n+1/2} - \underset{\sim}{u}^n}{\Delta t/2} - \frac{\nu}{2}\Delta \underset{\sim}{u}^{n+1/2} + \underset{\sim}{\nabla} p^{n+1/2} \\ &\qquad = \underset{\sim}{f}^{n+1/2} + \frac{\nu}{2}\Delta \underset{\sim}{u}^n - (\underset{\sim}{u}^n . \underset{\sim}{\nabla})\underset{\sim}{u}^n \quad \text{in } \Omega, \\ &\underset{\sim}{\nabla}.\underset{\sim}{u}^{n+1/2} = 0 \quad \text{in } \Omega, \end{aligned}\right. \tag{3.41}$$

$$\underset{\sim}{u}^{n+1/2} = \underset{\sim}{g}^{n+1/2} \quad \text{on } \Gamma,$$

and

$$\left\{\begin{aligned} &\frac{\underset{\sim}{u}^{n+1} - \underset{\sim}{u}^{n+1/2}}{\Delta t/2} - \frac{\nu}{2}\Delta \underset{\sim}{u}^{n+1/2} + (\underset{\sim}{u}^{n+1}.\underset{\sim}{\nabla})\underset{\sim}{u}^{n+1} \\ &\qquad = \underset{\sim}{f}^{n+1} + \frac{\nu}{2}\Delta \underset{\sim}{u}^{n+1/2} - \underset{\sim}{\nabla} p^{n+1/2} \quad \text{in } \Omega, \\ &\underset{\sim}{u}^{n+1} = \underset{\sim}{g}^{n+1} \quad \text{on } \Gamma, \end{aligned}\right. \tag{3.42}$$

respectively.

3.3.2. The Second Operator–Splitting Method

This method is derived from the scheme (3.9)–(3.12) and is the following:

$$\underset{\sim}{u}^0 = \underset{\sim}{u}_0 ; \tag{3.43}$$

then for $n \geq 0$ and starting from $\underset{\sim}{u}^n$ we solve

$$\left|\begin{aligned} &\frac{\underset{\sim}{u}^{n+\theta} - \underset{\sim}{u}^n}{\theta \Delta t} - \alpha\nu\Delta \underset{\sim}{u}^{n+\theta} + \underset{\sim}{\nabla} p^{n+\theta} \\ &\qquad = \underset{\sim}{f}^{n+\theta} + \beta\nu\Delta \underset{\sim}{u}^n - (\underset{\sim}{u}^n . \underset{\sim}{\nabla})\underset{\sim}{u}^n \quad \text{in } \Omega \\ &\underset{\sim}{\nabla}.\underset{\sim}{u}^{n+\theta} = 0 \quad \text{in } \Omega, \\ &\underset{\sim}{u}^{n+\theta} = \underset{\sim}{g}^{n+\theta} \quad \text{on } \Gamma, \end{aligned}\right. \tag{3.44}$$

$$\left|\begin{aligned} &\frac{\underset{\sim}{u}^{n+1-\theta} - \underset{\sim}{u}^{n+\theta}}{(1-2\theta)\Delta t} - \beta\nu\Delta \underset{\sim}{u}^{n+1-\theta} + (\underset{\sim}{u}^{n+1-\theta}.\underset{\sim}{\nabla})\underset{\sim}{u}^{n+1-\theta} \\ &\qquad = \underset{\sim}{f}^{n+1-\theta} + \alpha\nu\Delta \underset{\sim}{u}^{n+\theta} - \underset{\sim}{\nabla} p^{n+\theta} \quad \text{in } \Omega, \\ &\underset{\sim}{u}^{n+1-\theta} = g^{n+1-\theta} \quad \text{on } \Gamma, \end{aligned}\right. \tag{3.45}$$

$$\left|\begin{aligned} &\frac{\underset{\sim}{u}^{n+1} - \underset{\sim}{u}^{n+1-\theta}}{\theta\Delta t} - \alpha\nu\Delta\underset{\sim}{u}^{n+1} + \underset{\sim}{\nabla}p^{n+1} \\ &\qquad = \underset{\sim}{f}^{n+1} + \beta\nu\Delta\underset{\sim}{u}^{n+1-\theta} - (\underset{\sim}{u}^{n+1-\theta}.\underset{\sim}{\nabla})\underset{\sim}{u}^{n+1-\theta} \quad \text{in } \Omega\,, \\ &\underset{\sim}{\nabla}.\underset{\sim}{u}^{n+1} = 0 \quad \text{in } \Omega\,, \\ &\underset{\sim}{u}^{n+1} = \underset{\sim}{g}^{n+1} \quad \text{on } \Gamma\,. \end{aligned}\right. \tag{3.46}$$

For the choice of α and β, see section 3.3.3, below.

3.3.3. Some Remarks Concerning the Schemes (3.40)–(3.42) and (3.43)–(3.46)

Using the two operator–splitting methods described above, we have been able to decouple the nonlinearity and the incompressibility in the Navier–Stokes equations (2.1), (2.2). In sections 4 and 5, we will describe—briefly—the specific treatment of the subproblems encountered at each step of (3.40)–(3.42) and (3.43)–(3.46).

We note that $\underset{\sim}{u}^{n+1/2}$ and $\underset{\sim}{u}^{n+\theta}$, $\underset{\sim}{u}^{n+1}$ are obtained from the solution of linear problems very close to the steady Stokes problem. Despite its greater complexity, the scheme (3.43)–(3.46) is (per step) almost as economical, due to the fact that the "quasi"–steady Stokes problems (3.41) and (3.44), (3.46) (actually, convenient finite–element approximations of them) can be solved by quite efficient solvers, so that most of the computer time used to solve a full step is in fact used to solve the nonlinear subproblem. The good choice for α and β is given by (3.36) if one uses the scheme (3.43)–(3.46); with such a choice, many computer subprograms can be used for both the linear and nonlinear subproblems, saving thereby quite a substantial amount of core memory.

3.4. THE EIGENVALUE CALCULATIONS

3.4.1. Generalities. Synopsis

In this section our main objective is to show that the concepts introduced in section 3.1 apply also to eigenvalue calculations, at least for symmetric matrices (or operator). Since the resulting methods belong to the class of the so–called *inverse power methods*, the new approach brings very little to the linear eigenvalue problem (for which a basic reference is [23]), but it is nicely suited to solve nonlinear eigenvalue problems—such as the Hartree equation in quantum physics (see [24], [25] for more details).

3.4.2. The Statement of the Problem

Let $\underset{\sim}{A}$ be a symmetric $N \times N$ real matrix; we denote by λ_i the eigenvalues of $\underset{\sim}{A}$ and suppose that $\lambda_1 \leq \lambda_2 \leq \cdots \leq \lambda_N$.

We concentrate on the calculation of the smallest eigenvalue of $\underset{\sim}{A}$ (i.e., λ_1). It is well known that λ_1 satisfies

$$\lambda_1 = \min_{\underset{\sim}{v} \in S} (\underset{\sim}{A}\underset{\sim}{v},\underset{\sim}{v}) , \tag{3.47}$$

where

$$S = \{\underset{\sim}{v} | \underset{\sim}{v} \in \mathbf{R}^N, \ \|\underset{\sim}{v}\| = 1\} , \tag{3.48}$$

$$\begin{cases} (\underset{\sim}{v},\underset{\sim}{w}) = \sum_{i=1}^{N} v_i w_i, \ \forall \ \underset{\sim}{v} = \{v_i\}_{i=1}^N, \ \underset{\sim}{w} = \{w_i\}_{i=1}^N , \\ \|\underset{\sim}{v}\| = (\underset{\sim}{v},\underset{\sim}{v})^{1/2} . \end{cases} \tag{3.49}$$

Let us introduce now the functional I_S defined by

$$I_S(\underset{\sim}{v}) = \begin{cases} 0 & \text{if } \underset{\sim}{v} \in S , \\ +\infty & \text{if } \underset{\sim}{v} \notin S ; \end{cases} \tag{3.50}$$

I_S is the *indicator functional* of S. We clearly have

$$\lambda_{1/2} = \min_{\underset{\sim}{v} \in \mathbf{R}^N} \{\tfrac{1}{2}(\underset{\sim}{A}\underset{\sim}{v},\underset{\sim}{v}) + I_S(\underset{\sim}{v})\} . \tag{3.51}$$

Suppose that I_S is differentiable (which is definitely not the case) and denote by ∂I_S its differential; if $\underset{\sim}{u}$ is a minimizer in the problems (3.47), (3.51), i.e., an eigenvector of norm one, associated to λ_1, $\underset{\sim}{u}$ satisfies

$$\underset{\sim}{A}\underset{\sim}{u} + \partial I_S(\underset{\sim}{u}) = \underset{\sim}{0} . \tag{3.52}$$

It is then quite natural to associate to the nonlinear "equation" (3.52) the initial value problem:

$$\begin{cases} \dfrac{\partial \underset{\sim}{u}}{\partial t} + \underset{\sim}{A}\underset{\sim}{u} + \partial I_S(\underset{\sim}{u}) = \underset{\sim}{0} \\ \underset{\sim}{u}(0) = \underset{\sim}{u}_0 , \end{cases} \tag{3.53}$$

and to seek the steady-state solutions of (3.53), i.e., $\lim_{x \to +\infty} \underset{\sim}{u}(t)$, if such a limit exists. Noting the special form of (3.53), it is tempting to solve it using the operator–splitting methods discussed in sections 3.1 and 3.2. The resulting algorithms will be discussed next.

3.4.3. Solution of (3.52) Via (3.53), Using the Operator–Splitting Methods

We now apply the operator–splitting methods of section 3.1, with $A_1 = \partial I_S$, $A_2 = \underset{\sim}{A}$ and $f = \underset{\sim}{0}$.

Application of the Peaceman–Rachford Scheme (3.3)–(3.5):

$$\underset{\sim}{u}^0 = \underset{\sim}{u}_0 ; \tag{3.54}$$

then for $n \geq 0$ with u^n known we compute successively $\underset{\sim}{u}^{n+1/2}$ and $\underset{\sim}{u}^{n+1}$ by

$$\frac{\underset{\sim}{u}^{n+1/2} - \underset{\sim}{u}^n}{\Delta t/2} + \partial I_S(\underset{\sim}{u}^{n+1/2}) + \underset{\sim}{A}\underset{\sim}{u}^n = \underset{\sim}{0}, \tag{3.55}$$

$$\frac{\underset{\sim}{u}^{n+1} - \underset{\sim}{u}^{n+1/2}}{\Delta t/2} + \partial I_S(\underset{\sim}{u}^{n+1/2}) + \underset{\sim}{A}\underset{\sim}{u}^{n+1} = \underset{\sim}{0}. \tag{3.56}$$

Application of the Douglas–Rachford Scheme (3.6)–(3.8):

$$\underset{\sim}{u}^0 = \underset{\sim}{u}_0 ; \tag{3.57}$$

then for $n \geq 0$, with $\underset{\sim}{u}^n$ known we compute successively $\hat{\underset{\sim}{u}}^{n+1}$ and $\underset{\sim}{u}^{n+1}$ by

$$\frac{\hat{\underset{\sim}{u}}^{n+1} - \underset{\sim}{u}^n}{\Delta t} + \partial I_S(\hat{\underset{\sim}{u}}^{n+1}) + \underset{\sim}{A}\underset{\sim}{u}^n = \underset{\sim}{0}, \tag{3.58}$$

$$\frac{\underset{\sim}{u}^{n+1} - \underset{\sim}{u}^n}{\Delta t} + \partial I_S(\hat{\underset{\sim}{u}}^{n+1}) + \underset{\sim}{A}\underset{\sim}{u}^{n+1} = \underset{\sim}{0}, \tag{3.59}$$

Application of the Three–Stage Scheme (3.9)–(3.12):

$$\underset{\sim}{u}^0 = \underset{\sim}{u}_0 ; \tag{3.60}$$

then for $n \geq 0$, with $\underset{\sim}{u}^n$ known we compute successively $\underset{\sim}{u}^{n+\theta}$, $\underset{\sim}{u}^{n+1-\theta}$ and $\underset{\sim}{u}^{n+1}$ by

$$\frac{\underset{\sim}{u}^{n+\theta} - \underset{\sim}{u}^n}{\theta\Delta t} + \partial I_S(\underset{\sim}{u}^{n+\theta}) + \underset{\sim}{A}\underset{\sim}{u}^n = \underset{\sim}{0}, \tag{3.61}$$

$$\frac{\underset{\sim}{u}^{n+1-\theta} - \underset{\sim}{u}^{n+\theta}}{(1-2\theta)\Delta t} + \partial I_S(\underset{\sim}{u}^{n+\theta}) + \underset{\sim}{A}\underset{\sim}{u}^{n+1-\theta} = \underset{\sim}{0}, \tag{3.62}$$

$$\frac{\underset{\sim}{u}^{n+1} - \underset{\sim}{u}^{n+1-\theta}}{\theta\Delta t} + \partial I_S(\underset{\sim}{u}^{n+1}) + \underset{\sim}{A}\underset{\sim}{u}^{n+1-\theta} = \underset{\sim}{0}. \tag{3.63}$$

In order to derive more practical formulations of the above algorithms, let us consider the algorithm (3.54)–(3.56) (the result will hold also for the other two methods).

We observe that (3.55) is in fact a necessary condition of optimality for the following minimization problem:

$$\begin{cases} \textit{Find } \underset{\sim}{u}^{n+1/2} \in S \textit{ such that} \\ J_n(\underset{\sim}{u}^{n+1/2}) \le J_n(\underset{\sim}{v}), \ \forall\, \underset{\sim}{v} \in S, \end{cases} \tag{3.64}$$

with

$$J_n(\underset{\sim}{v}) = \frac{1}{2}\|v\|^2 - (\underset{\sim}{u}^n - \frac{\Delta t}{2}\underset{\sim}{A}\underset{\sim}{u}^n, \underset{\sim}{v}).$$

Since $\|\underset{\sim}{v}\| = 1$, $\forall\, \underset{\sim}{v} \in S$, the solution of (3.64) is given by

$$\underset{\sim}{u}^{n+1/2} = \frac{\underset{\sim}{u}^n - \frac{\Delta t}{2}\underset{\sim}{A}\underset{\sim}{u}^n}{\|\underset{\sim}{u}^n - \frac{\Delta t}{2}\underset{\sim}{A}\underset{\sim}{u}^n\|}.$$

On the other hand, it follows from (3.55) that

$$\frac{\Delta t}{2}\partial I_S(\underset{\sim}{u}^{n+1/2}) = \underset{\sim}{u}^n - \frac{\Delta t}{2}\underset{\sim}{A}\underset{\sim}{u}^n - \underset{\sim}{u}^{n+1/2}$$

which, combined with (3.56), implies

$$(\mathrm{I} + \frac{\Delta t}{2}\underset{\sim}{A})\underset{\sim}{u}^{n+1} = 2\underset{\sim}{u}^{n+1/2} - (\underset{\sim}{u}^n - \frac{\Delta t}{2}\underset{\sim}{A}\underset{\sim}{u}^n).$$

Collecting the above results, we obtain the following practical formulation for algorithm (3.54)–(3.56).

Practical formulation of algorithm (3.54)–(3.56):

$$\underset{\sim}{u}^0 = u_0, \tag{3.65}$$

then for $n \ge 0$, compute $\underset{\sim}{p}^n$ and $\underset{\sim}{u}^{n+1}$, from $\underset{\sim}{u}^n$, by

$$\underset{\sim}{p}^n = \underset{\sim}{u}^n - \frac{\Delta t}{2}\underset{\sim}{A}\underset{\sim}{u}^n, \tag{3.66}$$

$$\underset{\sim}{u}^{n+1} = (I + \frac{\Delta t}{2}\underset{\sim}{A})^{-1}\left(\frac{2}{\|\underset{\sim}{p}^n\|} - 1\right)\underset{\sim}{p}^n. \tag{3.67}$$

Using similar calculations yields the following formulations for (3.57)–(3.59) and (3.60)–(3.63).

Practical formulation of the algorithm (3.57)–(3.59):

$$\underset{\sim}{u}^0 = \underset{\sim}{u}_0 . \tag{3.68}$$

Then for $n \geq 0$, compute $\underset{\sim}{p}^n$ $\underset{\sim}{u}^{n+1}$ from $\underset{\sim}{u}^n$, using

$$\underset{\sim}{p}^n = \underset{\sim}{u}^n - \Delta t \underset{\sim}{A} \underset{\sim}{u}^n , \tag{3.69}$$

$$\underset{\sim}{u}^{n+1} = (I + \Delta t \underset{\sim}{A})^{-1} \left\{ \underset{\sim}{u}^n + \left(\frac{1}{\| \underset{\sim}{p}^n \|} - 1 \right) \underset{\sim}{p}^n \right\} . \tag{3.70}$$

Practical formulation of the algorithm (3.60)–(3.63):

$$\underset{\sim}{u}^0 = \underset{\sim}{u}_0 . \tag{3.71}$$

Then for $n \geq 0$, compute $\underset{\sim}{p}^n$, $\underset{\sim}{u}^{n+\theta}$, $\underset{\sim}{u}^{n+1-\theta}$, $\underset{\sim}{p}^{n+1-\theta}$, $\underset{\sim}{u}^{n+1}$ from $\underset{\sim}{u}^n$, using

$$\underset{\sim}{p}^n = \underset{\sim}{u}^n - \theta \Delta t \underset{\sim}{A} \underset{\sim}{u}^n , \tag{3.72}$$

$$\underset{\sim}{u}^{n+\theta} = \frac{\underset{\sim}{p}^n}{\| \underset{\sim}{p}^n \|} , \tag{3.73}$$

$$\left\{ \begin{aligned} \underset{\sim}{u}^{n+1-\theta} &= (\underset{\sim}{I} + (1-2\theta)\Delta t \underset{\sim}{A})^{-1} \left(\frac{1-\theta}{\theta} \underset{\sim}{u}^{n+\theta} - \frac{1-2\theta}{\theta} \underset{\sim}{p}^n \right) \\ &= (\underset{\sim}{I} + (1-2\theta)\Delta t \underset{\sim}{A})^{-1} \left(\frac{1-\theta}{\theta} \frac{1}{\| \underset{\sim}{p}^n \|} - \frac{1-2\theta}{\theta} \right) \underset{\sim}{p}^n , \end{aligned} \right. \tag{3.74}$$

$$\underset{\sim}{p}^{n+1-\theta} = \underset{\sim}{u}^{n+1-\theta} - \theta \Delta t \underset{\sim}{A} \underset{\sim}{u}^{n+1-\theta} , \tag{3.75}$$

$$\underset{\sim}{u}^{n+1} = \frac{\underset{\sim}{p}^{n+1-\theta}}{\| \underset{\sim}{p}^{n+1-\theta} \|} . \tag{3.76}$$

□

These algorithms are variations of the well–known inverse power methods (see, e.g., [23] for a detailed analysis of such methods). In the numerical experiments, various vector sequences generated by the above algorithms converge *linearly* to an eigenvector associated with the smallest eigenvalue λ_1, whereas $(\underset{\sim}{A}\underset{\sim}{u}^n, \underset{\sim}{u}^n)$ converges *quadratically* to λ_1. Indeed, the convergence is still good if λ_1 is a *multiple* eigenvalue. It is interesting to note that the fastest algorithm is (3.71)–(3.76), then (3.65)–(3.67), then (3.68)–(3.70); these results agree with the analysis done for the trivial linear problem that we considered in section 3.2.

In the following sections we go back to the Navier–Stokes equations and their numerical treatment.

4. Least squares conjugate gradient solution of the nonlinear subproblems obtained from the time discretization of the Navier–Stokes equations by the methods of section 3.3

4.1. CLASSICAL AND VARIATIONAL FORMULATION. SYNOPSIS

At each full step of the operator–splitting methods (3.40)–(3.42) and (3.43)–(3.46) we have to solve a nonlinear elliptic system of the following type:

$$\begin{cases} \alpha \underset{\sim}{u} - \nu \Delta \underset{\sim}{u} + (\underset{\sim}{u}.\underset{\sim}{\nabla})\underset{\sim}{u} = \underset{\sim}{f} \text{ in } \Omega , \\ \underset{\sim}{u} = \underset{\sim}{g} \text{ on } \Gamma , \end{cases} \tag{4.1}$$

where α and ν are two positive constants and where $\underset{\sim}{f}$ and $\underset{\sim}{g}$ are two given functions defined on Ω and Γ, respectively. We do not discuss here the existence and uniqueness of solutions for (4.1). We now introduce the following functional spaces of the Sobolev type:

$$H^1(\Omega) = \{\phi | \phi \in L^2(\Omega), \frac{\partial \phi}{\partial x_i} \in L^2(\Omega), \forall\, i = 1,\dots,N\} , \tag{4.2}$$

$$H_0^1(\Omega) = \{\phi | \phi \in H^1(\Omega),\ \phi = 0 \text{ on } \Gamma\} , \tag{4.3}$$

$$V_0 = (H_0^1(\Omega))^N , \tag{4.4}$$

$$V_g = \{\underset{\sim}{v} | \underset{\sim}{v} \in (H^1(\Omega))^N,\ \underset{\sim}{v} = \underset{\sim}{g} \text{ on } \Gamma\} ; \tag{4.5}$$

if $\underset{\sim}{g}$ is sufficiently smooth, then V_g is nonempty.

We shall use the following notation:

$$dx = dx_1,\dots,dx_N ,$$

and if $\underset{\sim}{u} = \{u_i\}_{i=1}^N$, $\underset{\sim}{v} = \{v_i\}_{i=1}^N$, then

$$\underset{\sim}{u}.\underset{\sim}{v} = \sum_{i=1}^N u_i v_i ,$$

$$\underset{\sim}{\nabla}\underset{\sim}{u}.\underset{\sim}{\nabla}\underset{\sim}{v} = \sum_{i=1}^N \underset{\sim}{\nabla} u_i.\underset{\sim}{\nabla} v_i = \sum_{i=1}^N \sum_{j=1}^N \frac{\partial u_i}{\partial x_j}\frac{\partial v_i}{\partial x_j} .$$

Using the Green formula, we can prove that for sufficiently smooth functions $\underset{\sim}{u}$ and $\underset{\sim}{v}$ belonging to $(H^1(\Omega))^N$ and V_0, respectively, we have

$$-\int_{\Omega} \Delta \underset{\sim}{u} . \underset{\sim}{v} \, dx = \int_{\Omega} \nabla \underset{\sim}{u} . \nabla \underset{\sim}{v} \, dx . \tag{4.6}$$

It can also be proved that if $\underset{\sim}{u}$ is a solution of (4.1) belonging to V_g, it is also a solution of the following nonlinear variational problem:

$$\left\{ \begin{aligned} & \underset{\sim}{u} \in V_g , \\ & \alpha \int_{\Omega} \underset{\sim}{u} . \underset{\sim}{v} \, dx + \nu \int_{\Omega} \nabla \underset{\sim}{u} . \nabla \underset{\sim}{v} \, dx + \int_{\Omega} ((\underset{\sim}{u} . \underset{\sim}{\nabla}) \underset{\sim}{u}) . \underset{\sim}{v} \, dx \\ & \qquad = \int_{\Omega} \underset{\sim}{f} . \underset{\sim}{v} \, dx, \ \forall \, \underset{\sim}{v} \in V_0 , \end{aligned} \right. \tag{4.7}$$

and conversely. We note that (4.1),(4.7) is not equivalent to a problem in Calculus of Variations since there is no functional of $\underset{\sim}{v}$ with $(\underset{\sim}{v} . \underset{\sim}{\nabla}) \underset{\sim}{v}$ as differential; however, using a convenient least squares formulation we shall be able to solve (4.1), (4.7) by iterative methods originating from nonlinear programming, such as the conjugate–gradient method.

4.2. LEAST SQUARES FORMULATION OF (4.1), (4.7)

Let $\underset{\sim}{v} \in V_g$; from $\underset{\sim}{v}$ we define $\underset{\sim}{y} = \underset{\sim}{y}(\underset{\sim}{v}) \in V_0$ as the solution of

$$\left\{ \begin{aligned} & \alpha \underset{\sim}{y} - \nu \Delta \underset{\sim}{y} = \alpha \underset{\sim}{v} - \nu \Delta \underset{\sim}{v} + (\underset{\sim}{v} . \underset{\sim}{\nabla}) \underset{\sim}{v} - \underset{\sim}{f} \quad \text{in } \Omega , \\ & \underset{\sim}{y} = \underset{\sim}{0} \quad \text{on } \Gamma . \end{aligned} \right. \tag{4.8}$$

Note that $\underset{\sim}{y}$ is obtained from $\underset{\sim}{v}$ via the solution of N uncoupled linear Poisson problems (one for each component of $\underset{\sim}{y}$); using (4.6) it can be shown that (4.8) is equivalent to the linear variational problem:

$$\left\{ \begin{aligned} & \text{Find } \underset{\sim}{y} \in V_0 \text{ such that } \forall \, \underset{\sim}{z} \in V_0, \\ & \alpha \int_{\Omega} \underset{\sim}{y} . \underset{\sim}{z} \, dx + \nu \int_{\Omega} \nabla \underset{\sim}{y} . \nabla \underset{\sim}{z} \, dx \\ & \quad = \alpha \int_{\Omega} \underset{\sim}{v} . \underset{\sim}{z} \, dx + \nu \int_{\Omega} \nabla \underset{\sim}{v} . \nabla \underset{\sim}{z} \, dx + \int_{\Omega} ((\underset{\sim}{v} . \underset{\sim}{\nabla}) \underset{\sim}{v}) . \underset{\sim}{z} \, dx - \int_{\Omega} \underset{\sim}{f} . \underset{\sim}{z} \, dx, \end{aligned} \right. \tag{4.9}$$

which has a unique solution. Suppose now that $\underset{\sim}{v}$ is a solution of the nonlinear problem (4.1), (4.7); the corresponding $\underset{\sim}{y}$ (obtained from the solution of (4.8), (4.9)) is clearly $\underset{\sim}{y} = \underset{\sim}{0}$; from this observation it is quite natural to introduce the following (nonlinear) least squares formulation of (4.1), (4.7):

$$\begin{aligned} & \text{Find } \underset{\sim}{u} \in V_g \text{ such that} \\ & J(\underset{\sim}{u}) \le J(\underset{\sim}{v}), \quad \forall \, \underset{\sim}{v} \in V_g , \end{aligned} \tag{4.10}$$

where $J: (H^1(\Omega))^N \to \mathbf{R}$ is the function of $\underset{\sim}{v}$ defined by

$$J(\underset{\sim}{v}) = \frac{1}{2}\int_\Omega \{\alpha|\underset{\sim}{y}|^2 + \nu|\underset{\sim}{\nabla}\underset{\sim}{y}|^2\}\, dx\,, \tag{4.11}$$

where $\underset{\sim}{y}$ is defined from $\underset{\sim}{v}$ by (4.8), (4.9). Note that if $\underset{\sim}{u}$ is the solution of (4.1), (4.7), then it is also a solution of (4.10) such that $J(\underset{\sim}{u}) = 0$; conversely, if $\underset{\sim}{u}$ is a solution of (4.10) such that $J(\underset{\sim}{u}) = 0$, then it is also a solution of (4.1), (4.7).

4.3. CONJUGATE–GRADIENT SOLUTION OF THE LEAST SQUARES PROBLEM (4.10)

4.3.1. Description of the algorithm

We use the *Polak–Ribiere* version (see [26]) of the conjugate–gradient method to solve the minimization problem (4.10); we have then (with $J'(\underset{\sim}{v})$ the differential of J at $\underset{\sim}{v}$)

Step 0: Initialization

$$\underset{\sim}{u}^0 \in V_g, \quad \text{given}\,; \tag{4.12}$$

we then define $\underset{\sim}{g}^0, \underset{\sim}{w}^0 \in V_0$ by

$$\left|\begin{aligned} &\underset{\sim}{g}^0 \in V_0\,, \\ &\alpha\int_\Omega \underset{\sim}{g}^0.\underset{\sim}{z}\, dx + \nu\int_\Omega \underset{\sim}{\nabla}\underset{\sim}{g}^0.\underset{\sim}{\nabla}\underset{\sim}{z}\, dx \\ &\qquad = \langle J'(\underset{\sim}{u}^0),\underset{\sim}{z}\rangle, \quad \forall\, \underset{\sim}{z} \in V_0\,, \end{aligned}\right. \tag{4.13}$$

$$\underset{\sim}{w}^0 = \underset{\sim}{g}^0\,, \tag{4.14}$$

respectively. □

Then for $n \geq 0$, assuming that $\underset{\sim}{u}^n$, $\underset{\sim}{w}^n$, $\underset{\sim}{g}^n$ are known, we obtain $\underset{\sim}{u}^{n+1}$, $\underset{\sim}{g}^{n+1}$, $\underset{\sim}{w}^{n+1}$ by

Step 1: Descent

$$\begin{aligned} &\text{Find } \lambda_n \in \mathbf{R}\,, \\ &J(\underset{\sim}{u}^n - \lambda_n \underset{\sim}{w}^n) \leq J(\underset{\sim}{u}^n - \lambda\underset{\sim}{w}^n), \quad \forall\, \lambda \in \mathbf{R}\,, \end{aligned} \tag{4.15}$$

$$\underset{\sim}{u}^{n+1} = \underset{\sim}{u}^n - \lambda_n \underset{\sim}{w}^n\,. \tag{4.16}$$

Step 2: Calculation of the new descent direction

$$\left\{\begin{aligned} &\text{Find } \underset{\sim}{g}^{n+1} \in V_0, \text{ such that} \\ &\alpha \int_\Omega \underset{\sim}{g}^{n+1}.\underset{\sim}{z}\, dx + \nu \int_\Omega \nabla \underset{\sim}{g}^{n+1}.\nabla \underset{\sim}{z}\, dx \\ &\qquad = \langle J'(\underset{\sim}{u}^{n+1}),\underset{\sim}{z}\rangle, \quad \forall\, \underset{\sim}{z} \in V_0\,, \end{aligned}\right. \tag{4.17}$$

$$\gamma_n = \frac{\alpha\int_\Omega \underset{\sim}{g}^{n+1}.(\underset{\sim}{g}^{n+1}-\underset{\sim}{g}^n)dx + \nu\int_\Omega \nabla\underset{\sim}{g}^{n+1}.\nabla(\underset{\sim}{g}^{n+1}-\underset{\sim}{g}^n)dx}{\alpha\int_\Omega |\underset{\sim}{g}^n|^2 dx + \nu\int_\Omega |\nabla\underset{\sim}{g}^n|^2 dx}\,, \tag{4.18}$$

$$\underset{\sim}{w}^{n+1} = \underset{\sim}{g}^{n+1} + \gamma_n \underset{\sim}{w}^n\,. \tag{4.19}$$

Do $n = n+1$, go to (4.15).

As we shall see, applying the algorithm (4.12)–(4.19), solving the least squares problem (4.10) requires solving at each iteration of exactly three Dirichlet systems (i.e., $3N$ scalar Dirichlet problems) associated to the elliptic operator $\alpha I - \nu\Delta$.

4.3.2. Calculation of J'

A most important step when making use of (4.12)–(4.19) to solve (4.10) is the calculation of $\langle J'(\underset{\sim}{u}^{n+1}),\underset{\sim}{z}\rangle$ at each iteration; we should easily prove (see, e.g., [5], [22]) that $J'(\underset{\sim}{v})$ can be identified with the linear functional from V_0 to $\mathbf{R}$, defined by

$$\begin{aligned} \langle J'(\underset{\sim}{v}),\underset{\sim}{z}\rangle &= \alpha \int_\Omega \underset{\sim}{y}.\underset{\sim}{z}\, dx + \nu \int_\Omega \nabla\underset{\sim}{y}.\nabla\underset{\sim}{z}\, dx \\ &\quad + \int_\Omega \underset{\sim}{y}.(\underset{\sim}{v}.\nabla)\underset{\sim}{z}\, dx + \int_\Omega \underset{\sim}{y}.(\underset{\sim}{z}.\nabla)\underset{\sim}{v}\, dx, \quad \forall\, \underset{\sim}{z} \in V_0\,, \end{aligned} \tag{4.21}$$

where

$$(\underset{\sim}{v}.\nabla)\underset{\sim}{w} = \{\sum_{j=1}^{N} v_j \frac{\partial w_i}{\partial x_j}\}_{i=1}^{N}, \quad \forall\, \underset{\sim}{v},\underset{\sim}{w}\,;$$

$\langle J'(\underset{\sim}{v}),\underset{\sim}{z}\rangle$ has therefore a *purely integral representation*, which is of major importance in view of finite–element (or spectral) implementations of (4.12)–(4.19). From the above results, to obtain $\langle J'(\underset{\sim}{u}^{n+1}),\underset{\sim}{z}\rangle$ we should proceed as follows:

(a) Compute $\underset{\sim}{y}^{n+1}$, associated to $\underset{\sim}{u}^{n+1}$ by (4.8), (4.9) as indicated in section 4.3.3, below.
(b) We then obtain $\langle J'(\underset{\sim}{u}^{n+1}),\underset{\sim}{z}\rangle$ by taking $\underset{\sim}{v} = \underset{\sim}{u}^{n+1}$ and $\underset{\sim}{y} = \underset{\sim}{y}^{n+1}$ in (4.21).

4.3.3. Calculation of λ_n. Comments on the Algorithm (4.12)–(4.19)

A problem of practical importance is the calculation of λ_n. Let us denote by $\underset{\sim}{y}^n(\lambda)$ the solution of (4.8), (4.9) associated to $\underset{\sim}{v} = \underset{\sim}{u}^n - \lambda\underset{\sim}{w}^n$; we clearly have

$$\underset{\sim}{y}^n(0) = \underset{\sim}{y}^n, \quad \underset{\sim}{y}^n(\lambda_n) = \underset{\sim}{y}^{n+1}, \tag{4.22}$$

and also

$$\underset{\sim}{y}^n(\lambda) = \underset{\sim}{y}^n - \lambda\underset{\sim}{y}_1^n + \lambda^2\underset{\sim}{y}_2^n, \tag{4.23}$$

where $\underset{\sim}{y}_1^n$, $\underset{\sim}{y}_2^n$ are the solutions of

$$\begin{cases} \alpha\underset{\sim}{y}_1^n - \nu\Delta\underset{\sim}{y}_1^n = \alpha\underset{\sim}{w}^n - \nu\Delta\underset{\sim}{w}^n + (\underset{\sim}{u}^n.\underset{\sim}{\nabla})\underset{\sim}{w}^n \\ \qquad\qquad + (\underset{\sim}{w}^n.\underset{\sim}{\nabla})\underset{\sim}{u}^n \text{ in } \Omega, \\ \underset{\sim}{y}_1^n = \underset{\sim}{0} \text{ on } \Gamma, \end{cases} \tag{4.24}$$

$$\begin{cases} \alpha\underset{\sim}{y}_2^n - \nu\Delta\underset{\sim}{y}_2^n = (\underset{\sim}{w}^n.\underset{\sim}{\nabla})\underset{\sim}{w}^n \text{ in } \Omega, \\ \underset{\sim}{y}_2^n = \underset{\sim}{0} \text{ on } \Gamma, \end{cases} \tag{4.25}$$

respectively. Since

$$J(\underset{\sim}{u}^n - \lambda\underset{\sim}{w}^n) = \frac{1}{2}\int_\Omega \{\alpha|\underset{\sim}{y}^n(\lambda)|^2 + \nu|\underset{\sim}{\nabla}\underset{\sim}{y}^n(\lambda)|^2\}dx, \tag{4.26}$$

the function $\lambda \to J(\underset{\sim}{u}^n - \lambda\underset{\sim}{w}^n)$ is, from (4.23), a *quartic* polynomial in λ that we shall denote by $j_n(\lambda)$; λ_n is therefore a solution of the *cubic* equation

$$j_n'(\lambda) = 0. \tag{4.27}$$

We shall use the standard Newton method to compute λ_n from (4.27), starting from $\lambda = 0$. The resulting algorithm is given by

$$\lambda^0 = 0, \tag{4.28}$$

then for $k \geq 0$, we obtain λ^{k+1} from λ^k by

$$\lambda^{k+1} = \lambda^k - \frac{j_n'(\lambda^k)}{j_n''(\lambda^k)}. \tag{4.29}$$

In our calculations, we always observed fast convergence of (4.28), (4.29). Once λ_n is known, we know $\underset{\sim}{y}^{n+1}$ since (from (4.22)) $\underset{\sim}{y}^{n+1} = \underset{\sim}{y}^n(\lambda_n)$.

If we now count the number of Dirichlet systems for $\alpha I - \nu\Delta$ to be solved at each iteration, we observe that we have to solve only three such systems, namely (4.24), (4.25) and then (4.17) (to obtain $\underset{\sim}{g}^{n+1}$); this number is optimal for a nonlinear problem since the solution of a linear problem by the least square–preconditioned conjugate–gradient method requires the solution at each iteration of two linear systems associated to the preconditioning operator.

From the above remarks, it is apparent that the practical implementation of (4.12)–(4.19) will require an efficient (direct or iterative) elliptic solver, like one of those discussed in [27], [28]. To conclude, we would like to mention that (4.12)–(4.19) (in fact, its finite–dimensional variants) is quite efficient; when used in combination with the operator–splitting methods of section 3, three to five iterations suffice to reduce the value of the cost function by a factor of 10^4 to 10^6. However, in view of other applications we are now testing some of those methods combining the features of conjugate gradients and quasi–Newton algorithms, such as the methods discussed in [29], [30] (the results recently obtained for the calculation of transonic potential flows containing shocks are very promissing).

5. Solution of the "quasi" Stokes linear subproblems

5.1. GENERALITIES. SYNOPSIS

At each full step of the splitting methods discussed in section 3.3 we have to solve one or two linear problems of the following type:

$$\begin{cases} \alpha \underset{\sim}{u} - \nu\Delta\underset{\sim}{u} + \underset{\sim}{\nabla} p = \underset{\sim}{f} \quad \text{in } \Omega, \\ \underset{\sim}{\nabla}.\underset{\sim}{u} = 0 \quad \text{in } \Omega, \\ \underset{\sim}{u} = \underset{\sim}{g} \quad \text{on } \Gamma \ \left(\text{with } \int_\Gamma \underset{\sim}{g}.\underset{\sim}{n}\, d\Gamma = 0\right), \end{cases} \tag{5.1}$$

where α and ν are two positive constants and f and g are two given functions defined on Ω and Γ, respectively. We recall that if $\underset{\sim}{f}$ and $\underset{\sim}{g}$ are sufficiently smooth, then (5.1) has a unique solution in $V_g \times (L^2(\Omega)/\mathbf{R})$ (with V_g still defined by (4.5); $p \in (L^2(\Omega)/\mathbf{R})$ means that p is defined only to within an arbitrary constant). We shall describe below two iterative methods for solving (5.1), which are quite easy to implement using finite element or spectral methods. (More details are given in [5], [22], including the proofs of convergence; more methods are discussed in [5].)

5.2. A CONJUGATE–GRADIENT ALGORITHM FOR SOLVING (5.1)

A complete justification of this algorithm is given in [5]; we can say briefly that eliminating $\underset{\sim}{u}$ in (5.1), it appears that p is a solution of a linear functional equation associated to an operator which is self–adjoint and strongly elliptic from H onto H, where

$$H = \{q | q \in L^2(\Omega), \int_\Omega q \, dx = 0\} .$$

Such properties justify a conjugate–gradient solution of (5.1) and lead to the algorithm below:

$$p^0 \in L^2(\Omega) , \quad given , \tag{5.2}$$

$$\begin{cases} \alpha \underset{\sim}{u}^0 - \nu \Delta \underset{\sim}{u}^0 = \underset{\sim}{f} - \underset{\sim}{\nabla} p^0 , \\ \underset{\sim}{u}^0 = \underset{\sim}{g} \quad \text{on } \Gamma , \end{cases} \tag{5.3}$$

$$g^0 = \underset{\sim}{\nabla} . \underset{\sim}{u}^0 , \tag{5.4}$$

$$w^0 = g^0 . \tag{5.5}$$

Then for $n \geq 0$, p^n, g^n, w^n being known, compute p^{n+1}, g^{n+1}, w^{n+1} as follows:
Solve

$$\begin{cases} \alpha \underset{\sim}{\chi}^n - \nu \Delta \underset{\sim}{\chi}^n = -\underset{\sim}{\nabla} w^n , \\ \underset{\sim}{\chi}^n = \underset{\sim}{0} \quad \text{on } \Gamma , \end{cases} \tag{5.6}$$

$$\rho_n = \frac{\int_\Omega | g^n |^2 \, dx}{\int_\Omega \underset{\sim}{\nabla} . \underset{\sim}{\chi}^n w^n \, dx} , \tag{5.7}$$

$$p^{n+1} = p^n - \rho_n w^n , \tag{5.8$_1$}$$

$$\underset{\sim}{u}^{n+1} = \underset{\sim}{u}^n - \rho_n \underset{\sim}{\chi}_n , \tag{5.8$_2$}$$

$$g^{n+1} = \underset{\sim}{g}^n - p_n \underset{\sim}{\nabla} \cdot \underset{\sim}{\chi}_n , \tag{5.8$_3$}$$

$$\gamma_n = \frac{\int_\Omega | g^{n+1} |^2 dx}{\int_\Omega | g^n |^2 dx} , \tag{5.9}$$

$$w^{n+1} = g^{n+1} + \gamma_n w^n . \tag{5.10}$$

Do $n = n+1$, go to (5.6).

We note that the algorithm (5.2)–(5.10) requires the solution at each iteration of only one Dirichlet system, namely (5.6). It can be proved that

$$\lim_{n \to +\infty} \{\underset{\sim}{u}^n, p^n\} = \{\underset{\sim}{u}, p_0\} \tag{5.11}$$

where $\{\underset{\sim}{u}, p_0\}$ is a solution of (5.1) such that

$$\int_\Omega p_0 \, dx = \int_\Omega p^0 \, dx .$$

5.3. THE SECOND ITERATIVE METHOD FOR SOLVING (5.1)

This method is defined as follows (r being a nonnegative parameter):

$$p^0 \in L^2(\Omega) , \text{ given .} \tag{5.12}$$

Then for $n \geq 0$, define $\underset{\sim}{u}^{n+1}$ and p^{n+1}, from p^n by

$$\begin{cases} \alpha \underset{\sim}{u}^n - \nu \Delta \underset{\sim}{u}^n - r \underset{\sim}{\nabla}(\underset{\sim}{\nabla} . \underset{\sim}{u}^n) = \underset{\sim}{f} - \underset{\sim}{\nabla} p^n , \\ \underset{\sim}{u}^n = \underset{\sim}{g} \quad \text{on } \Gamma , \end{cases} \tag{5.13}$$

$$p^{n+1} = p^n - \rho \underset{\sim}{\nabla} . \underset{\sim}{u}^n . \tag{5.14}$$

The above method is related to the *artificial–compressibility* methods of Chorin and Yanenko since (5.14) can be considered as the discretization of

$$\frac{\partial p}{\partial t} + \underset{\sim}{\nabla} . \underset{\sim}{u} = 0$$

(ρ then plays the role of a time step).

For the convergence of (5.12)–(5.14), we should prove (see, e.g., [5, chapter 7] for such a proof) the following

Proposition 5.1. *Suppose that*

$$0 < \rho < 2(r + \frac{\nu}{N}) ; \tag{5.15}$$

we have then

$$\lim_{n \to +\infty} \{\underset{\sim}{u}^n, p^n\} = \{\underset{\sim}{u}, p_0\} \textit{ strongly in } (H^1(\Omega))^N \times L^2(\Omega) , \tag{5.16}$$

where $\{\underset{\sim}{u}, p_0\}$ *is the solution of* (5.1) *such that*

$$\int_\Omega p_0 \, dx = \int_\Omega p^0 \, dx .$$

Moreover, the convergence is linear (i.e., $\|\underset{\sim}{u}^n-\underset{\sim}{u}\|_{(H^1(\Omega))^N}$ *and* $\|p^n-p_0\|_{L^2(\Omega)}$ *converges to zero as least as fast as geometric sequences).*

Remark 5.1. (*The choice of* ρ *and* r). We should use $\rho = r$ in practice, since it can then be proved that the convergence ratio of algorithm (5.12)–(5.14) is $0(r^{-1})$ for large values of r. In most applications, taking $r = 10^2\nu$ to $10^4\nu$ yields a practical convergence of (5.12)–(5.14) in 3 to 4 iterations. There is, however, a practical upper bound for r, since, for too large values of r, (5.13) will be ill–conditioned and its practical solution sensitive to roundoff errors.

Remark 5.2. If $r = 0$, (5.13) reduces to the solution of N uncoupled (one for each component of $\underset{\sim}{u}^n$) scalar Dirichlet problems for $\alpha I - \nu\Delta$; if $r > 0$ the N components of $\underset{\sim}{u}^n$ are coupled by $\underset{\sim}{\nabla}(\underset{\sim}{\nabla}.\underset{\sim}{u}^n)$, making the solution of (5.13) much more costly. In fact, the elliptic operator on the left–hand side of (5.13) is very close to the linear elasticity operator, and its close variants occur naturally in compressible and/or turbulent viscous flow problems.

Remark 5.3. Other methods for solving (5.1) are discussed in [5], [31], [32].

6. Finite element approximation of the time dependent Navier–Stokes equations

We shall describe in this section a specific class of finite–element approximations for the time–dependent Navier–Stokes equations. Actually, these methods, which lead to continuous approximations for both pressure and velocity, are fairly simple, and some of them have been known for years. They have been advocated, for example, by Hood and Taylor (see [33]). Other finite–element approximations of the incompressible Navier–Stokes equations can be found in [1], [2], [4], [5], [34] (see also the references therein).

6.1. BASIC HYPOTHESES. FUNDAMENTAL DISCRETE SPACES

We suppose that Ω is a bounded polygonal domain of $\mathbf{R}^2$. With $\mathscr{C}_h$ a standard finite element triangulation of Ω, and h the maximal length of the edges of the triangles of $\mathscr{C}_h$, we introduce the following discrete spaces (with P_k = space of the polynomials in two variables of degree $\leq k$):

$$H_h^1 = \{q_h | q_h \in C^0(\overline{\Omega}),\ q_{h|T} \in P_1,\ \forall\, T \in \mathscr{C}_h\}\,, \tag{6.1}$$

$$V_h = \{\underset{\sim}{v}_h | \underset{\sim}{v}_h \in C^0(\overline{\Omega}) \times C^0(\overline{\Omega}),\ \underset{\sim}{v}_{h|T} \in P_2 \times P_2,\ \forall\, T \in \mathscr{C}_h\}\,, \tag{6.2}$$

$$V_{0h} = \{\underset{\sim}{v}_h \in V_h,\ \underset{\sim}{v}_h = \underset{\sim}{0} \text{ on } \Gamma\} = V_h \cap V_0 . \tag{6.3}$$

Two useful variants of V_h (and V_{0h}) are obtained as follows: either

$$V_h = \{\underset{\sim}{v}_h | \underset{\sim}{v}_h \in C^0(\overline{\Omega}) \times C^0(\overline{\Omega}),\ \underset{\sim}{v}_{h|T} \in P_1 \times P_1,\ \forall\, T \in \tilde{\mathscr{C}}_h\} , \tag{6.4}$$

or (this space has been introduced in [35])

$$V_h = \{\underset{\sim}{v}_h | \underset{\sim}{v}_h \in C^0(\overline{\Omega}) \times C^0(\overline{\Omega}),\ \underset{\sim}{v}_{h|T} \in P_{1T}^* \times P_{1T}^*,\ \forall\, T \in \mathscr{C}_h\} . \tag{6.5}$$

In (6.4), $\tilde{\mathscr{C}}_h$ is the triangulation of Ω obtained from $\mathscr{C}_h$ by joining the midpoints of the edges of $T \in \mathscr{C}_h$, as shown in figure 6.1; we have the same global number of unknowns if we use V_h defined by either (6.2) or (6.4). However, the matrices encountered in the latter case are more compact and sparse. In (6.5), P_{1T}^* is the subspace of P_3 defined as follows:

$$P_{1T}^* = \{q | q = q_1 + \lambda\phi_T, \text{ with } q_1 \in P_1, \lambda \in \mathbf{R}, \text{ and } \phi_T \in P_3,$$
$$\phi_T = 0 \text{ on } \partial T,\ \phi_T(G_T) = 1\} , \tag{6.6}$$

where, in (6.6), G_T is the *centroid* of T (see figure 6.2 below). A function like ϕ_T is usually called a *bubble function.*

Fig. 6.1

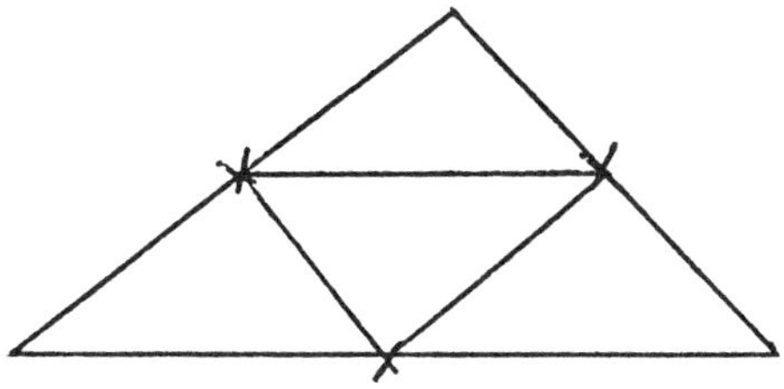

Fig. 6.2

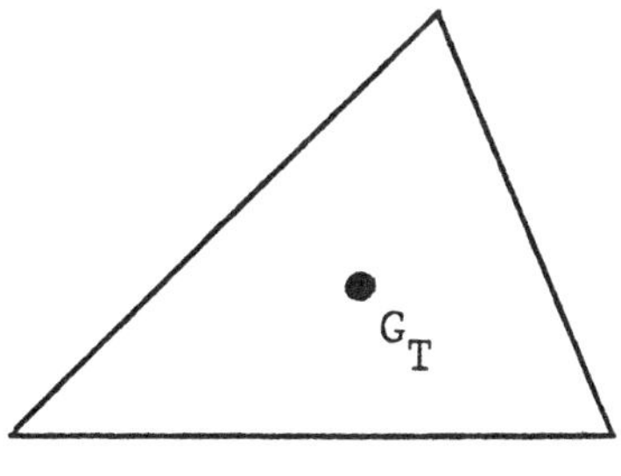

6.2. APPROXIMATION OF THE BOUNDARY CONDITIONS

If the boundary conditions are defined by

$$\mathbf{u} = \mathbf{g} \text{ on } \Gamma \quad \text{with } \int_\Gamma \mathbf{g}.\mathbf{n}\, d\Gamma = 0 , \tag{6.7}$$

it is of fundamental importance to approximate $\mathbf{g}$ by $\mathbf{g}_h$ such that $\int_\Gamma \mathbf{g}_h.\mathbf{n}\, d\Gamma = 0$. The construction of such $\mathbf{g}_h$ is discussed in [5, appendix 3].

6.3. SPACE APPROXIMATIONS OF THE TIME–DEPENDENT NAVIER–STOKES EQUATIONS

Using the spaces H_h^1, V_h and V_{0h}, we approximate the time–dependent Navier–Stokes equations as follows:

Find $\{\mathbf{u}_h(t),p_h(t)\} \in V_h \times H_h^1$, $\forall$ t ≥ 0, such that

$$\begin{cases} \int_\Omega \frac{\partial \mathbf{u}_h}{\partial t}.\mathbf{v}_h\, dx + \nu \int_\Omega \nabla \mathbf{u}_h.\nabla \mathbf{v}_h\, dx + \int_\Omega (\mathbf{u}_h.\nabla)\mathbf{u}_h.\mathbf{v}_h\, dx \\ \qquad + \int_\Omega \nabla p_h.\mathbf{v}_h\, dx = \int_\Omega \mathbf{f}_h.\mathbf{v}_h\, dx, \quad \forall\, \mathbf{v}_h \in V_{0h} , \end{cases} \tag{6.8}$$

$$\int_\Omega \nabla.\mathbf{u}_h q_h\, dx = 0, \quad \forall\, q_h \in H_h^1 , \tag{6.9}$$

$$\mathbf{u}_h = \mathbf{g}_h \text{ on } \Gamma , \tag{6.10}$$

$$\mathbf{u}_h(x,0) = \mathbf{u}_{0h} \text{ (with } \mathbf{u}_{0h} \in V_h) ; \tag{6.11}$$

in (6.8)–(6.11), $\mathbf{f}_h$, $\mathbf{u}_{0h}$ and $\mathbf{g}_h$ are convenient approximations of $\mathbf{f}$, $\mathbf{u}_0$ and $\mathbf{g}$, respectively.

6.4. TIME DISCRETIZATION OF (6.8)–(6.11) BY OPERATOR–SPLITTING METHODS

We consider now a fully discrete version of the scheme (3.40)– (3.42) discussed in section 3.3; it is defined as follows (with Δt as in section 3.3):

$$\mathbf{u}_h^0 = \mathbf{u}_{0h} . \tag{6.12}$$

Then for $n \geq 0$, compute (from $\mathbf{u}_h^n$) $\{\mathbf{u}_h^{n+1}, p_h^{n+1}\} \in V_h \times H_h^1$, and then $\mathbf{u}_h^{n+1} \in V_h$, by solving

$$\left\{\begin{array}{l} \displaystyle\int_\Omega \frac{\underset{\sim}{u}_h^{n+1/2} - \underset{\sim}{u}_h^n}{\Delta t/2} . \underset{\sim}{v}_h \, dx + \frac{\nu}{2}\int_\Omega \underset{\sim}{\nabla} \underset{\sim}{u}_h^{n+1/2} . \underset{\sim}{\nabla} \underset{\sim}{v}_h \, dx + \int_\Omega \underset{\sim}{\nabla} p_h^{n+1/2} . \underset{\sim}{v}_h \, dx \\ \displaystyle \quad = \int_\Omega \underset{\sim}{f}_h^{n+1/2} . \underset{\sim}{v}_h \, dx - \frac{\nu}{2}\int_\Omega \underset{\sim}{\nabla} \underset{\sim}{u}_h^n . \underset{\sim}{\nabla} \underset{\sim}{v}_h \, dx - \int_\Omega (\underset{\sim}{u}_h^n . \underset{\sim}{\nabla}) \underset{\sim}{u}_h^n . \underset{\sim}{v}_h \, dx , \\ \quad \forall\, \underset{\sim}{v}_h \in V_{0h} , \end{array}\right. \tag{6.13$_1$}$$

$$\int_\Omega \underset{\sim}{\nabla} . \underset{\sim}{u}_h^{n+1/2} q_h \, dx = 0 , \quad \forall\, q_h \in H_h^1 , \tag{6.13$_2$}$$

$$\underset{\sim}{u}_h^{n+1/2} \in V_h, \ p_h^{n+1/2} \in H_h^1, \ \underset{\sim}{u}_h^{n+1/2} = \underset{\sim}{g}_h^{n+1/2} \ \text{on}\ \Gamma , \tag{6.13$_3$}$$

and

$$\left\{\begin{array}{l} \displaystyle\int_\Omega \frac{\underset{\sim}{u}_h^{n+1} - \underset{\sim}{u}_h^{n+1/2}}{\Delta t/2} . \underset{\sim}{v}_h \, dx + \frac{\nu}{2}\int_\Omega \underset{\sim}{\nabla} \underset{\sim}{u}_h^{n+1} . \underset{\sim}{\nabla} \underset{\sim}{v}_h \, dx \\ \displaystyle \quad + \int_\Omega (\underset{\sim}{u}_h^{n+1} . \underset{\sim}{\nabla}) \underset{\sim}{u}_h^{n+1} . \underset{\sim}{v}_h \, dx = \int_\Omega \underset{\sim}{f}_h^{n+1} . \underset{\sim}{v}_h \, dx \\ \displaystyle \quad - \frac{\nu}{2}\int_\Omega \underset{\sim}{\nabla} \underset{\sim}{u}_h^{n+1/2} . \underset{\sim}{\nabla} \underset{\sim}{v}_h \, dx - \int_\Omega \underset{\sim}{\nabla} p_h^{n+1/2} . \underset{\sim}{v}_h \, dx, \ \forall\, \underset{\sim}{v}_h \in V_{0h} , \end{array}\right. \tag{6.14}$$

$$\underset{\sim}{u}_h^{n+1} \in V_h, \ \underset{\sim}{u}_h^{n+1} = \underset{\sim}{g}_h^{n+1} \ \text{on}\ \Gamma , \tag{6.15}$$

respectively.

The same techniques apply to the space discretization of the scheme (3.43)–(3.46) (see [5] for more details).

Various subproblems encountered at each step of (6.12)–(6.15) can be solved by the discrete variants of the method discussed in sections 4 and 5; see, again, [5] for more details.

7. Numerical experiments

We illustrate the numerical methods described in the above sections by the results of numerical experiments where these methods have been applied to simulate some incompressible viscous flows of practical interest. All the calculations which follow have been made, using the finite–element method associated with the discrete space defined by (6.1), (6.3), (6.4) (some preliminary and promissing results have been obtained recently, using V_h defined by (6.5), (6.6)).

7.1. THE FIRST CLASS OF TEST PROBLEMS

We consider the solution of the Navier–Stokes equations for the flow of an incompressible viscous fluid in the channel with a step in figure 7.1. We have selected this problem since it is quite a classical and significant test problem for Navier–Stokes solvers (see [34] for a comparison of various methods for solving this test problem). The finite–element triangulations used for these calculations are shown in figure 7.1; the coarse (respectively, fine) one is used for approximating the pressure (respectively, velocity).

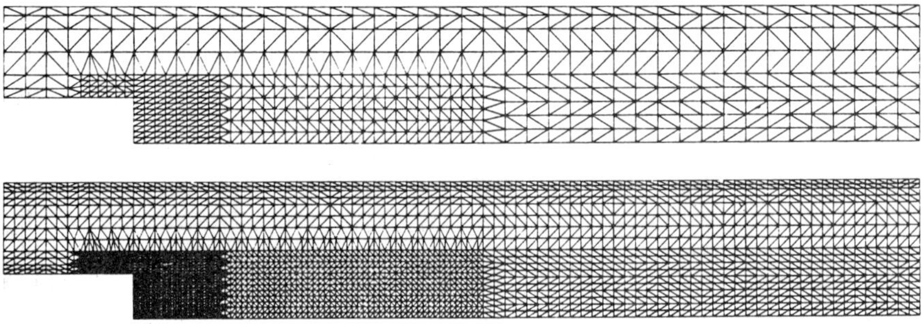

	$\mathcal{T}_h$	$\tilde{\mathcal{T}}_h$
Nodes	619	2346
Triangles	1109	4436
Cholesky's coefficients	21654	154971

Fig. 7.1

We have also indicated in figure 7.1 the number of nodes, triangles and nonzero Cholesky coefficients of the matrix approximating Δ (respectively, $\alpha I - \nu\Delta$) on $\mathcal{C}_h$ (respectively, $\tilde{\mathcal{C}}_h$). The methods described in the preceding sections have been used to compute the steady–state solutions of (2.1), (2.2) for the following boundary conditions:

$$\text{$\underset{\sim}{u}$ satisfies Poiseuille velocity profiles at the entrance and exit of the channel and is equal to $\underset{\sim}{0}$ elsewhere on Γ.} \tag{7.1}$$

We have taken Re = 100 and 191. The numerical results agree quite well with those in [34], [36] and show a clear superiority of the schemes derived from (3.43)–(3.46) over the schemes derived from (3.40)–(3.42). For the scheme (3.43)–(3.46) we have tested $\theta = .25$ and $1-\sqrt{2}/2$ (for the same Δt); the convergence to the steady state is faster with the second value of θ (for this class of problems at least). We have shown in figure 7.2 (respectively, figure 7.3) the stream lines (respectively, bar lines), of the steady–state solution corresponding to Re = 100 and 191. We note that the size of the recirculation region increases with Re.

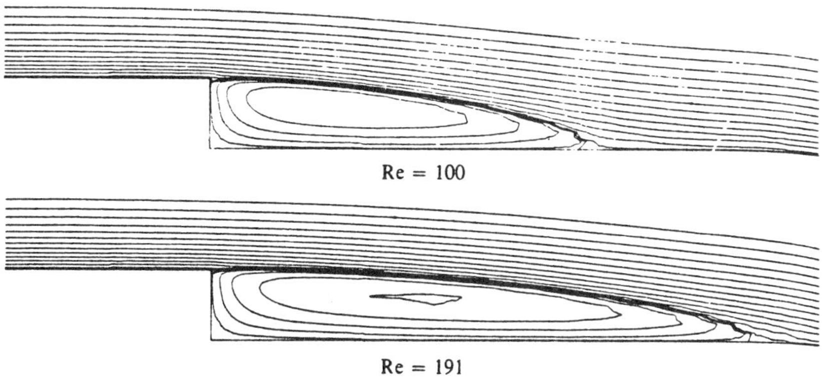

Fig. 7.2. Stream lines

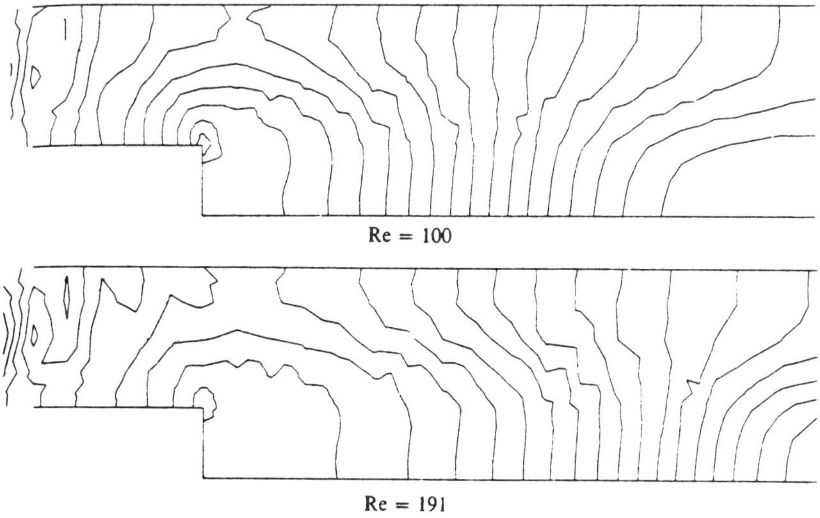

Fig. 7.3. Isopressure lines

7.2. THE SECOND CLASS OF PROBLEMS

The second test problem that we considered is much more complicated than the first one, since it concerns the simulation of an incompressible viscous flow around and inside a (two-dimensional) nozzle at high incidence (40 degrees), at Re = 750 (the characteristic length being the distance between the walls of the nozzle). We used the same kind of finite-element approximation as in section 7.1. Figures 7.4 and 7.5 show the details of the triangulations $\mathcal{C}_h$ and $\tilde{\mathcal{C}}_h$, respectively, close to the air intake. Figures 7.6 and 7.10 show the stream lines and the vortex pattern of the flow at t = 0, 0.2, 0.4, 0.6, 0.8, the initial velocity being associated to the corresponding steady Stokes flow, and a suction phenomenon being simulated inside the nozzle.

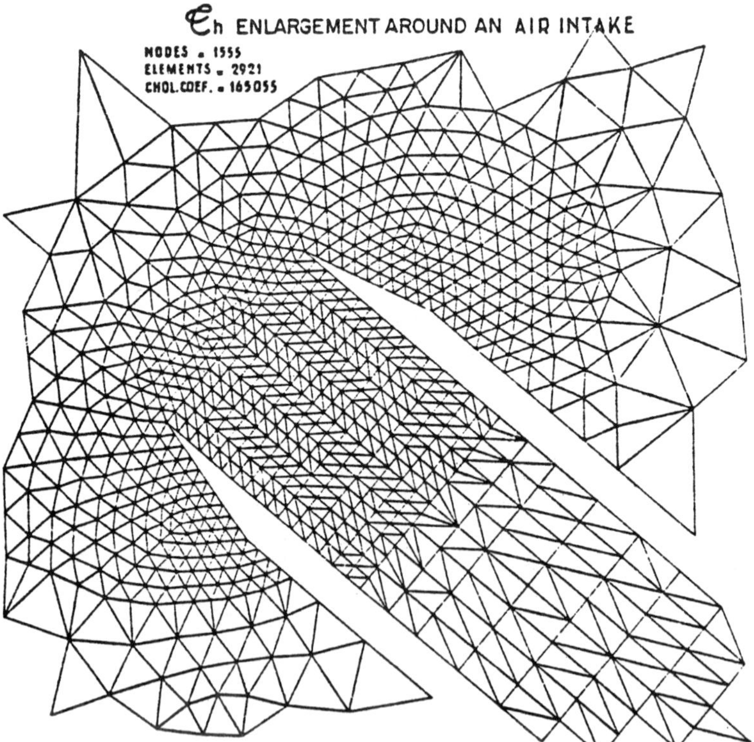

Fig. 7.4. Pressure grid

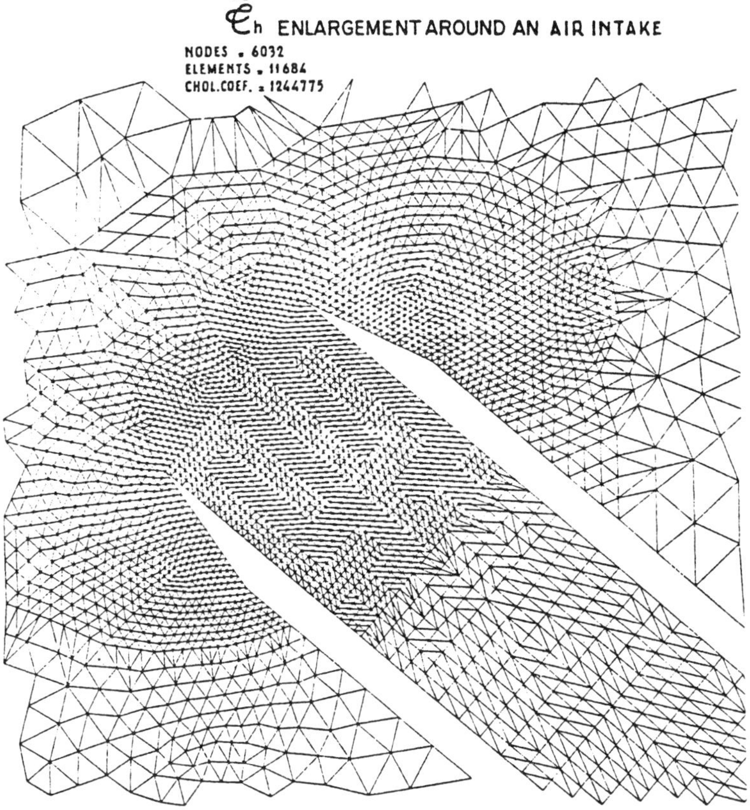

Fig. 7.5. Velocity grid

8. Conclusion

We have presented in this paper numerical methods for solving the time–dependent incompressible Navier–Stokes equations. One of the key ingredients to make the solution process faster and to minimize computer storage, was undoubtedly the use of operator–splitting methods in order to decouple the two main difficulties of the problem, namely the nonlinearity and the incompressibility. Other splitting methods for the incompressible Navier–Stokes equations are discussed in [37]–[40], [1], [17]. Another important reference for operator–splitting methods is [41].

Application of these splitting methods to nonlinear eigenvalue problems will be discussed in a forthcoming paper.

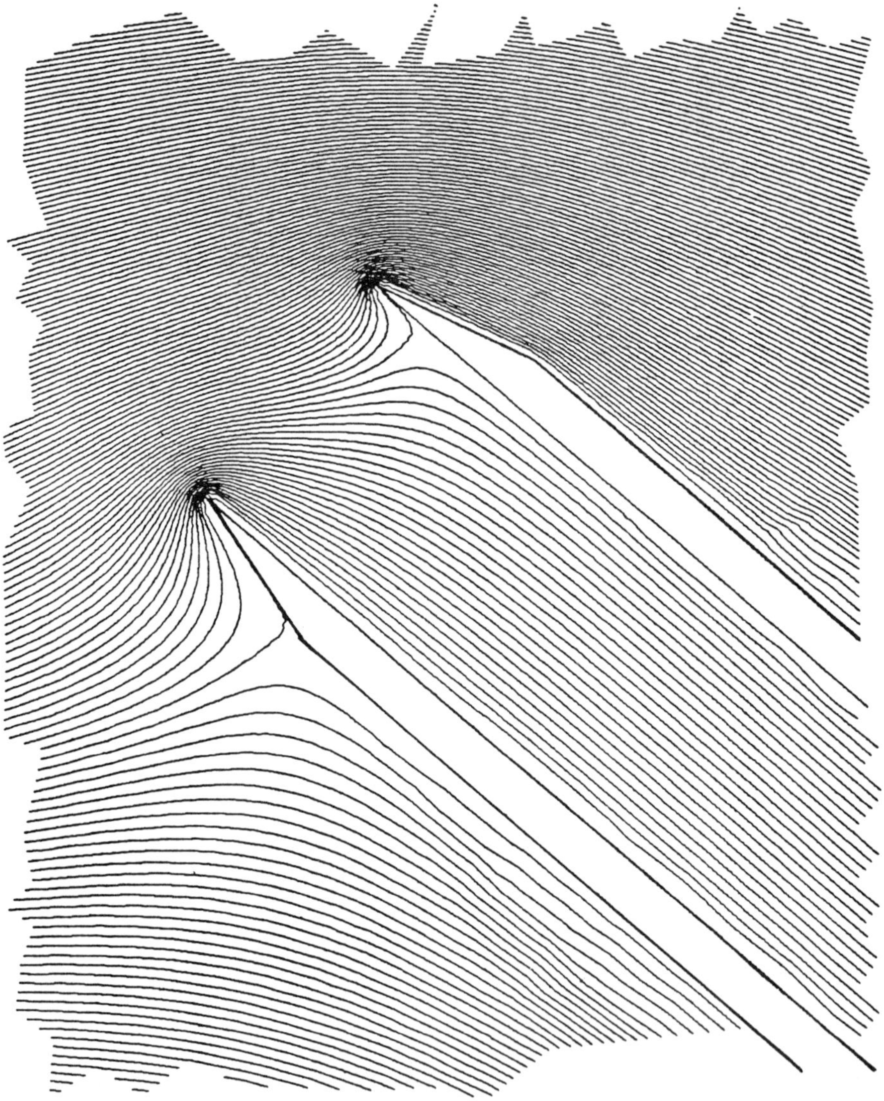

Fig. 7.6. Re = 750, $t = 0.0$

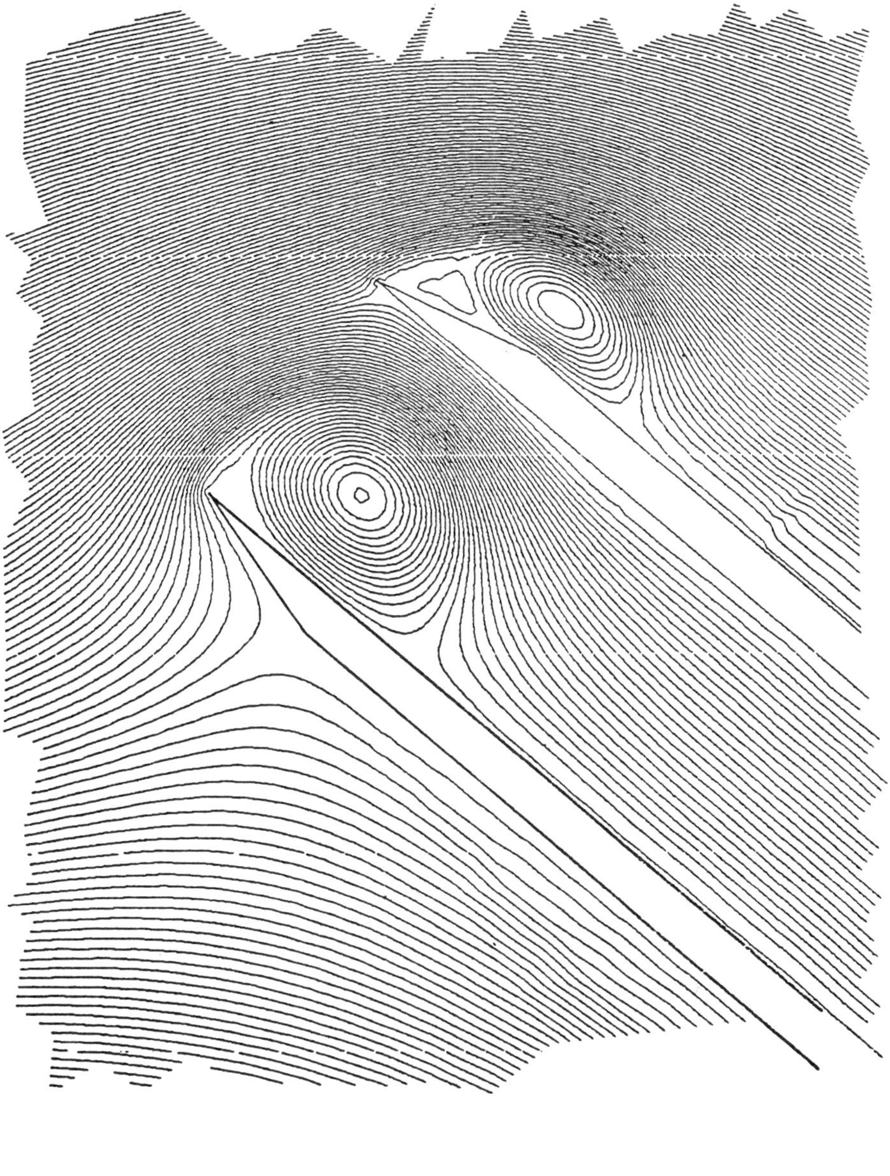

Fig. 7.7. Re = 750, $t = 0.2$

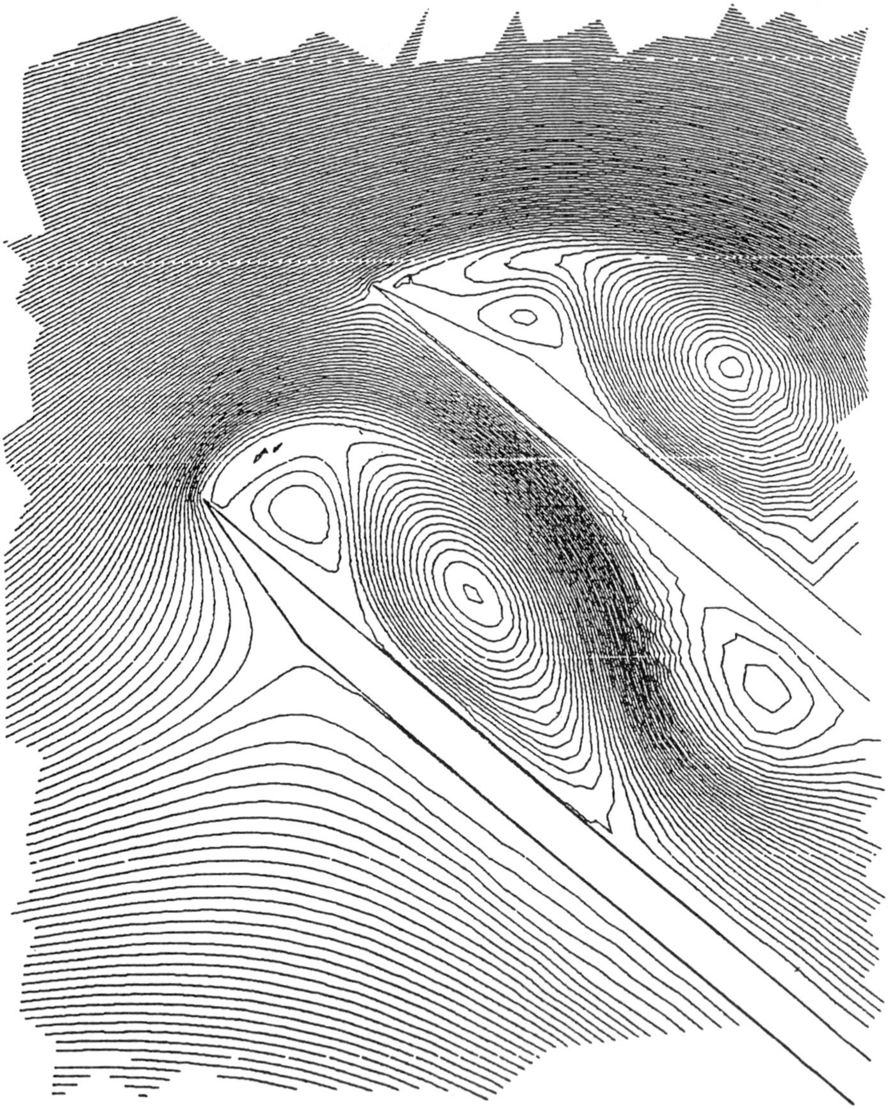

Fig. 7.8. Re = 750, t = 0.4

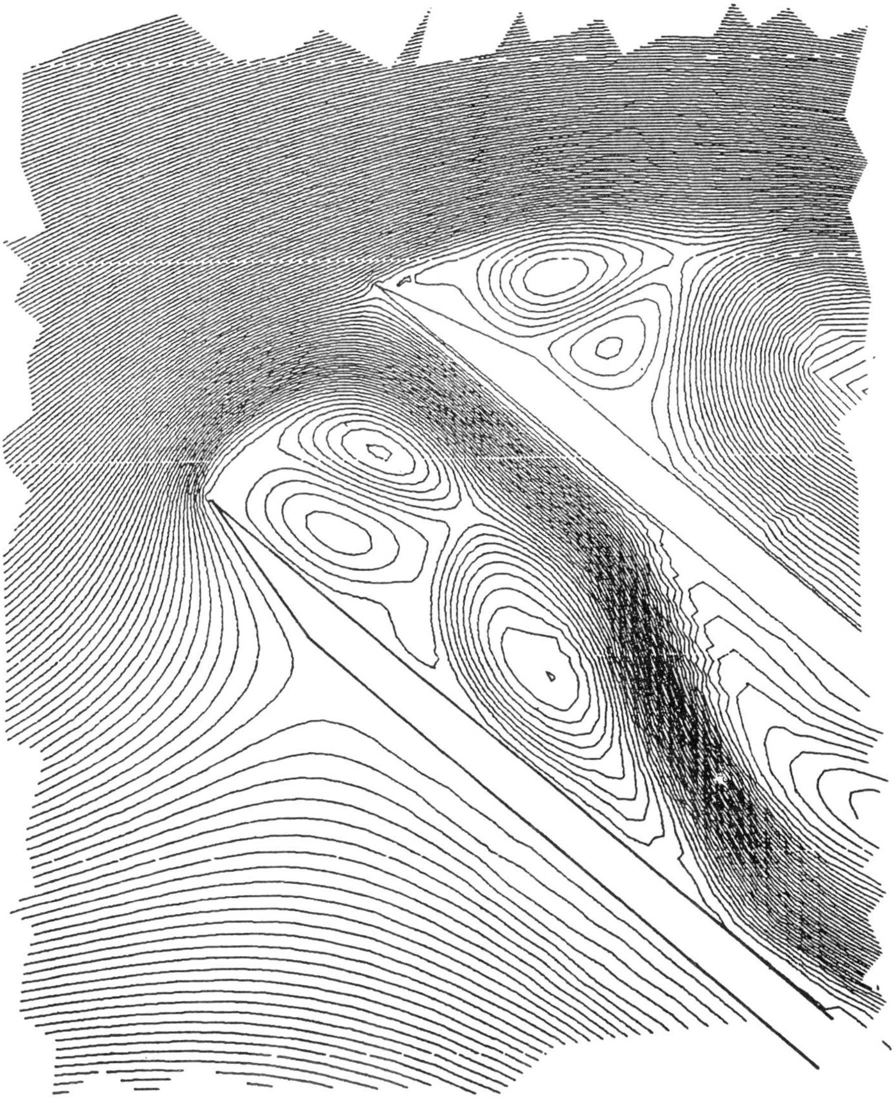

Fig. 7.9. Re = 750, $t = 0.6$

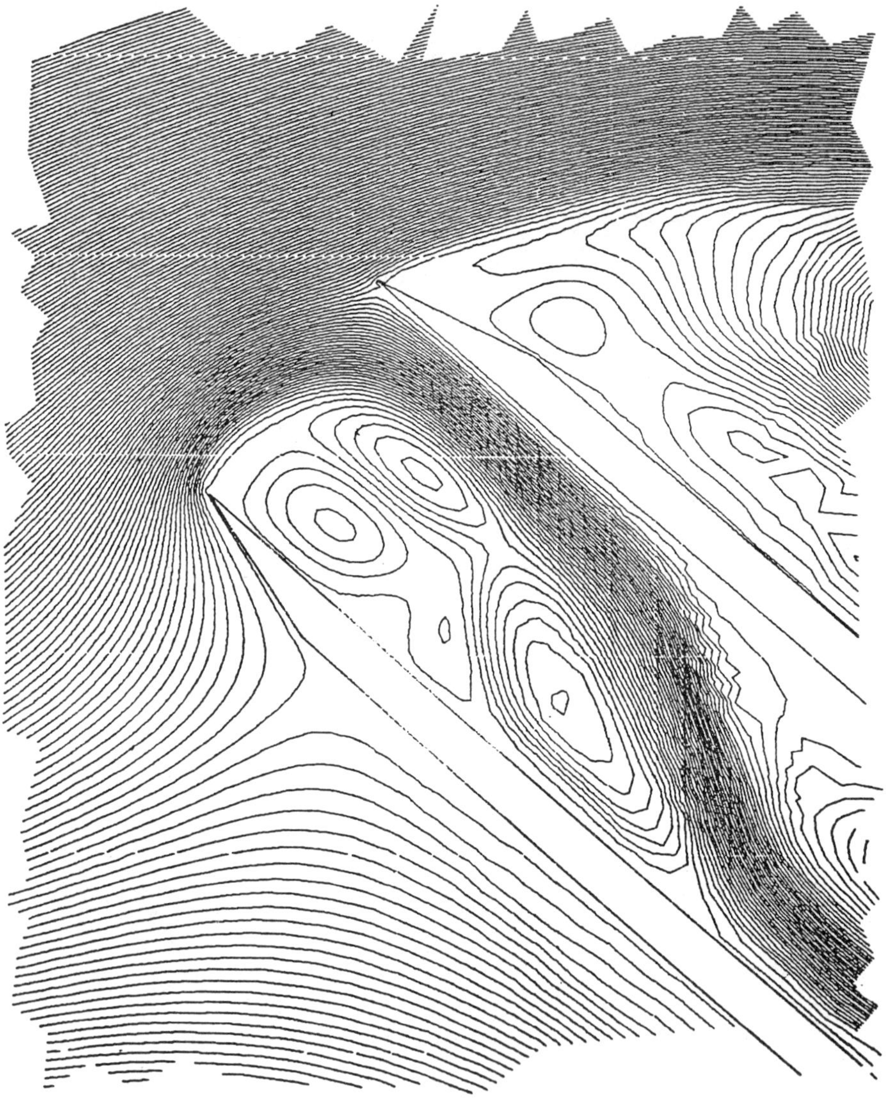

Fig. 7.10. Re = 750, t = 0.8

REFERENCES

[1] Temam, R. *Navier–Stokes Equations*. Amsterdam New York: North-Holland, 1977.
[2] Girault, V., and P.A. Raviart. *Finite-Element Approximation of Navier–Stokes Equations*. Lecture Notes in Mathematics 749. Berlin New York Heidelberg Tokyo: Springer–Verlag, 1979.
[3] Rautmann, R., ed. *Approximation Methods for Navier–Stokes Problems*. Lecture Notes in Mathematics 771. Berlin New York Heidelberg Tokyo: Springer–Verlag, 1981.
[4] Thomasset, F. *Implementation of Finite–Element Methods for Navier–Stokes Equations*. New York Berlin Heidelberg Tokyo: Springer–Verlag, 1981.
[5] Glowinski, R. *Numerical Methods for Nonlinear Variational Problems*. New York Berlin Heidelberg Tokyo: Springer–Verlag, 1984.
[6] Marchuk, G.I. *Methods of Numerical Mathematics*. New York Berlin Heidelberg Tokyo: Springer–Verlag, 1975.
[7] Fortin, M., and F. Thomasset. 1979. Mixed finite–element methods for incompressible flow problems. *J. Comput. Phys*. 310: 173–215.
[8] Glowinski, R., and O. Pironneau. 1979. Numerical methods for the first biharmonic equation and for the two–dimensional Stokes problem. *SIAM Review* 21:167–212.
[9] Reinhart, L. 1980. Sur la résolution numérique de problèmes aux limites nonlinéaires par des méthodes de continuation. Thèse de 3e cycle, Université Pierre et Marie Curie, Paris.
[10] Keller, H.B., and S. Schreiber. 1983. Spurious solutions in driven cavity calculations. *J. Comp. Phys*. 49:165–72.
[11] Glowinski, R., H.B. Keller, and L. Reinhart. 1985. Continuation–conjugate–gradient methods for the least squares solution of nonlinear boundary value problems. *SIAM J. Sci. Stat. Comp*. 6:793–832.
[12] Roache, P.J. 1972. *Computational fluid dynamics*. Albuquerque, NM: Hermosa Publ. Co.
[13] Lions, J.L. *Quelques méthodes de résolution des problèmes aux limites nonlinéaires*. Paris: Dunod, 1969.
[14] Ladyzhenskaia, O.A. *The Mathematical Theory of Viscous Incompressible Flow*. New York: Gordon and Breach, 1963.
[15] Tartar, L. *Topics in Nonlinear Analysis*. Publications Mathématiques d'Orsay, Université de Paris–Sud, Département de Mathématiques, Paris, 1978.
[16] Strang, S.G. 1968. On the construction and comparison of difference schemes. *SIAM J. Num. Anal*. 5:506–17.
[17] Beale, J.T., and A. Majda. 1981. Rates of convergence for viscous splitting of the Navier–Stokes equations. *Math. Comp*. 37:243–60.
[18] Leveque, R. 1982. *Time–split methods for partial differential equations*. Ph.D. diss., Computer Science Department, Stanford University.

[19] Leveque, R., and J. Oliger. 1981. Numerical methods based on additive splitting for hyperbolic partial differential equations. Manuscript NA–81–16, Numerical Analysis Project, Computer Science Department, Stanford University.

[20] Lions, J.L., and B. Mercier. 1979. Splitting algorithms for the sum of two nonlinear operators. *SIAM J. Num. Anal.* 16:964–79.

[21] Godlewsky, E. 1980. Méthodes à pas multiples et de directions alternées pour la discrétisation d'équations d'évolution. Thèse de 3e cycle, Université Pierre et Marie Curie, Paris.

[22] Glowinski, R., B. Mantel, and J. Periaux. Numerical solution of the time–dependent Navier–Stokes equations for incompressible viscous fluids, by finite element and alternating direction methods. In *Numerical Methods in Aeronautical Fluid Dynamics*, ed. P.L. Roe, 309–36. London: Academic Press, 1982.

[23] Parlett, B.N. *The Symmetric Eigenvalue Problem.* Englewood Cliffs, NJ: Prentice Hall, 1980.

[24] Loura, L.C. de. 1983. Résolution numérique de l'équation de Hartree. Thèse de 3e cycle, Université Pierre et Marie Curie, Paris.

[25] Glowinski, R., and P. Le Tallec. *Augmented Lagrangian methods in nonlinear mechanics*. Forthcoming.

[26] Polak, E. *Computational Methods in Optimization.* New York: Academic Press, 1971.

[27] Glowinski, R., B. Mantel, J. Periaux, P. Perrier, and O. Pironneau. On an efficient new preconditioned conjugate–gradient method. Application to the incore solution of the Navier–Stokes equations. In *Finite Elements in Fluids*, ed. R.H. Gallagher, D.H. Norrie, J.T. Oden, and O.C. Zienkiewicz, vol. 4, 365–401. London New York: John Wiley & Sons Publ. Co., 1982.

[28] Birkhoff, G., and A. Schoenstadt. *Elliptic Problem Solvers*, vol. 2. New York: Academic Press, 1984.

[29] Shanno, D.F. 1978. Conjugate–gradient method with inexact line search. *Math. Oper. Research* 13:244–55.

[30] Buckley, A., and A. Lenir. 1983. QN–like variable storage conjugate gradients. *Math. Programming* 27:155–80.

[31] Bristeau, M.O., R. Glowinski, J. Periaux, P. Perrier, O. Pironneau, and G. Poirier. Application of optimal control and finite–element methods to the calculation of transonic flows and incompressible viscous flows. In *Numerical Methods in Applied Fluid Dynamics*, ed. B. Hunt, 203–312. London: Academic Press, 1980.

[32] Bristeau, M.O., R. Glowinski, B. Mantel, J. Periaux, P. Perrier, and O. Pironneau. A finite–element approximation of Navier–Stokes equations for incompressible viscous fluids. Iterative methods of solution. In *Approximation Methods for Navier–Stokes Problems*, ed. R. Rautmann, 78–128. Lecture Notes in Mathematics 771. Berlin New York Heidelberg Tokyo: Springer–Verlag, 1980.

[33] Hood, P., and C. Taylor. 1973. A numerical solution of the Navier–Stokes equations using the finite–element technique. *Comput. Fluids*, 73–100.

[34] Morgan, K., J. Periaux, and F. Thomasset, eds. *Numerical Analysis of Laminar Flow Over a Step*. GAAM Workshop, Bievres, France, January 1983. Braunschweig–Weisbaden: Vieweg–Verlag, 1983.

[35] Arnold, D.N., F. Brezzi, and M. Fortin. 1983. A stable finite–element for the Stokes equations. Report 362, Istituto di Analisi Numerica del CNR, Pavia, Italy.

[36] Hutton, A.G. 1975. A general finite–element method for vorticity and stream function applied to a laminar separated flow. Central Electricity–Generating Board Report, Research Department, Berkeley Nuclear Lab., U.K.

[37] Chorin, A.J. 1967. A numerical method for solving incompressible viscous flow problems. *J. Comput. Phys.* 2:12–26.

[38] ————. 1968. Numerical solution of incompressible flow problems. In *Studies in Numerical Analysis*, 2; *Numerical Solution of Nonlinear Problems*, 64–71. The SIAM Symposium, Philadelphia. SIAM, PA, 1970.

[39] ————. 1968. On the convergence and approximation of discrete aprroximations to the Navier–Stokes equations. *Math. Comp.* 23:341–53.

[40] ————. 1973. Numerical study of slightly viscous flows. *J. Fluid Mech.* 57:785–96.

[41] Yanenko, N.N. *The Method of Fractional Steps*. New York Berlin Heidelberg Tokyo: Springer–Verlag, 1971.

ITERATIVE METHODS IN SUBSPACES FOR EIGENVALUE PROBLEMS

Yurij A. Kuznetsov
Department of Numerical Mathematics
The USSR Academy of Sciences
Moscow, USSR

Introduction

During the last 10 to 15 years iterative methods in subspaces for solving linear algebraic systems have been greatly improved [7], [8], [9], [10], [12]. Among them, the most effective methods are based on the notions of the fictitious–component method [11] and the domain–decomposition method [3], [5], [7]. In this paper, methods in subspaces are used for the computation of the minimal eigenvalue for a generalized eigenvalue problem. These methods have been described for the first time in [6], where they have been used for solving spectral problems in transport theory. In [2] and [9], the methods for spectral problems for the Laplacian, using domain decomposition, have been discussed.

1. A simple example of the domain decomposition method

Let us consider the spectral problem

$$\begin{aligned} -\Delta u &= \lambda u \quad \text{in } \Omega , \\ u &= 0 \quad \text{on } \partial\Omega , \end{aligned} \tag{1}$$

where Δ is a two–dimensional Laplacian in the simplest domain Ω shown in figure 1. Let us construct in Ω a square mesh with step $h = 1/2(n+1)$, where n is some positive integer and next approximate (1), using an ordinary five–point difference scheme. As a result, we obtain an algebraic eigenvalue problem

$$\mathbf{A}\mathbf{u} = \lambda \mathbf{u} \tag{2}$$

with a symmetric positive definite $N \times N$ matrix $\mathbf{A}$, where $N = (2n+1)^2 - (n+1)^2$. We wish to find the minimal eigenvalue $\lambda_1 = 1/\rho(\mathbf{A}^{-1})$; here ρ is the spectral radius. This problem can be equivalently formulated as follows: find a maximal λ_1 such that the matrix

$$\mathbf{A}_\lambda = \mathbf{A} - \lambda \mathbf{I} \tag{3}$$

is positive definite for any $\lambda < \lambda_1$, i.e., find λ_1 so that $\det \mathbf{A}_{\lambda_1} = 0$ and $\mathbf{A}_\lambda > 0$ for every $\lambda < \lambda_1$. Here and in the sequel $\mathbf{I}$ will denote a unit matrix.

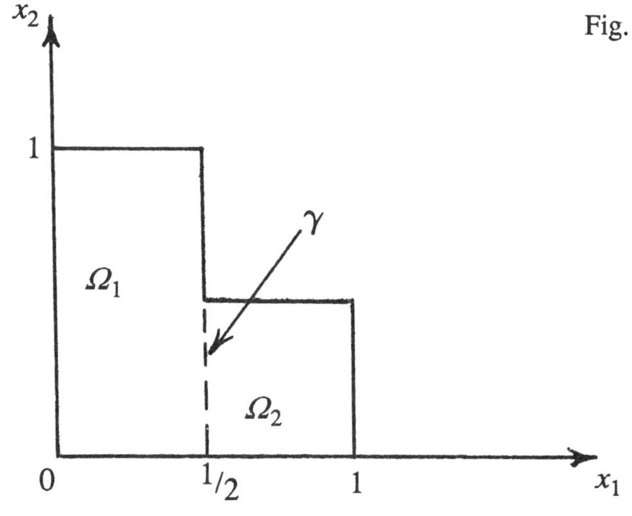

Fig. 1

To solve the problem (3) let us use the bisection method. We suppose that for any given integer $k \geq 1$ the boundaries a_{k-1}, b_{k-1} $(0 \leq a_{k-1} < b_{k-1})$ of an interval $(a_{k-1}, b_{k-1}]$, which contain the minimal eigenvalue λ_1 (which is to be found), are known and that $\lambda^{(k)} = (a_{k-1} + b_{k-1})/2$. Then the kth step of the bisection method is realized as follows:

$$\begin{cases} \text{if } \mathbf{A}_{\lambda^{(k)}} > 0, \text{ then set } a_k = \lambda^{(k)},\ b_k = b_{k-1} \\ \quad \text{or otherwise } a_k = a_{k-1},\ b_k = \lambda^{(k)}\ . \end{cases} \tag{4}$$

It is obvious that

$$|\lambda_1 - \lambda^{(k)}| \leq (b_0 - a_0)/2^k\ . \tag{5}$$

Thus the implementation of the bisection method gives rise to two main questions: 1) how to choose initial boundaries of the interval and 2) how to determine whether the matrix $\mathbf{A}$ is positive definite for a given λ.

The answer to the first question is to put $a_0 = 0$ and $b_0 = \|\mathbf{A}\|_*$ for any given matrix norm $\|\cdot\|_*$, in particular for $\|\cdot\|_* = \|\cdot\|_\infty$. As we proceed, we will give some other ways to choose b_0. The answer to the second question will be given by the iterative method which is an inner iterative process with respect to (4).

According to figure 1, $\Omega = \Omega_1 \cup \gamma \cup \Omega_2$, where Ω_1 and Ω_2 are rectangular nonintersecting subdomains of Ω and $\gamma = (\overline{\Omega}_1 \cap \overline{\Omega}_2) \backslash \partial\Omega$. We divide the inner mesh points into three groups: the first group includes the mesh points of Ω_1, the second group includes those of Ω_2 and the third contains all the remaining mesh points which belong to γ. We equip all of the vectors and matrices associated with the points of the third group with an index on γ. Now the matrix $\mathbf{A}$ can be written in the block form corresponding to the groups of the mesh points:

$$\mathbf{A} = \begin{bmatrix} \mathbf{A}_1 & 0 & -\mathbf{A}_{1\gamma} \\ 0 & \mathbf{A}_2 & -\mathbf{A}_{2\gamma} \\ -\mathbf{A}_{\gamma 1} & -\mathbf{A}_{\gamma 2} & \mathbf{A}_\gamma \end{bmatrix}, \tag{6}$$

where $N_i \times N_i$ matrices $\mathbf{A}_i$ correspond to the difference Laplacian for subdomains Ω_i with the Dirichlet boundary conditions on $\partial\Omega_i$, i=1,2 and $\mathbf{A}_\gamma$ is a tridiagonal $n \times n$–matrix ($N = N_1 + N_2 + n$).

Let us introduce the matrices

$$\mathbf{B} = \begin{bmatrix} \mathbf{A}_1 & 0 & -\mathbf{A}_{1\gamma} \\ 0 & \mathbf{A}_2 & -\mathbf{A}_{2\gamma} \\ 0 & 0 & \mathbf{A}_\gamma \end{bmatrix}, \quad \mathbf{C} = \mathbf{B} - \mathbf{A} = \begin{bmatrix} 0 & 0 & 0 \\ 0 & 0 & 0 \\ \mathbf{A}_{1\gamma} & \mathbf{A}_{2\gamma} & 0 \end{bmatrix}, \tag{7}$$

$\mathbf{B}_\lambda = \mathbf{B} - \lambda\mathbf{I}$ and $\mathbf{T} = \mathbf{B}_\lambda^{-1}\mathbf{C}$. Now let d be the minimal eigenvalue of the matrix $\mathbf{B}$; in our case d is the minimal eigenvalue of the matrix $\mathbf{A}_1$ and can be computed using the explicit expression. Obviously, $\lambda_1 < d$. Then, Lemma 1 follows from the Ostrowski–Reich theorem [16].

Lemma 1. *For any* $\lambda \in (0,d)$ *the matrix* $\mathbf{A}_\lambda$ *is positive definite iff* $\rho(\mathbf{T}_\lambda) < 1$.

Throughout the remainder of this section we assume that $\lambda \in (0,d)$. Then, to find out whether $\mathbf{A}_\lambda$ is positive definite, it suffices, according to Lemma 1, to compute $\rho(\mathbf{T}_\lambda)$ with some accuracy. It is easy to see that

$$\rho(\mathbf{T}_\lambda) = \rho(\mathbf{B}_\lambda \mathbf{T}_\lambda \mathbf{B}_\lambda^{-1}) = \rho(\mathbf{Q}_\lambda), \tag{8}$$

where the matrix

$$\mathbf{Q}_\lambda = [\sum_{i=1}^{2} \mathbf{A}_{\gamma i}(\mathbf{A}_i - \lambda\mathbf{I}_i)^{-1}\mathbf{A}_{i\gamma}](\mathbf{A}_\gamma - \lambda\mathbf{I}_\gamma)^{-1} \tag{9}$$

is similar to the symmetric positive definite matrix

$$\mathbf{S}_\lambda = (\mathbf{A}_\gamma - \lambda \mathbf{I}_\gamma)^{-1/2}\, \mathbf{Q}_\lambda (\mathbf{A}_\gamma - \lambda \mathbf{I}_\gamma)^{-1/2} \tag{10}$$

with positive elements (here we have used the condition $\lambda \in (0,d)$). In particular, all the eigenvalues of the matrix $\mathbf{Q}_\lambda$ are real and positive and the matrix $\mathbf{Q}_\lambda$ possesses the complete system of the $\mathbf{R}_\lambda \equiv (\mathbf{A}_\gamma - \lambda \mathbf{I}_\gamma)^{-1}$ orthonormal eigenvectors. Moreover, it follows from the Perron–Frobenius theorem [16] that the maximal eigenvalue $\rho(\mathbf{Q}_\lambda)$ of the matrix $\mathbf{Q}_\lambda$ is a monotonically increasing function of λ and for any $\lambda \in (0,d)$ a positive eigenvector corresponds to it.

Let a nonzero, nonnegative vector $\mathbf{v}^0 \in \mathbf{E}^n$ be given with $\|\mathbf{v}^0\|_{\mathbf{R}_\lambda} = 1$, where $\mathbf{E}^n$ is the space of real n–dimensional vectors equipped with usual scalar product $(\cdot,\cdot)$ and norm $\|\cdot\| = (\cdot,\cdot)^{1/2}$.

Since the matrix $\mathbf{Q}_\lambda$ is $\mathbf{R}_\lambda$–self–adjoint and $\mathbf{R}_\lambda$–positive definite in $\mathbf{E}^n$, i.e., it possesses the foregoing properties in the sense of scalar product induced by the matrix $\mathbf{R}_\lambda = \mathbf{R}_\lambda^T > 0$, one can use the standard power method to compute $\rho(\mathbf{Q}_\lambda)$:

$$\psi^\ell = \mathbf{Q}_\lambda v^{\ell-1}, \mu^\ell = (\psi^\ell, v^{\ell-1})_{\mathbf{R}_\lambda}, v^\ell = \frac{\psi^\ell}{\|\psi^\ell\|}, \ell = 1,2,... \tag{11}$$

or the generalized minimized iterative method of Lanczos [12]:

$$\begin{gathered} v^\ell = \mathbf{Q}_\lambda v^{\ell-1} - \alpha_\ell v^{\ell-1} - \beta_\ell v^{\ell-2}, \\ \alpha_\ell = \frac{(\mathbf{Q}_\lambda v^{\ell-1}, v^{\ell-1})_{\mathbf{R}_\lambda}}{\|v^{\ell-1}\|^2_{\mathbf{R}_\lambda}}, \ \beta_\ell = \frac{\|v^{\ell-1}\|^2_{\mathbf{R}_\lambda}}{\|v^{\ell-2}\|^2_{\mathbf{R}_\lambda}}, \ \ell = 1,2,... \end{gathered} \tag{12}$$

(with $v^{-1} = 0$ and $\beta_1 = 0$), where $\mu^{(\ell)}$ is chosen equal to the maximal eigenvalue of the Jacobi matrix

$$\begin{bmatrix} \alpha_1 & 1 & & 0 \\ \beta_2 & \ddots & \ddots & \\ & \ddots & \ddots & 1 \\ 0 & & \beta_\ell & \alpha_\ell \end{bmatrix} \tag{13}$$

In both cases $\mu^{(\ell)} \leq \rho(\mathbf{Q}_\lambda)$ and $\mu^{(\ell)}$ tend to $\rho(\mathbf{Q}_\lambda)$, monotonically increasing with the growth of κ. Of course we can use some other methods to compute $\rho(\mathbf{Q}_\lambda)$, for example the method of the subspace iterations [15]. It is important to note that if for any $\ell \geq 1$ we obtain $\mu^{(\ell)}$ 1, then the corresponding process (11) or (12) can be stopped, since it corresponds to the case $\lambda > \lambda_1$, i.e., the matrix $\mathbf{A}_\lambda$ is not positive definite for given λ. It means for the values $\lambda > \lambda_1$ we may not compute $\rho(\mathbf{Q}_\lambda)$ using the bisection method (4) as the outer iterative process, but we have only to ob–

tain the inequality $\mu^{(\ell)} > 1$ for some $\ell \geq 1$. Thus the above-mentioned method includes outer and inner iterative processes. The outer iterative process is the bisection method (4) with the initial interval boundaries $a_0 = 0$ and $b_0 = d$. The computation of λ_1 with the accuracy $\varepsilon > 0$ requires $k_\varepsilon = 0(\ln 1/\varepsilon)$ steps. The minimized iterative method [12] will be used as the inner iterative process which requires in this case $n = 0(h^{-1})$ steps. In practice, the number of steps in the inner process can be considerably less than n. The multiplication of the vector v by the matrix $\mathbf{R}_\lambda$ means the solution of a linear system with the matrix $\mathbf{R}_\lambda^{-1} = \mathbf{A}_\gamma - \lambda \mathbf{I}_\gamma$ with $o(h^{-1})$ arithmetic operations. The most expensive procedure with respect to the number of operations of the methods (4) and (12) is to find the vector

$$\mathbf{w} = \sum_{i=1}^{2} \mathbf{A}_{\gamma i}(\mathbf{A}_i - \lambda \mathbf{I}_i)^{-1} \mathbf{A}_{i\gamma}\mathbf{v} \tag{14}$$

for a given vector $\mathbf{v} \in \mathbf{E}^n$. During the computation this procedure is not repeated more than $0(h^{-1} \ln 1/\varepsilon)$ times. All the other computations require at one step of the inner iterative process only $0(h^{-1})$ arithmetic operations. Let us describe a method for the solution of the problem (14) which requires only $0(h^{-1} \ln 1/h)$ arithmetic operations with a simultaneous use of only $0(h^{-1})$ memory locations.

Let a vector $\mathbf{v} \in \mathbf{E}^n$ be given and a vector

$$\mathbf{w}^{(1)} = \mathbf{A}_{\gamma 1}(\mathbf{A}_1 - \lambda \mathbf{I}_1)^{-1} \mathbf{A}_{1\gamma}\mathbf{v} \tag{15}$$

is to be found. Let us consider a linear system

$$(\mathbf{A}_1 - \lambda \mathbf{I}_1)\mathbf{z}^{(1)} = \mathbf{A}_{1\gamma}\mathbf{v} \tag{16}$$

with symmetric positive definite $N_1 \times N_1$-matrix $\mathbf{A}_1 - \lambda \mathbf{I}_1$. This algebraic system is the difference Laplace equation in the rectangular domain Ω_1 with nonhomogeneous Dirichlet boundary conditions on the right side of Ω_1 and with homogeneous Dirichlet boundary conditions on the other sides. The most important thing for us in this problem is that for computing the vector $\mathbf{w}^{(1)}$ from (15) we have to use only those components of the vector $\mathbf{z}^{(1)}$ which correspond to the nonzero columns of the matrix $\mathbf{A}_{\gamma 1}$. But the nonzero columns of the matrix $\mathbf{A}_{\gamma 1}$ correspond to the nodes (not all) of Ω_1 which are not more than one grid step h away from the right side of Ω_1, i.e., they correspond to the adjacent nodes. That is why it is sufficient to find only $2n+1$ components of the vector $\mathbf{z}^{(1)}$ from (16) which correspond to the aforementioned mesh points. The formulated problem has been called "the partial problem." The methods for solving it for systems with matrices which allow the use of the method of separation of variables have been studied in [1], [5], [8]. In particular, the method suggested in [5] allows us to solve the partial problem at the expense of $0(h^{-1} \ln 1/h)$ arithmetic operations. This algorithm uses the fast Fourier transform in the variable x_2 (see figure 1) and some special formulas for solving partial problems for the systems with tridiagonal matrices. It should be noted that the realization of this algorithm requires using only $0(h^{-1})$ memory locations. The problem of finding the vector $\mathbf{w}^{(2)} = \mathbf{A}_{\gamma 2}(\mathbf{A}_2 - \lambda \mathbf{I}_2)^{-1}\mathbf{A}_{2\gamma}\mathbf{v}$ can be solved in a similar way.

Thus we have proved the following theorem.

Theorem 1. *The computation of the minimal eigenvalue* λ_1 *of the matrix* **A** *from* (2) *by the aforementioned variant of the domain decomposition method* (4), (12) *requires not more than* $0(h^{-2}(\ln 1/h)^2)$ *arithmetical operations with the simultaneous use of only a finite number of vectors of dimension* $0(h^{-1})$.

The second proposition of the theorem seems to be more interesting since there are methods involving fewer arithmetic operations. It is worth noting that to obtain this estimation we do not use estimations of the rate of convergence of the method (12) (used as the iterative process), which strongly influences the final result.

The bisection method is a simple but not very effective outer iterative process. In our case, it may be replaced by a more effective method if the following fact is used.

Lemma 2. *The function*

$$\mu(\lambda) = \rho(\mathbf{Q}_\lambda) \tag{17}$$

is continuous and monotonically increasing in the interval $(0,d)$.

The proof of this lemma uses the Peron–Frobenius theorem as well as the properties of blocks of the matrix **A**. It follows from Lemma 2 that the problem of finding λ_1 is equivalent to the problem of finding in the interval $(0,d)$ the unique root of the equation

$$\mu(\lambda) = 1 \tag{18}$$

with the implicit function μ (as in figure 2). To solve (18) one can use a large number of methods, in particular the secant method. In methods for solving equation (18) the rate of convergence is greater than in the method (4). Still, we must take into account the following facts: first, the values of the function μ must be computed by means of the method (12) with higher accuracy than in the bisection method; second, we have according to [5] that $\mu(0) \sim 1-ch$, where c is a positive constant not depending on h, and that leads to a decrease of the rate of convergence of the iterative methods for the solution of (18) as $h \to 0$.

We can formulate the method (12) in a different way if we view it as a computational process in a subspace of $\mathbf{E}^N$; this will serve as a base for our study of more general methods in the subsequent sections and will make them more obvious and clear to the reader.

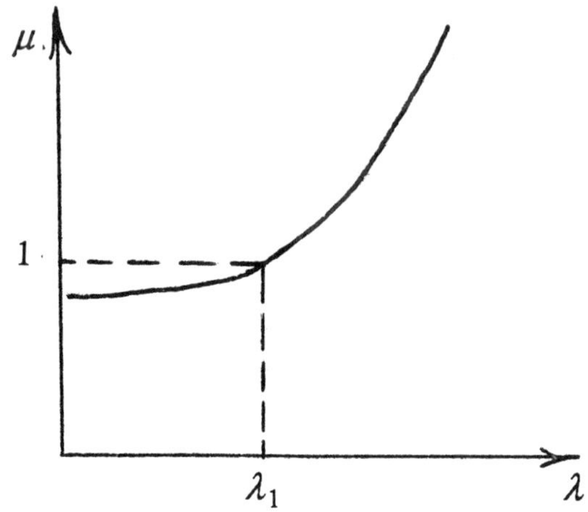

Fig. 2

Thus, the spectral radius of the matrix $B_\lambda^{-1}C$ or, equivalently, of the matrix CB_λ^{-1} is to be found. Let us introduce the subspace $U = \text{Im}C$, the image of the matrix C, which is invariant with respect to the matrix CB_λ^{-1}. It is easy to see that the matrix $R_\lambda = B_\lambda^{-1}$ is self–adjoint and positive definite in the subspace U, i.e., $(R_\lambda\xi,\eta) = (\xi,R_\lambda\eta)$ for all $\xi, \eta \in U$, and $(R_\lambda\xi,\xi) > 0$ for every nonzero $\xi \in U$. Then one can introduce in U the scalar product $(\cdot,\cdot)_{R_\lambda}$ induced by the matrix R_λ and the corresponding norm $\|\cdot\|_{R_\lambda}$. Again, it is easy to see that the matrix $B_\lambda^{-1}CB_\lambda^{-1}$ is self–adjoint and positive definite in the subspace U or, equivalently, the matrix CB_λ^{-1} is R_λ–self–adjoint and R_λ–positive definite in this subspace.

The above implies that the generalized minimal iterations method of Lanczos can be used in the subspace U for computing $\rho(CB_\lambda^{-1})$:

$$\begin{gathered} \xi^\ell = CB_\lambda^{-1}\xi^{\ell-1} - \alpha_\ell\xi^{\ell-1} - \beta_\ell\xi^{\ell-2}, \\ \alpha_\ell = \frac{(CB_\lambda^{-1}\xi^{\ell-1},\ B_\lambda^{-1}\xi^{\ell-1})}{\|\xi^{\ell-1}\|_{R_\lambda}^2}, \quad \beta_\ell = \frac{\|\xi^{\ell-1}\|_{R_\lambda}^2}{\|\xi^{\ell-2}\|_{R_\lambda}^2} \end{gathered} \tag{19}$$

and that allows us, for any nonzero nonnegative vector $\xi^0 \in U$, to compute the maximal eigenvalue of the matrix (13) for the corresponding ℓ with at most n steps ($\ell \le \dim U = n$).

Let us represent the vectors ξ^ℓ of the method (19) in the form $\xi^\ell = \begin{bmatrix} 0 \\ v_\ell \end{bmatrix}$ where $v^\ell \in E^n$. One can see that the methods (12) and (19) completely coin–cide when the initial vectors v^0 are the same, i.e., the corresponding vectors and the coefficients α_ℓ and β_ℓ coincide. This proves the equiva–lence of both formulations of the given variant of the domain–decomposition method.

Let us now consider diagonal matrices $\mathbf{P}_1$ and $\mathbf{P}_2$ with zeros and ones in the diagonals. Let the diagonal element of $\mathbf{P}_1$ be unity if the corresponding component of any vector $\xi \in \mathbf{U}$ is nonzero and let it be zero otherwise. Obviously,

$$\mathbf{P}_1 = \begin{bmatrix} 0 & 0 \\ 0 & \mathbf{I}_\gamma \end{bmatrix}, \tag{20}$$

where $\mathbf{I}_\gamma$ is a unit $n\times n$–matrix. On the other hand, let the diagonal element of $\mathbf{P}_2$ be unity if in the corresponding column of matrix $\mathbf{C}$ there is at least one nonzero element; let it be zero otherwise. The constructed matrices $\mathbf{P}_1$ and $\mathbf{P}_2$ have the following property: $\mathbf{Cw} = \mathbf{CP}_2\mathbf{w}$ for any $\mathbf{w} \in \mathbf{E}^n$ and for all $\mathbf{w} \in \mathbf{E}^n$ and $\xi \in \mathbf{U}$ the equality $(\mathbf{w},\xi) = (\mathbf{P}_1\mathbf{w},\xi)$ holds. Taking into account the previous remarks, the formulas for the coefficients α_ℓ and β_ℓ from (19) can be rewritten as

$$\alpha_\ell = \frac{(\mathbf{CP}_2\mathbf{B}_\lambda^{-1}\xi^{\ell-1}, \mathbf{P}_1\mathbf{B}_\lambda^{-1}\xi^{\ell-1})}{(\xi^{\ell-1}, \mathbf{P}_1\mathbf{B}_\lambda^{-1}\xi^{\ell-1})},$$

$$\beta_\ell = \frac{(\xi^{\ell-1}, \mathbf{P}_1\mathbf{B}_\lambda^{-1}\xi^{\ell-1})}{(\xi^{\ell-2}, \mathbf{P}_1\mathbf{B}_\lambda^{-1}\xi^{\ell-2})}. \tag{21}$$

Hence it follows at once that, as in (12), the scalar products can be computed at the expense of only $0(h^{-1})$ arithmetic operations. Moreover, one does not need to know all the vectors $\mathbf{B}_\lambda^{-1}\xi^{\ell-1}$ but only those components of vectors $\mathbf{P}_1\mathbf{B}_\lambda^{-1}\xi^{\ell-1}$ and $\mathbf{P}_2\mathbf{B}_\lambda^{-1}\xi^{\ell-1}$ which correspond to the nonzero diagonal elements of $\mathbf{P}_1$ and $\mathbf{P}_2$. That leads to two partial problems for the system

$$\mathbf{B}_\lambda \mathbf{z}^\ell = \xi^{\ell-1}; \tag{22}$$

namely, to the problems of finding the projections $\mathbf{P}_1\mathbf{z}^\ell$ and $\mathbf{P}_2\mathbf{z}^\ell$ on the solution $\mathbf{z}^\ell$ of this system. Such partial problems have been discussed above. They can be solved via the method [5] at the expense of $0(h^{-1}\ln 1/h)$ arithmetic operations.

2. Block–relaxation methods

Let us consider a generalized eigenvalue problem

$$\mathbf{Au} = \lambda\mathbf{Su} \tag{23}$$

with symmetric positive definite N×N–matrices $\mathbf{A}$ and $\mathbf{S}$.

We have to find the minimal eigenvalue λ_1 of the problem (23), which can be formulated equivalently as: find the maximal λ_1 such that the matrix

$$\mathbf{A}_\lambda = \mathbf{A} - \lambda \mathbf{S} \tag{24}$$

would be positive definite for any $\lambda < \lambda_1$.

To solve this problem we apply the two-stage iterative method which uses (as the outer iterative process) the bisection method (4).

Let the matrices **A** and **S** be represented in the following block form:

$$\mathbf{A} = \begin{bmatrix} \mathbf{A}_{1\,1} & \cdots & \mathbf{A}_{1\,m} \\ \vdots & & \vdots \\ \mathbf{A}_{m\,1} & \cdots & \mathbf{A}_{m\,m} \end{bmatrix}, \quad \mathbf{S} = \begin{bmatrix} \mathbf{S}_{1\,1} & \cdots & \mathbf{S}_{1\,m} \\ \vdots & & \vdots \\ \mathbf{S}_{m\,1} & \cdots & \mathbf{S}_{m\,m} \end{bmatrix}, \tag{25}$$

where m is a positive integer with the square blocks $\mathbf{A}_{ii}$, $\mathbf{S}_{ii}$, $i = 1,\dots,m$ of the same dimension.

Then the matrix $\mathbf{A}_\lambda$ also has the block representation

$$\mathbf{A}_\lambda = \begin{bmatrix} \mathbf{A}_{1\,1}-\lambda\mathbf{S}_{1\,1} & \cdots & \mathbf{A}_{1\,m}-\lambda\mathbf{S}_{1\,m} \\ \vdots & & \vdots \\ \mathbf{A}_{m\,1}-\lambda\mathbf{S}_{m\,1} & \cdots & \mathbf{A}_{m\,m}-\lambda\mathbf{S}_{m\,m} \end{bmatrix}. \tag{26}$$

Let us introduce a block diagonal matrix

$$\mathring{\mathbf{B}}_\lambda = (\mathbf{A}_{11} - \lambda\mathbf{S}_{11}) \oplus \cdots \oplus (\mathbf{A}_{m\,m} - \lambda\mathbf{S}_{m\,m}) \tag{27}$$

and a quantity

$$d = \min_{1 \le i \le m} 1/\rho(\mathbf{A}_{ii}^{-1}\mathbf{S}_{ii}) . \tag{28}$$

It follows from the properties of the Rayleigh quotient for the problem (23) that $\lambda_1 \le d$. We set $a_0 = 0$ and $b_0 = d$ for the bisection method, and hence in the sequel we assume that $\lambda \in (0,d)$.

It is obvious that for any $\lambda < d$ the matrix $\mathring{\mathbf{B}}_\lambda$ is positive definite. It follows that all the eigenvalues of the matrix $\mathring{\mathbf{B}}_\lambda^{-1}\mathbf{A}_\lambda$ (when λ is fixed) are real and the matrix has the complete system of eigenvectors, and all the eigenvalues of this matrix will be positive if and only if $\lambda < \lambda_1$ (therefore we assume that $\lambda \in (0,d)$). Hence, for a generalized eigenvalue problem

$$\mathring{\mathbf{C}}_\lambda \mathbf{w} = \mu \mathring{\mathbf{B}}_\lambda \mathbf{w} , \tag{29}$$

where $\mathring{\mathbf{C}}_\lambda = \mathring{\mathbf{B}}_\lambda - \mathring{\mathbf{A}}_\lambda$ or for the equivalent generalized eigenvalue problem

$$\mathbf{A}_\lambda \mathbf{w} = (1-\mu)\mathring{\mathbf{B}}_\lambda \mathbf{w}$$

we have that all the eigenvalues μ will be less than one if and only if $\lambda < \lambda_1$, i.e., the matrix $\mathbf{A}_\lambda$ is positive definite.

Let us introduce a quantity

$$r(\mathring{\mathbf{T}}_\lambda) = \max_{\mathbf{w} \in \mathbf{E}^n} \frac{(\mathring{\mathbf{C}}_\lambda \mathbf{w},\mathbf{w})}{(\mathring{\mathbf{B}}_\lambda \mathbf{w},\mathbf{w})}, \tag{30}$$

where $\mathring{\mathbf{T}}_\lambda = \mathring{\mathbf{B}}_\lambda^{-1} \mathring{\mathbf{C}}_r$.

Obviously $r(\mathring{\mathbf{T}}_\lambda)$ is the maximal eigenvalue of the problem (29). Then the inner iterative process must provide the answer to the question whether $r(\mathring{\mathbf{T}}_\lambda)$ is less than one for given λ. Naturally we would like to use, as in the previous section, the power method (11) or the generalized iterative method of Lanczos (12). Unfortunately, their utilization demands an additional assumption that $r(\mathring{\mathbf{T}}_\lambda)$ is not less than the module of the minimal eigenvalue of the matrix $\mathring{\mathbf{T}}_\lambda$, i.e., $r(\mathring{\mathbf{T}}_\lambda) = \rho(\mathring{\mathbf{T}}_\lambda)$.

We consider next two important practical cases where this condition is satisfied.

Case 1. **A** is an M–matrix [16] and **S** is a matrix with nonnegative elements.

In this case, $\mathring{\mathbf{T}}_\lambda$ is a matrix with nonnegative elements and therefore its spectral radius is equal to the module of its maximal eigenvalue. If in addition it is supposed that the matrix **A** is irreducible, then the eigenvalue $\rho(\mathring{\mathbf{T}}_\lambda) = r(\mathring{\mathbf{T}}_\lambda)$ of the matrix $\mathring{\mathbf{T}}_\lambda$ is simple and the positive eigenvector corresponds to it.

From the previous discussion and from the theory of regular splittings of M–matrices [16] we have the following lemma.

Lemma 3. *The matrix* $\mathbf{A}_\lambda$ *is positive definite if and only if* $\rho(\mathring{\mathbf{T}}_\lambda) < 1$.

Thus, to compute (or estimate) $\rho(\mathring{\mathbf{T}}_\lambda)$ one can use the generalized minimized iterative method of Lanczos (19), replacing the matrix $\mathring{\mathbf{B}}_\lambda$ and the matrix $\mathbf{C}_\lambda$ by the matrix $\mathring{\mathbf{C}}_\lambda$.

From the form of $\mathring{\mathbf{B}}_\lambda$, $\mathring{\mathbf{C}}_\lambda$ and from the theory of regular splittings of M–matrices we have the following lemma.

Lemma 4. *If the matrix* **A** *is irreducible, then the function* $\mu(\lambda) = \rho(\mathring{\mathbf{T}}_\lambda)$ *is monotonically increasing in the interval* $(0,d)$.

This lemma implies that, as in the previous section, we can consider the problem of finding the unique root of equation (18) in the interval $(0,d)$, using appropriate methods.

Case 2. $\mathbf{A}_\lambda$ is a 2–cyclic matrix. We assume without loss of generality that in (26) m=2. Indeed, by the definition of a 2–cyclic matrix there exists a block permutation matrix **P** such that

$$\tilde{A}_\lambda = PA_\lambda P^T = \begin{bmatrix} \tilde{A}_{11}-\lambda\tilde{S}_{11} & \tilde{A}_{12}-\lambda\tilde{S}_{12} \\ \tilde{A}_{21}-\lambda\tilde{S}_{21} & \tilde{A}_{22}-\lambda\tilde{S}_{22} \end{bmatrix},$$

where

$$(\tilde{A}_{11} - \lambda\tilde{S}_{11}) \oplus (\tilde{A}_{22} - \lambda\tilde{S}_{22})$$
$$= P_\lambda(A_{11} - \lambda S_{11}) \oplus \cdots \oplus (A_{mm} - \lambda S_{mm})_\lambda P^T .$$

In particular, for the matrix A_λ from the previous section we have

$$\tilde{A}_{11} - \lambda\tilde{S}_{11} = (A_1 - \lambda I_1) \oplus (A_2 - \lambda I_2),$$
$$\tilde{A}_{22} - \lambda\tilde{S}_{22} = A_\gamma - \lambda I_\gamma .$$

Here $\mathring{T}_\lambda$ is a weak 2–cyclic matrix and, according to the theory of such matrices, all the eigenvalues lie symmetrically with respect to zero in the segment $[-\rho(\mathring{T}_\lambda),\rho(\mathring{T}_\lambda)]$. This means that to find $\rho(\mathring{T}_\lambda)$ it is sufficient to compute the maximal eigenvalue of the matrix $[\mathring{T}_\lambda]^2$ with nonnegative eigen–values (recall that in process (25) it is sufficient to find whether the eigenvalue is less than one or not). It is easy to see that the nonzero eigenvalues of the matrix $[\mathring{T}_\lambda]^2$ coincide (and may differ only by their mul–tiplicities) with the eigenvalues of the matrices $T_\lambda = B_\lambda^{-1}C_\lambda$ and $B_\lambda T_\lambda B_\lambda^{-1} = C_\lambda B_\lambda^{-1}$, where

$$B_\lambda = \begin{bmatrix} A_{11}-\lambda S_{11} & A_{12}-\lambda S_{12} \\ 0 & A_{22}-\lambda S_{22} \end{bmatrix},$$
$$C_\lambda = B_\lambda - A_\lambda = \begin{bmatrix} 0 & 0 \\ -A_{21}+\lambda S_{21} & 0 \end{bmatrix}. \tag{31}$$

As in the previous section, it can easily be proved that the matrix B_λ^{-1} is self–adjoint positive definite in the subspace $\mathrm{Im}C_\lambda$ and the matrix $C_\lambda B_\lambda^{-1}$ is B_λ^{-1}–self–adjoint and B_λ^{-1}–positive definite in the same subspace. Then it follows that to compute the maximal eigenvalue $\rho(T_\lambda)$ of the matrix T_λ one can use the generalized minimized iterative method of Lanczos (19) with the matrices B_λ and $C = C_\lambda$ from (31) in the subspace $U = \mathrm{Im}C_\lambda$, which is invariant with respect to the matrix $C_\lambda B_\lambda^{-1}$. Of course we need to assume that the initial vector ξ^0 belongs to U and has the necessary non–zero component in the decomposition by the eigenvectors of the matrix $C_\lambda B_\lambda^{-1}$. It is worth noting that the vector $\xi \in U$ may be constructed by the formula $\xi = C_\lambda B_\lambda^{-1} w$ for any vector $w \in E^N$.

Now we have to identify $\rho(T_\lambda)$ with the property of positive definite–ness of the matrix A_λ. The answer to this question is given by the follow–ing lemma.

Lemma 5. *The matrix* **A** *is positive definite if and only if* $\rho(\mathbf{T}_\lambda) < 1$. *Moreover,* $\rho(\mathbf{T}_\lambda) > 1$ *for all* $\lambda > \lambda_1$.

As above, the proof of this lemma follows from the Ostrowski–Reich theorem [16]. It follows from Lemma 5 that the eigenvalue λ_1 sought is the unique solution in the interval $(0,d)$ of equation (18) with the continuous function $\mu(\lambda) = \rho(\mathbf{T}_\lambda)$.

The question of properties of the function μ is more complex in this case than in case 1. Let us make an additional assumption that $\mathbf{S}_{12} = \mathbf{S}_{21}^* = 0$. Then it is easy to see that the following representation holds true:

$$\tilde{\mu}(\lambda) = \max_{\mathbf{v} \in \mathbf{E}^n} \frac{(\mathring{\mathbf{C}}\mathbf{v},\mathbf{v})}{(\mathring{\mathbf{B}}_\lambda \mathbf{v},\mathbf{v})},$$

where $\mathring{\mathbf{C}} \equiv \mathring{\mathbf{C}}_\lambda$ is a matrix not depending on λ. From this we obtain that $\mu(\lambda)$ in the interval $(0,d)$ is a continuous, nondecreasing function of the variable λ. Taking into consideration that (18) has a unique solution, it is possible to see that $\mu(\lambda)$ is a monotonically increasing function in the neighborhood of λ_1.

The question of the implementation of the methods in the subspace $\mathbf{U} = \mathrm{Im}\mathbf{C}_\lambda$, i.e., the methods using the partial solution of systems with the matrix $\mathbf{B}_\lambda$, are worthy of interest only in the context of concrete applied problems, as was done in the previous section. The questions as to when the block decomposition (25) corresponds to the domain–decomposition method have been studied in [3], [5] and [7].

3. Fictitious component method

Let symmetric positive semidefinite N×N matrices **A** and **S** be given such that ker **A** = ker **S**. Here we shall consider the generalized eigenvalue problem

$$\mathbf{A}\mathbf{u} = \lambda \mathbf{S}\mathbf{u}, \quad \mathbf{u} \in \mathrm{Im}\mathbf{A}, \tag{32}$$

for which the minimal eigenvalue λ_1 is to be found. As in the previous sections, this problem can be equivalently formulated as follows: find such maximal λ_1 that the matrix $\mathbf{A}_\lambda = \mathbf{A} - \lambda\mathbf{S}$ would be positive definite in the subspace ImA. If the interval $(a_{k-1}, b_{k-1}]$, containing λ_1, is given and $\lambda^{(k)} = (a_{k-1} + b_{k-1})/2$, then the corresponding modification of the bisection method can be realized as follows: if $\mathbf{A}_{\lambda^{(k)}} > 0$ in ImA, then $a_k = \lambda^{(k)}$, $b_k = b_{k-1}$; otherwise $a_k = a_{k-1}$, $b_k = \lambda^{(k)}$.

Let a symmetric matrix $\mathbf{B}_\lambda$ depending on λ as a parameter correspond to the generalized eigenvalue problem (32). We suppose that for the bisection method an interval (a_0, b_0) containing the eigenvalue λ_1 (which is to be found) is given and that the matrix $\mathbf{B}_\lambda$ is positive definite for any $\lambda \in (a_0, b_0)$. In addition, let for any $\lambda \in (a_0, b_0)$ a quantity τ_λ be known such that

$$r(\mathbf{T}_\lambda) = \max_{\mathbf{v} \in \mathrm{Im}\, \mathbf{B}^{-1}\mathbf{A}} \frac{(\mathbf{T}_\lambda \mathbf{v}, \mathbf{v})_{\mathbf{B}_\lambda}}{(\mathbf{v}, \mathbf{v})_{\mathbf{B}_\lambda}} \tag{33}$$

would not be less than the module of the minimal eigenvalue of the matrix

$$\mathbf{T}_\lambda = \mathbf{I} - \tau_\lambda \mathbf{B}_\lambda^{-1} \mathbf{A}_\lambda , \tag{34}$$

where the matrix $\mathbf{A}_\lambda$ has been defined above. For instance, we may choose $\tau_\lambda = 1/\|\mathbf{B}_\lambda^{-1}\mathbf{A}\|_*$ for an arbitrary matrix norm $\|\cdot\|_*$. It is obvious that the matrix $\mathbf{A}_\lambda$ is positive definite in ImA if and only if $\tau(\mathbf{T}_\lambda) < 1$.

With respect to the previous assumption, it is possible to use the minimized iterative method of Lanczos to compute $\tau(\mathbf{T}_\lambda)$:

$$\begin{gathered} \xi^\ell = \tilde{\mathbf{T}}_\lambda \xi^{\ell-1} - \alpha_\ell \xi^{\ell-1} - \beta_\ell \xi^{\ell-2} , \\ \alpha_\ell = \frac{(\mathbf{T}_\lambda \xi^{\ell-1}, \xi^{\ell-1})_{\mathbf{R}_\lambda}}{\| \xi^{\ell-1} \|^2_{\mathbf{R}_\lambda}} , \quad \beta_\ell = \frac{\|\xi^{\ell-1}\|^2_{\mathbf{R}_\lambda}}{\|\xi^{\ell-2}\|^2_{\mathbf{R}_\lambda}} , \end{gathered} \tag{35}$$

where $\tilde{\mathbf{T}}_\lambda = \mathbf{B}_\lambda \mathbf{T}_\lambda \mathbf{B}_\lambda^{-1}$ and $\mathbf{R}_\lambda = \mathbf{B}_\lambda^{-1}$ with the conditions $\xi^0 \in$ ImA and in the decomposition of ξ^0 by the eigenvectors of the matrix $\tilde{\mathbf{T}}_\lambda$ the component corresponding to the eigenvalue $r(\tilde{\mathbf{T}}_\lambda)$ is not zero. The second condition is necessary and the first one, $\xi^0 \in$ ImA, can be changed; namely, we may choose the vector ξ^0 from any subspace **U** which possesses the following properties: it is invariant with respect to the matrix $\tilde{\mathbf{T}}_\lambda$, it belongs to ImA and it contains at least one eigenvector of the matrix $\tilde{\mathbf{T}}_\lambda$ corresponding to its eigenvalue $r(\tilde{\mathbf{T}}_\lambda)$. Naturally, we would like to construct a subspace of smaller dimension, as small as possible. Later we shall point out the matrix $\mathbf{B}_\lambda$ and the corresponding subspace **U** for a concrete applied problem (for a simple case) based on the notion of the fictitious–component method.

Let us again consider the spectral problem (1) in the domain Ω with piecewise linear boundary $\partial\Omega$, as shown in figure 3. Let us then imbed the rectangle Π with the sides parallel to the coordinates and construct in Π a uniform square mesh Π_h with step h so that all the ends of the linear sections of the $\partial\Omega$ would lie in the set of its nodes (it is supposed that the coordinates of the ends permit such a construction of mesh). The intersection of the domain $\overline{\Omega}$ with the mesh lines and the boundary $\partial\Omega$ will give a mesh Ω_h consisting of mesh rectangles and right isosceles triangles with hypotenuses belonging to the set of inclined sections of $\partial\Omega$.

To approximate a differential problem, we introduce the finite-dimensional subspace H_{N_0} of the Sobolev space $\overset{\circ}{W}{}^1_2(\Omega)$, including all the continuous functions which are bilinear in each rectangle and linear in each triangle of the mesh Π_h. Here N_0 is the number of nodes of the mesh Ω_h belonging to Ω and, also, it is the dimension of H_{N_0}. Then, using the following variant of the finite–element method, namely finding the quantities λ as functions $\mathbf{u}^h \in H_{N_0}$ such that

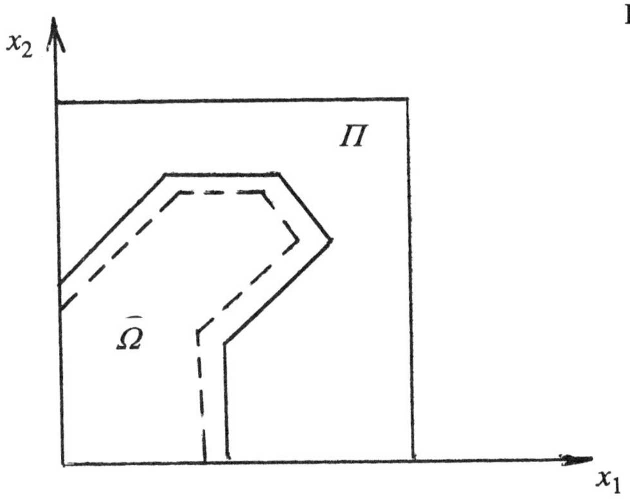

Fig. 3

$$\int_{\Omega} \text{grad } \mathbf{u}^h \text{ grad } \mathbf{v}^h \, d\Omega = \lambda \int_{\Omega} \mathbf{u}^h \mathbf{v}^h \, d\Omega \;\; \forall \; \mathbf{v}^h \in H_{N_0} , \tag{36}$$

we arrive at the generalized algebraic eigenvalue problem

$$\mathbf{A}_0 \mathbf{u} = \lambda \mathbf{S}_0 \mathbf{u} \tag{37}$$

with symmetric positive definite $N_0 \times N_0$ matrices $\mathbf{A}_0$ and $\mathbf{S}_0$.

Using the notion of the fictitious–component method [11], we can replace (37) by (32), supposing that $N > N_0$ and there exists a permutation matrix $\mathbf{P}$ such that

$$\mathbf{PAP}^{\top} = \begin{bmatrix} \mathbf{A}_0 & \mathbf{0} \\ \mathbf{0} & \mathbf{0} \end{bmatrix} , \quad \mathbf{PSP}^{\top} = \begin{bmatrix} \mathbf{S}_0 & \mathbf{0} \\ \mathbf{0} & \mathbf{0} \end{bmatrix} . \tag{38}$$

Obviously, ker $\mathbf{A}$ = ker $\mathbf{S}$ and the set of eigenvalues of (32) coincide with the set of eigenvalues of (37).

Now we can construct the matrix $\mathbf{B}_{\lambda}$. Let us consider the problem (1), but this time in the new domain $\Omega = \Pi$, where (1) is approximated by the following variant of the finite–element method, namely, to find the quantities λ and the functions $\mathbf{v}^h \in V_N$ so that

$$\int_{\Pi} \text{grad } \mathbf{v}^h \text{ grad } \mathbf{w}^h \, d\Pi = \int_{\Pi} \lambda \, \mathbf{v}^h \, \mathbf{w}^h \, d\Pi , \;\; \forall \; \mathbf{w}^h \in V_N . \tag{39}$$

Here $V_N \subset \overset{\circ}{W}{}^1_2(\Pi)$ and contains all those functions which are continuous in Π and bilinear in every rectangle of Π_h.

The problem (39) is equivalent to the algebraic eigenvalue problem

$$\mathbf{K}\mathbf{v} = \lambda \mathbf{R}\mathbf{v} \tag{40}$$

with symmetric positive definite matrices

$$\mathbf{K} = \mathbf{K}_1 \otimes \mathbf{R}_2 + \mathbf{R}_1 \otimes \mathbf{K}_2 , \qquad \mathbf{R} = \mathbf{R}_1 \otimes \mathbf{R}_2 , \tag{41}$$

where

$$\mathbf{K}_\alpha = \frac{1}{h}\begin{bmatrix} 2 & -1 & & 0 \\ -1 & \ddots & \ddots & \\ & \ddots & \ddots & -1 \\ 0 & & -1 & 2 \end{bmatrix}, \quad \mathbf{R}_\alpha = \frac{h}{6}\begin{bmatrix} 4 & 1 & & 0 \\ 1 & \ddots & \ddots & \\ & \ddots & \ddots & 1 \\ 0 & & 1 & 4 \end{bmatrix} \tag{42}$$

are $N_\alpha \times N_\alpha$–matrices, $\alpha = 1,2$.

We assume we can find a positive d such that $\lambda_1 < d$. Let us choose a maximal positive N_d so that the minimal eigenvalue of the generalized eigenvalue problem

$$\mathbf{B}_d(\lambda)\mathbf{w} \equiv (\mathbf{K}_d \otimes \mathbf{R}_2 + \mathbf{R}_d \otimes \mathbf{S}_2 - \lambda \mathbf{R}_d \otimes \mathbf{R}_2)\mathbf{w} = 0 \tag{43}$$

is less than d, where $\mathbf{K}_d$ *and* $\mathbf{R}_d$ are $N_d \times N_d$–matrices of the form (42). It is easy to see that this eigenvalue increases monotonically with decreasing N_d, and is larger than $3/h^2$ when $N_d = 1$, i.e., N always exists.

Without loss of generality let N_1 be divisible by N_d or otherwise extend the rectangle Π in the positive direction of the x_1 axis so that this condition is satisfied. Let us put

$$\mathbf{B}_\lambda = \mathbf{B}_d(\lambda) \otimes \mathbf{I}_m, \tag{44}$$

where $\mathbf{I}_m$ is a unit matrix of the order $m = N_1/N_d$. There is another way of constructing $\mathbf{B}_\lambda$, namely decomposition of the matrix $\mathbf{K}-\lambda\mathbf{R}$ into blocks of dimension $N_d \times N_2$ and the choice of $\mathbf{B}_\lambda$ as a block–diagonal matrix composed of the diagonal blocks of $\mathbf{K}-\lambda\mathbf{R}$. It is natural to suppose that the rows with the same indices of all the matrices correspond to the same mesh nodes.

It is possible to interpret every diagonal block of $\mathbf{B}_\lambda$ as follows: the rectangle Π can be represented as the union of rectangles $\Pi_1,\dots,\Pi_m$ (as shown in figure 4) so that the width of the intersection of adjacent rectangles would be equal to h (here left sides of the rectangles $\Pi_2,\dots,\Pi_m$ are dashed lines). Then the blocks of $\mathbf{B}_\lambda$ can be constructed when the problem (39) is considered for every rectangle Π_α $(1 \le \alpha \le m)$.

Fig. 4

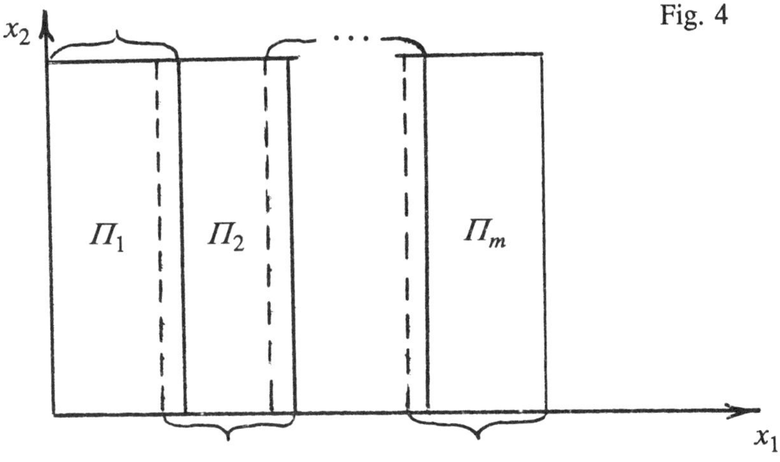

The matrix $\mathbf{B}_\lambda$ thus obtained satisfies all the demands formulated at the beginning of this section. It has several other remarkable properties. First, the method of separation of variables is applicable to the solution of this system. Second, the matrix $\mathbf{C}_\lambda = \mathbf{B}_\lambda - \mathbf{A}_\lambda$ has nonzero rows only for those mesh points of Π_h which belong to G. Here the set G contains all those nodes Ω_h which either belong to the intersection of Ω with the vertical sides of rectangles Π_α, $\alpha = 1,...,m$, or adjacent to the boundary $\partial\Omega$, but never adjacent to the boundary $\partial\Pi$ (such a set has been marked by a dotted line in figure 3). Then it follows that if we define a subspace

$$U = \mathrm{Im}\mathbf{C} \cap \mathrm{Im}\mathbf{A} \,,$$

which is, obviously, invariant with respect to the matrix $\tilde{\mathbf{T}}_\lambda$ from this section, then any vector $\xi \in \mathbf{U}$ has at most $0(h^{-1})$ nonzero components (it is assumed that $m \sim$ const. > 0).

Define the diagonal matrices $\mathbf{P}_1$ and $\mathbf{P}_2$ as in the first section. Let a diagonal element of $\mathbf{P}_1$ be unity if this element corresponds to a mesh point of G. Next, let a diagonal element of $\mathbf{P}_2$ be unity if this element corresponds to a mesh point of Π_h belonging either to the set G or to the boundary $\partial\Omega$. We put all the other diagonal elements of $\mathbf{P}_1$ and $\mathbf{P}_2$ equal to zero.

It is easy to see that $\mathbf{U} = \mathrm{Im}\mathbf{P}_1$ and the equality $\mathbf{C}_\lambda \mathbf{w} = \mathbf{C}_\lambda \mathbf{P}_2 \mathbf{w}$ holds true for any $\mathbf{w} \in \mathbf{B}_\lambda^{-1}\mathrm{Im}\mathbf{A}$. Then it follows that the coefficients α_ℓ and β_ℓ can be computed with the help of (21) with the constructed matrices $\mathbf{P}_1$ and $\mathbf{P}_2$ for the realization of (35). Since in this case m is a constant not depending on the mesh step, then (rank $\mathbf{P}_1$) $\sim$ (rank $\mathbf{P}_2$) $\sim h^{-1}$.

Thus, since $\mathrm{Im}\mathbf{P}_1 \subseteq \mathrm{Im}\mathbf{P}_2$, the main computational procedure is solving the following partial problem:

$$\begin{array}{c}\text{find the vector } \mathbf{P}_2 \mathbf{B}_\lambda^{-1} \xi^{\ell-1} \\ \text{for the given vector } \xi^{\ell-1} \in \mathrm{Im}\mathbf{P}_1\end{array} \tag{45}$$

According to [1] and [8], we can solve this problem at the expense of $0(h^{-2})$ arithmetic operations with simultaneous storage of $0(h^{-1})$ memory locations.

One of the most important problems in the implementation of this method is the choice of parameters τ_λ. It can be shown [14] that $\tau_\lambda \sim h$ for spectral problems of type (1). This problem is worthy of further study; we note only that, for the sake of identification of the quantity $\tau(\mathbf{T}_\lambda)$ one can use the generalized conjugate–gradient method in the same subspace U, but this time for the matrix $\mathbf{A}_\lambda \mathbf{B}_\lambda^{-1}$ [7], [10], [12].

REFERENCES

[1] Banegas, A. 1978. Fast Poisson solvers for problems with sparsity. *Math. Comp.* 32:441–46.

[2] Bespalov, A.N., and Yu.A. Kuznetsov. 1984. The block–relaxation method in the subspace of computation of the minimal eigenvalue of the Laplace difference operator (in Russian). In *Chislennoe Modelirovanie Fizicheskikh Protsessov Okruzhayushchej Sredy*, 59–67, Department of Numerical Mathematics of the USSR Academy of Sciences, Moscow.

[3] D'yakonov, E.G. 1979. On some primal and iterative methods based on bordered matrices (in Russian). In *Chislennye Metody v Matematicheskoj Fizike*, 45–68. Computing Center of the USSR Academy of Sciences, Siberian Branch, Novosibirsk.

[4] Kuznetsov, Yu.A. (Kuznecov, Ju.A.) 1969. On the theory of iteration processes. *Soviet Math. Doklady* 10, no. 1:59–62. (English transl.)

[5] ————. 1978. The block–relaxation methods in subspaces: optimization and applications (in Russian). In *Variatsionno–raznostnye Methody v Matematicheskoj Fizike*, 178–222. Computing Center of the USSR Academy of Sciences, Siberian Branch, Novosibirsk.

[6] ————. 1978. Sur la symmetrization des problems approches de la theorie du transport. In *Etude numerique des grands systèmes*, 182–97. Paris: Dunod–Gauthier–Villars.

[7] ————. 1984. Matrix iterative methods in subspaces. In *Proceedings of the International Congress of Mathematicians*, August 16–24, 1983, Warszawa, vol. 2, 1509–21. Warszawa: Polish Scientific Publishers/ Amsterdam New York Oxford: North–Holland.

[8] ————. 1984. Computational methods in subspaces (in Russian). In *Vychislitel'nye Protsessy i Sistemy*, vol. 2, 265–354. Moscow: Nauka.

[9] ————. 1984. Matrix computational processes in subspaces. In *Computing Methods in Applied Sciences and Engineering*, VI, 15–31. Amsterdam New York Oxford: North–Holland.

[10] Marchuk, G.I., and Yu.A. Kuznetsov (Marcuk, G.I., and Ju.A. Kuznecov). 1968. On optimal iteration processes. *Soviet Math. Doklady* 9, no. 4:1041–45. (English transl.)
[11] ————. 1972. Some problems involving iterative methods (in Russian). *Vychislitel'nye Metody Linejnoj Algebry*, 4–20. Computing Center of the USSR Academy of Sciences, Siberian Branch, Novosibirsk.
[12] ————. 1972. Iterative methods and quadratic functionals (in Russian). Computing Center of the USSR Academy of Sciences, Siberian Branch, Novosibirsk, 205. (Methodes iteratives et fonctionelles quadratiques. *Sur les methodes numeriques en sciences physiques et economiques*, 1–132. Paris: Dunod.)
[13] ————. 1974. Stationary iterative methods for solving systems of linear equations with singular matrices. The 6th Gatlinburg Symposium on Numerical Algebra, Munich.
[14] Matsokin, A.M. 1973. On the development of the method of fictitious domains (in Russian). In *Vychislitel'nye Methody Linejnoj Algebry*, 48–56. Computing Center of the USSR Academy of Sciences, Siberian Branch, Novosibirsk.
[15] Parlett, B.N. *The Symmetric Eigenvalue Problem*. Englewood Cliffs, NJ: Prentice–Hall, 1980.
[16] Varga, R.S. *Matrix Iterative Analysis*. Englewood Cliffs, NJ: Prentice–Hall, 1962.

A REMARK ON THE APPROXIMATION OF NONHOMOGENEOUS HYPERBOLIC BOUNDARY VALUE PROBLEMS

Jacques–Louis Lions

College de France and I.N.R.I.A.
Paris, France

Introduction

A large number of applications lead to the control of systems governed by hyperbolic partial differential equations, where the control is applied by way of the boundary conditions. This leads to nonhomogeneous boundary value problems for hyperbolic equations.

We consider here the simplest situation one can think of in this setting, namely the wave equation

$$\frac{\partial^2 u}{\partial t^2} - \Delta u = f \quad \text{in a domain } \Omega \times (0,T) , \tag{1}$$

where u is subject to

$$u = g \quad \text{on } \Sigma = \Gamma \times (0,T) , \ \Gamma = \partial\Omega \tag{2}$$

and where the initial data for u are given, say

$$u(x,0) = 0 , \ \frac{\partial u}{\partial t}(x,0) = 0 \ \text{ in } \Omega . \tag{3}$$

This is hardly a new problem! But if we think of g as the control variable, a natural setting in this framework is to take

$$g \in L^2(\Sigma) \tag{4}$$

without extra regularity assumptions.

This leads to the question: What are the properties of u, defined as the weak solution of (1), (2), (3)?

Properties of u have been given in Lions and Magenes [1]; these properties, obtained by the transposition of nonoptimal regularity results for the wave equation, are far from being optimal.

But, by using a priori estimates derived from an appropriate modification of a classical Rellich's idea, a more precise result has been obtained in Lions [1] (cf. also Govorov [1] by a rather different method); *if* g *satisfies* (4), *then* u *is continuous from* $[0,T] \to L^2(\Omega)$.

We want to address here the next, natural question: *What are the "good" numerical schemes for the approximation of* u?†

This paper does not pretend, by any means, to settle this question! We confine ourselves to a particular case of this question: one of the difficulties in finding numerical algorithms for (1), (2), (3) is the fact that it can be written in variational form only *after* subtracting from u a smooth function which satisfies (2) on the boundary Σ. This presents two difficulties: first of all such a smooth function *does not exist* if g is only in $L^2(\Sigma)$, and when g is smooth, this procedure is not intrinsic.

Hence the idea is to approximate (1), (2), (3) by a boundary value problem with a "simple variational formulation."

The natural candidate to such an approximation would be to consider the equations

$$\frac{\partial^2 u_\varepsilon}{\partial t^2} - \Delta u_\varepsilon = f \quad \text{in } Q\,, \tag{5}$$

$$\varepsilon \frac{\partial u_\varepsilon}{\partial \nu} + u_\varepsilon = g \quad \text{on } \Sigma\,, \quad \varepsilon > 0\,, \tag{6}$$

$$u_\varepsilon(x,0) = \frac{\partial u_\varepsilon}{\partial t}(x,0) = 0 \quad \text{in } \Omega\,. \tag{7}$$

The variational formulation of this problem is:

$$\int_\Omega \frac{\partial^2 u_\varepsilon}{\partial t^2} v\, dx + \frac{1}{\varepsilon}\int_\Gamma u_\varepsilon\, v\, d\Gamma + \sum_{i=1}^{n} \int_\Omega \frac{\partial u_\varepsilon}{\partial x_i}\frac{\partial v}{\partial x_i} dx = \int_\Omega fv\, dx + \frac{1}{\varepsilon}\int_\Gamma gv\, d\Gamma \tag{8}$$

for every test function v.

But it leads to (apparently) serious difficulties when g is only supposed to be in $L^2(\Sigma)$.

We introduce therefore a more complicated but smoother approximation, namely (using a variational formulation)

$$\int_\Omega \frac{\partial^2 u_\varepsilon}{\partial t^2} v\, dx + \frac{1}{\varepsilon}\int_\Gamma (\beta u_\varepsilon) v\, d\Gamma + \sum_{i=1}^{n} \int_\Omega \frac{\partial u_\varepsilon}{\partial x_i}\frac{\partial v}{\partial x_i} dx = \int_\Omega fv\, dx + \frac{1}{\varepsilon}\int_\Gamma (\beta g) v\, d\Gamma\,, \tag{9}$$

† We refer the reader to G.I. Marchuk [1] for related questions.

where β is a self-adjoint second-order elliptic operator on the variety Γ (assumed to be a C^2 variety).

Then one shows—and this is the main goal of this paper—*that, indeed,* (9) *is a "good" approximation of problems* (1), (2), (3).

The plan of this paper is as follows:

1. Some a priori estimates

1.1. THE NOTATION AND STATEMENT OF THE PROBLEM

Let Ω be an open set on $\mathbf{R}^n$, with smooth boundary Γ. We assume that Ω is bounded (although this is not essential).

Let $T > 0$ be given. We consider the wave equation in $Q = \Omega \times (0,T)$:

$$\frac{\partial^2 u}{\partial t^2} - \Delta u = f, \tag{1.1}$$

where u is subject to Dirichlet boundary conditions

$$u = 0 \quad \text{on } \Sigma = \Gamma \times (0,T) \tag{1.2}$$

and to the initial conditions

$$u(x,0) = \frac{\partial u}{\partial t}(x,0) = 0 \quad \text{in } \Omega . \tag{1.3}$$

We could as well consider nonzero initial data but confine ourselves to the slightly simpler case (1.3).

We assume that

$$f \in L^1(0,T; L^2(\Omega)) . ^{\dagger} \tag{1.4}$$

Then it is known that u is uniquely defined by (1.1), (1.2), (1.3) and that it satisfies

† All functions considered throughout are real valued.

$$\begin{cases} u \in C([0,T]; H_0^1(\Omega)) , \\ \dfrac{\partial u}{\partial t} \in C([0,T]; L^2(\Omega)) . \end{cases} \tag{1.5}$$

In (1.5), $C([0,T]; X)$ denotes the space of functions which are continuous from $[0,T] \to X$, where X is a (real) Banach space. We denote by $H^1(\Omega)$ the Sobolev space:

$$H^1(\Omega) = \{\varphi | \varphi, \frac{\partial \varphi}{\partial x_1}, \ldots, \frac{\partial \varphi}{\partial x_n} \in L^2(\Omega)\}$$

and by $H_0^1(\Omega)$ the subspace of $H^1(\Omega)$ defined by

$$H_0^1(\Omega) = \{\varphi | \varphi \in H^1(\Omega), \varphi = 0 \text{ on } \Gamma\} .$$

A property of regularity of u is as follows:

$$\frac{\partial u}{\partial \nu} \in L^2(\Sigma) ,^{\dagger} \tag{1.6}$$

and the mapping $f \to \partial u/\partial \nu$ is continuous from $L^1(0,T;L^2(\Omega))$ into $L^2(\Sigma)$.

For a proof of (1.6), cf. Lions [1], Th. 4.1, chapter 2††.

In this section we want to construct an approximation of u (solution of (1.1), (1.2), (1.3)) with a "Neumann's type" boundary condition and such that, if u denotes the solution of the approximate problem, then $\partial u_\varepsilon/\partial \nu \to \partial u/\partial \nu$ in $L^2(\Sigma)$ (at least weakly).

1.2. AN APPROXIMATE BOUNDARY VALUE PROBLEM

We introduce:

$$\beta = \text{second–order elliptic operator of the variety } \Gamma, \\ \beta \text{ being self–adjoint} . \tag{1.7}$$

For example, one can take

$$\beta = -\Delta_\Gamma + I , \tag{1.8}$$

where Δ_Γ is the Laplacian corresponding to the Riemann metric on Γ induced by $\mathbf{R}^n$, and where I = identity (we could also take $\beta = -\Delta_\Gamma$).

We denote by $H^1(\Gamma)$ the Sobolev space of order 1 on Γ and by $b(\varphi,\psi)$ the continuous bilinear form on $H^1(\Gamma)$ corresponding to β, i.e.,

† $\partial u/\partial \nu$ denotes the normal derivative on Γ, ν oriented toward the exterior of Ω to fix ideas.

†† The techniques of the proof will be used below.

$$b(\varphi,\psi) = \langle\beta\varphi,\psi\rangle_\Gamma \quad \forall\ \varphi,\psi \in H^1(\Gamma)\ , \tag{1.9}$$

where $\langle,\rangle_\Gamma$ denotes the duality between $H^{-1}(\Gamma)$ and $H^1(\Gamma)$; we have

$$\left| \begin{aligned} b(\varphi,\psi) &= b(\psi,\varphi) \quad \forall\ \varphi,\psi \in H^1(\Gamma)\ , \\ b(\varphi,\varphi) &\geq \beta\|\varphi\|^2_{H^1(\Gamma)}\ , \quad \beta > 0\ . \end{aligned} \right. \tag{1.10}$$

$$\frac{\partial^2 u_\varepsilon}{\partial t^2} - \Delta u_\varepsilon = f \quad \text{in } Q\ , \tag{1.11}$$

$$\varepsilon \frac{\partial u_\varepsilon}{\partial \nu} + \beta u_\varepsilon = 0 \quad \text{on } \Sigma\ , \quad (\varepsilon > 0)\ , \tag{1.12}$$

$$u_\varepsilon(x,0) = \frac{\partial u_\varepsilon}{\partial t}(x,0) = 0 \quad \text{in } \Omega\ . \tag{1.13}$$

Proposition 1.1. *Problem* (1.1), (1.2), (1.3) *admits a unique solution* u_ε *which satisfies*

$$\left| \begin{aligned} & u_\varepsilon \in C([0,T];\ H^1(\Omega))\ , \\ & \frac{\partial u_\varepsilon}{\partial t} \in C([0,T];\ L^2(\Omega))\ , \end{aligned} \right. \tag{1.14}$$

and u_ε *remains in a bounded set of these spaces when* $\varepsilon \to 0$. *Moreover,*

$$\frac{1}{\sqrt{\varepsilon}} u_\varepsilon|_\Gamma \ \textit{remains bounded in}\ C([0,T];\ H^1(\Gamma))\ . \tag{1.15}$$

Proof. Let us introduce the variational form of the problem. We define

$$a(\varphi,\psi) = \int_\Omega \frac{\partial\varphi}{\partial x_i}\frac{\partial\psi}{\partial x_i}\,dx\ ,$$

$$(\varphi,\psi) = \int_\Omega \varphi\psi\,dx\ ,$$

$$\varphi' = \frac{\partial\varphi}{\partial t}\ , \quad \varphi'' = \frac{\partial^2\varphi}{\partial t^2}\ , \quad \varphi(0) = \text{“}x \to \varphi(x,0)\text{”}\ , \ \ldots$$

Then (1.11), (1.12), (1.13) amount to finding u_ε with properties (1.14), such that

$$\left| \begin{aligned} & (u''_\varepsilon,v) + a(u_\varepsilon,v) + \frac{1}{\varepsilon} b(u_\varepsilon,v) = (f,v) \quad \forall\ v \in H^1(\Omega)\ , \\ & u_\varepsilon(0) = 0\ , \ u'_\varepsilon(0) = 0\ . \end{aligned} \right. \tag{1.16}$$

Taking $v = u_\varepsilon'$ in (1.16) gives

$$\frac{1}{2}\frac{d}{dt}[|u_\varepsilon'|^2 + a(u_\varepsilon) + \frac{1}{\varepsilon} b(u_\varepsilon)] = (f,u_\varepsilon') , \tag{1.17}$$

where we have set

$$|\varphi|^2 = (\varphi,\varphi) , \quad a(\varphi) = a(\varphi,\varphi) , \quad b(\varphi) = b(\varphi,\varphi) .$$

Results (1.14), (1.15) easily follow.

It follows immediately from (1.14) and (1.15) that, as $\varepsilon \to 0$,

$$\begin{aligned} &u_\varepsilon \to u \quad \text{in } L^\infty(0,T;\, H^1(\Omega)) \text{ weak star }, ^\dagger \\ &u_\varepsilon' \to u' \quad \text{in } L^\infty(0,T;\, L^2(\Omega)) , \end{aligned} \tag{1.18}$$

$$u_\varepsilon \to 0 \quad \text{in } L^\infty(0,T;\, H^1(\Gamma)) , \tag{1.19}$$

where u is the solution of (1.1), (1.2), (1.3).

We now want to prove

Theorem 1.1. *Let u_ε be the solution of* (1.11), (1.12), (1.13). *Then*

$$\frac{\partial u_\varepsilon}{\partial \nu} \in L^2(\Sigma) \tag{1.20}$$

and, as $\varepsilon \to 0$,

$$\frac{\partial u_\varepsilon}{\partial \nu} \to \frac{\partial u}{\partial \nu} \quad \text{in } L^2(\Sigma) \text{ weakly} , \tag{1.21}$$

where u is the solution of (1.1), (1.2), (1.3).

Remark 1.1. A more "natural" approximation would be to take instead of (1.12) the simpler boundary condition

$$\varepsilon \frac{\partial u_\varepsilon}{\partial \nu} + u_\varepsilon = 0 \quad \text{on } \Sigma . \tag{1.22}$$

But then the result analogous to (1.20), (1.21) is not proven (and could be false).

Proof. Step 1. It will be sufficient to prove that

$$\int_\Sigma (T-t)\left(\frac{\partial u_\varepsilon}{\partial \nu}\right)^2 d\Sigma \leq C\|f\|^2_{L^1(0,T;\, L^2(\Omega))} , \tag{1.23}$$

† We could do better, i.e., to prove convergence in $C([0,T];\, H^1(\Omega))$, but this will be sufficient for our objective in this paper.

where C does not depend on ε and where we can assume that f is smooth.

Indeed, since T does not play any role (we can extend f in, say, $L^1(0,2T; L^2(\Omega))$ and replace T by $2T$), we will then have (maybe with another con–stant!)

$$\int_\Sigma \left(\frac{\partial u_\varepsilon}{\partial \nu}\right)^2 d\Sigma \le C\|f\|^2_{L^1(0,T;\, L^2(\Omega))}; \tag{1.24}$$

and by extension by continuity, (1.24) will be valid for *every* f in $L^1(0,T; L^2(\Omega))$.

It follows from (1.24) that we can extract a sequence such that

$$\frac{\partial u_\varepsilon}{\partial \nu} \to \chi \quad \text{in } L^2(\Sigma) \text{ weakly}. \tag{1.25}$$

But if φ is a smooth function in $\overline{Q}$, such that $\varphi(x,T) = 0$, then (1.11) implies†

$$\int_Q (-u'_\varepsilon\varphi' + \frac{\partial u_\varepsilon}{\partial x_i}\frac{\partial \varphi}{\partial x_i})\, dx\, dt - \int_\Sigma \left(\frac{\partial u_\varepsilon}{\partial \nu}\right)\varphi\, d\Sigma = \int_Q f\varphi\, dx\, dt. \tag{1.26}$$

Passing to the limit in (1.26) gives

$$\int_Q (-u'\varphi' + \frac{\partial u}{\partial x_i}\frac{\partial \varphi}{\partial x_i})\, dx\, dt - \int_\Sigma \chi\varphi\, d\Sigma = \int_Q f\varphi\, dx\, dt \tag{1.27}$$

for every smooth function φ such that $\varphi(x,T)$. Then necessarily

$$\chi = \frac{\partial u}{\partial \nu}$$

and (1.25) proves (1.21).

Step 2. Proof of (1.21).

Let us introduce functions h_i such that

$$h_i \in C^1(\overline{\Omega}), \quad h_i = \nu_i \text{ on } \Gamma, \tag{1.28}$$

and let us multiply (1.11) by $(T-t)h_i \dfrac{\partial u_\varepsilon}{\partial x_i}$.

Integrating over Q leads to

$$-\int_Q u'_\varepsilon\, (T-t)h_i \frac{\partial u'_\varepsilon}{\partial x_i}\, dx\, dt + \int_Q u'_\varepsilon\, h_i \frac{\partial u_\varepsilon}{\partial x_i}\, dx\, dt$$

$$-\int_\Sigma \frac{\partial u_\varepsilon}{\partial \nu}(T-t)h_i \frac{\partial u_\varepsilon}{\partial x_i}\, d\Sigma + \int_Q \frac{\partial u_\varepsilon}{\partial x_j}\frac{\partial}{\partial x_j}((T-t)h_i \frac{\partial u_\varepsilon}{\partial x_i})\, dx\, dt \tag{1.29}$$

† We use the convention of summation with respect to repeated indices.

$$= \int_Q f(T-t) h_i \frac{\partial u_\varepsilon}{\partial x_i} dx\, dt .$$

We write $0(\|f\|)$ for any quantity which is bounded in absolute value by $C\|f\|_{L^1(0,T;\, L^2(\Omega))}$.

With this notation and using (1.14), we obtain

$$- \int_Q (T-t) \frac{h_i}{2} \frac{\partial}{\partial x_i} (u_\varepsilon')^2 dx\, dt - \int_\Sigma (T-t) \left(\frac{\partial u_\varepsilon}{\partial \nu}\right)^2 d\Sigma$$

$$+ \int_Q (T-t)\, h_i \frac{\partial u_\varepsilon}{\partial x_j} \frac{\partial^2 u_\varepsilon}{\partial x_i \partial x_j} dx\, dt = 0(\|f\|^2) . \tag{1.30}$$

Integrating by parts, (1.30) gives

$$- \int_\Sigma \frac{(T-t)}{2} (u_\varepsilon')^2\, d\Sigma - \int_\Sigma (T-t) \left(\frac{\partial u_\varepsilon}{\partial \nu}\right)^2 d\Sigma$$

$$+ \int_\Sigma \frac{(T-t)}{2} \left(\frac{\partial u_\varepsilon}{\partial x_j} \frac{\partial u_\varepsilon}{\partial x_j}\right) d\Sigma = 0(\|f\|^2) . \tag{1.31}$$

But using (1.15), one has

$$\int_\Sigma \frac{(T-t)}{2} \frac{\partial u_\varepsilon}{\partial x_j} \frac{\partial u_\varepsilon}{\partial x_j} d\Sigma + \int_\Sigma (T-t) \left(\frac{\partial u_\varepsilon}{\partial \nu}\right)^2 d\Sigma + \varepsilon 0(\|f\|^2) \tag{1.32}$$

so that (1.31) gives

$$- \int_\Sigma \frac{(T-t)}{2} (u_\varepsilon')^2\, d\Sigma - \int_\Sigma (T-t) \left(\frac{\partial u_\varepsilon}{\partial \nu}\right)^2 d\Sigma = \varepsilon 0(\|f\|^2) , \tag{1.33}$$

hence (1.23) follows.

Remark 1.2. It also follows from (1.33) that

$$\| u_\varepsilon' \|_{L^2(\Sigma)} \le C , \tag{1.34}$$

which implies that (also using (1.19))

$$u_\varepsilon' \to 0 \quad \text{in } L^2(\Sigma) \text{ weakly} . \tag{1.35}$$

2. Approximation of a nonhomogeneous boundary value problem

2.1. SETTING OF THE PROBLEM

As in the Introduction, we consider now the nonhomogeneous boundary value problem

$$\frac{\partial^2 u}{\partial t^2} - \Delta u = f \quad \text{in } Q\,, \tag{2.1}$$

$$u = g \quad \text{on } \Sigma\,, \tag{2.2}$$

$$u(0) = u'(0) = 0 \quad \text{in } \Omega\,. \tag{2.3}$$

In (2.1) we assume that

$$f \in L^1(0,T;\, L^2(\Omega)) \tag{2.4}$$

(we could assume more general situations!), and in (2.2) we assume that

$$g \in L^2(\Sigma)\,. \tag{2.5}$$

It was proven in Lions [1], loc. cit. using the transposition method as in Lions and Magenes [1], that (2.1), (2.2), (2.3) admits a unique solution which satisfies

$$u \textit{ is continuous from } [0,T] \to L^2(\Omega)\,. \tag{2.6}$$

We now consider the "approximate" problem:

$$\frac{\partial^2 u_\varepsilon}{\partial t^2} - \Delta u_\varepsilon = f \quad \text{in } Q\,, \tag{2.7}$$

$$\varepsilon \frac{\partial u_\varepsilon}{\partial \nu} + \beta u_\varepsilon = \beta g \quad \text{on } \Sigma\,, \tag{2.8}$$

$$u_\varepsilon(0) = u_\varepsilon'(0) \quad \text{in } \Omega\,. \tag{2.9}$$

We are going to show in Section 2.1 below that this problem admits a unique solution. We will show in Section 2.2 that, as $\varepsilon \to 0$, $u_\varepsilon \to u$ (in a sense to be made precise below), where u is the solution of (2.1), (2.2), (2.3).

2.2. SOLUTION OF THE APPROXIMATE PROBLEM

We use the transposition method.

Let ψ be given, such that

$$\psi \in L^1(0,T; L^2(\Omega)) . \tag{2.10}$$

Let φ_ε be the solution of

$$\left| \begin{aligned} \varphi_\varepsilon'' - \Delta\varphi_\varepsilon &= \psi \quad \text{in } Q , \\ \varepsilon \frac{\partial \varphi_\varepsilon}{\partial \nu} + \beta\varphi_\varepsilon &= 0 \quad \text{on } \Sigma , \\ \varphi_\varepsilon(T) = \varphi_\varepsilon'(T) &= 0 \quad \text{in } \Omega . \end{aligned} \right. \tag{2.11}$$

This is a problem analogous to (1.11), (1.12), (1.13) but where we have reversed time.

Let us assume first, in a formal way, that all data are smooth and all solutions are smooth. Taking the scalar product of (2.7) with φ_ε and integrating over Q leads to

$$\int_Q f\varphi_\varepsilon \, dx\, dt = \int_Q \psi u_\varepsilon \, dx\, dt - \int_\Sigma \frac{\partial u_\varepsilon}{\partial \nu} \varphi_\varepsilon \, d\Sigma + \int_\Sigma u_\varepsilon \frac{\partial \varphi_\varepsilon}{\partial \nu} \, d\Sigma . \tag{2.12}$$

But

$$\begin{aligned} \int_\Sigma u_\varepsilon \frac{\partial \varphi_\varepsilon}{\partial \nu} \, d\Sigma &= \text{(using } (2.11)_2\text{)} = -\frac{1}{\varepsilon} \int_\Sigma u_\varepsilon(\beta\varphi_\varepsilon) \, d\Sigma \\ &= \text{(since } \beta \text{ is self–adjoint)} = -\int_\Sigma (\beta u_\varepsilon)\varphi_\varepsilon \, d\Sigma \end{aligned}$$

so that

$$\begin{aligned} -\int_\Sigma \frac{\partial u_\varepsilon}{\partial \nu} \varphi_\varepsilon \, d\Sigma + \int_\Sigma u_\varepsilon \frac{\partial \varphi_\varepsilon}{\partial \nu} \, d\Sigma &= -\int_\Sigma \left(\frac{\partial u_\varepsilon}{\partial \nu} + \frac{1}{\varepsilon}\beta u_\varepsilon\right) \varphi_\varepsilon \, d\Sigma \\ &= \text{(using (2.8))} = -\int_\Sigma (\beta g) \frac{\varphi_\varepsilon}{\varepsilon} \, d\Sigma \\ &= \text{(since } \beta \text{ is self–adjoint)} = -\int_\Sigma g \frac{1}{\varepsilon} \beta\varphi_\varepsilon \, d\Sigma \\ &= \text{(using (2.11))} = \int_\Sigma g \frac{\partial \varphi_\varepsilon}{\partial \nu} \, d\Sigma , \end{aligned}$$

so that we finally obtain

$$\int_Q u_\varepsilon \psi \, dx\, dt = \int_Q f\varphi_\varepsilon \, dx\, dt - \int_\Sigma g \frac{\partial \varphi_\varepsilon}{\partial \nu} d\Sigma . \tag{2.13}$$

The identity (2.13) allows us to *define* u_ε. Indeed, using the result of Theorem 1.1 for φ_ε, we see that

$$\psi \to \int_Q f\varphi_\varepsilon \, dx\, dt - \int_\Sigma g \frac{\partial \varphi_\varepsilon}{\partial \nu} d\Sigma = L_\varepsilon(\psi) \tag{2.14}$$

defines a continuous linear form on $L^1(0,T; L^2(\Omega))$.

Therefore (2.13) defines u_ε in a unique fashion, and

$$u_\varepsilon \in L^\infty(0,T; L^2(\Omega)) . \tag{2.15}$$

In fact this shows that

$$|u_\varepsilon|_{L^\infty(0,T;\, L^2(\Omega))} \leq C[\|f\|_{L^1(0,T;\, L^2(\Omega))} + \|g\|_{L^2(\Sigma)}] \tag{2.16}$$

and passing to the limit with respect to smooth functions f and g, one obtains that

$$u_\varepsilon \text{ is continuous in } [0,T] \to L^2(\Omega) \tag{2.17}$$

and that, as $\varepsilon \to 0$, u_ε *remains in a bounded set of* $C([0,T]; L^2(\Omega))$.

2.3. CONVERGENCE RESULT

It is now a simple matter to prove the result we had in mind.

Let u be the solution of (2.1), (2.2), (2.3) and let u_ε be the solution of (2.7), (2.8), (2.9).

We have

Theorem 2.1. *When* $\varepsilon \to 0$ *one has*

$$u_\varepsilon \to u \quad \text{in } L^\infty(0,T; L^2(\Omega)) \text{ weak star} . \tag{2.18}$$

Proof. According to the result of Section 2.2 we can extract a sub-sequence still denoted by u_ε, such that

$$u_\varepsilon \to w \quad \text{in } L^\infty(0,T; L^2(\Omega)) \text{ weak star} . \tag{2.19}$$

Using Theorem 1.1, we see that

$$\mathrm{L}_\varepsilon(\psi) \to \mathrm{L}(\psi) , \tag{2.20}$$

where

$$L(\psi) = \int_Q f\varphi \, dx \, dt - \int_\Sigma g \frac{\partial \varphi}{\partial \nu} \, d\Sigma \,, \tag{2.21}$$

where φ is the solution of

$$\left| \begin{aligned} \frac{\partial^2 \varphi}{\partial t^2} - \Delta\varphi &= \psi \quad \text{in } Q \,, \\ \varphi &= 0 \quad \text{on } \Sigma \,, \\ \varphi(T) &= \varphi'(T) = 0 \quad \text{in } \Omega \,. \end{aligned} \right. \tag{2.22}$$

Therefore (2.13) gives

$$(w,\varphi) = L(\psi) \quad \forall \, \psi \in L^1(0,T; L^2(\Omega)) \,,$$

which is the definition of u. Hence (2.18) follows.

2.4. VARIOUS REMARKS

Remark 2.1. We can take f in a larger space than $L^1(0,T; L^2(\Omega))$. Indeed it suffices that

$$\psi \rightarrow \int_Q f\varphi \, dx \, dt$$

be continuous on $L^1(0,T; L^2(\Omega))$. This will be the case, if, for instance, we take $f = f_1 + f_2$, $f_1 \in L^1(0,T; L^2(\Omega))$ and $f_2 \in L^1(0,T; H^{-1}_K(\Omega))$, where $H^{-1}_K(\Omega)$ denotes the space of functions in $H^{-1}(\Omega)$ with support in K, an arbitrary compact set contained in Ω.

Remark 2.2. In all that has been said, one can replace $-\Delta$ by

$$A = -\frac{\partial}{\partial x_i}(a_{ij}(x,t) \frac{\partial}{\partial x_j}) \,, \tag{2.23}$$

where

$$\left\{ \begin{aligned} a_{ij} &= a_{ji} \in C^1(\overline{Q}) \,, \\ a_{ij}(x,t)\xi_i\xi_j &\geq \alpha \, \xi_i\xi_i \,, \quad \alpha > 0, \quad \forall \, \xi_i \in \mathbf{R}, \quad \forall \, x, t \in Q \,. \end{aligned} \right. \tag{2.24}$$

REFERENCES

Govorov, V.M. [1]. 1982. The initial-boundary value problem for a hyperbolic equation with boundary function in L^2. *Soviet Math. Doklady* 25, no. 1:158–62. (English transl.)

Lions, J.L. [1]. *Contrôle des systèmes distribués singuliers*. Paris: Gauthier Villars, 1983.

Lions, J.L., and E. Magenes [1]. *Problèmes aux limites nonhomogènes et applications*. Vol. 1, 2. Paris: Dunod, 1968.

Marchuk, G.I. [1]. *Methods of Numerical Mathematics*. New York Berlin Heidelberg Tokyo: Springer–Verlag, 1975.

METHOD OF FICTITIOUS COMPONENTS AND THE ALTERNATING-SUBDOMAINS METHOD

A.M. Matsokin
Computing Center
Siberian Branch of the USSR Academy of Sciences
Novosibirsk, USSR

The method of fictitious components as an iterative technique for solving systems of finite–difference or finite–element equations was suggested and investigated, for example, in [1]–[6]. This method may be considered as the finale of the method of fictitious domains [7]. One variant of the method of fictitious components is presented in this paper, the formulation of which is the same for elliptic boundary value problems and for their finite–element approximations [5], [8]. It should be noted that a special variant of the well–known Schwarz alternating–subdomain method is dual to the method of fictitious components [5], [8], [9]. The investigation of these methods in subspaces plays an important role in proving and implementing the finite–dimensional analogs of these methods [10].

1. The method of fictitious components

The concept of the fictitious–components method can be illustrated as follows. Let Ω_0, Ω_1 and Ω_2 be some bounded domains in $\mathbf{R}^n$, $n \geq 1$, such that

$$\overline{\Omega}_0 = \overline{\Omega}_1 \cup \overline{\Omega}_2 , \qquad \Omega_1 \cap \Omega_2 = \{\emptyset\} ,$$

$$\Omega_0 \supset \overline{\Omega}_1 , \quad \Gamma = \partial\Omega_0 , \quad S = \partial\Omega_1 ,$$

$$S \cup \Gamma = \partial\Omega_2 .$$

We shall denote by $\partial u(x)/\partial n_i$ the derivative of the function $u(x)$ in the direction n_i of the outward normal to $\partial\Omega_i$ at $x \in \partial\Omega_i$, $i = 0,1,2$. Let us consider the boundary value problems

$$\begin{aligned} -\Delta u_1(x) + u_1(x) &= f_1(x) , \quad x \in \Omega_1 , \\ u_1(x) &= 0 , \quad x \in S , \end{aligned} \tag{1.1}$$

and

$$-\Delta u_2(x) + u_2(x) = f_2(x)\,, \quad x \in \Omega_2\,,$$
$$\frac{\partial u_2(x)}{\partial n_2} = 0\,, \quad x \in S \cup \Gamma\,, \tag{1.2}$$

where $f_i(x) \in L_2(\Omega_i)$, $i = 1,2$, are some functions. For given $g_i(x) \in L_2(\Omega_i)$, $i = 1,2$, we will also consider the following problem:

$$-\Delta v_1(x) + v_1(x) = g_1(x)\,, \quad x \in \Omega_1\,,$$
$$-\Delta v_2(x) + v_2(x) = g_2(x)\,, \quad x \in \Omega_2\,,$$
$$v_1(x) = v_2(x)\,, \quad x \in S\,, \tag{1.3}$$
$$\frac{\partial v_2(x)}{\partial n_2} = 0\,, \quad x \in S \cup \Gamma\,.$$

We assume that the solution $u_1(x)$ of the problem (1.1) and the solution $v_1(x)$, $v_2(x)$ of (1.3) exist and are sufficiently smooth if

$$g_1(x) = f_1(x)\,, \quad g_2(x) \equiv 0\,; \tag{1.4}$$

therefore

$$v_2(x) \equiv 0\,, \quad v_1(x) = u_1(x)\,.$$

Similarly, for

$$g_2(x) = f_2(x) \tag{1.5}$$

we immediately obtain $v_2(x) = u_2(x)$, $x \in \Omega_2$ for any $g_1(x) \in L_2(\Omega_1)$, where $u_2(x)$ is the solution of the problem (1.2). Hence, to solve the problem (1.1) or (1.2) it is sufficient to find the solution of the problem (1.3), the right side of which is defined by (1.4) or (1.5).

Let $v(x)$ be any smooth function defined on Ω_0, for example, $v(x)$ belongs to a Sobolev space $W_2^1(\Omega_0)$. Multiplying the first two equations in (1.3) by the function $v(x)$ and integrating by parts (we assume that it is possible to do), we obtain the following identities:

$$\int_{\Omega_1} (\nabla v_1 \nabla v + v_1 v)dx = \int_S \frac{\partial v_1}{\partial n_1} v\, dS + \int_{\Omega_1} g_1 v\, dx\,, \tag{1.6}$$

$$\int_{\Omega_2} (\nabla v_2 \nabla v + v_2 v)dx = \int_{\Omega_2} g_2 v\, dx\,. \tag{1.7}$$

Since the solution $v_2(x)$ of (1.3) belongs to the Sobolev space $W_2^1(\Omega_2)$, and $v_1(x)$ is an extension of the function $v_2(x)$ to the subdomain Ω_1, we assume that the function

$$u(x) = \begin{cases} v_1(x), & x \in \Omega_1, \\ v_2(x), & x \in \Omega_2, \end{cases} \tag{1.8}$$

belongs to the Sobolev space $H = W_2^1(\Omega_0)$. Let

$$\begin{aligned} (u,v)_i &= \int_{\Omega_i} (\nabla u \nabla v + uv)\, dx, \quad i = 1,2, \\ (u,v) &= (u,v)_1 + (u,v)_2, \\ g_i(v) &= \int_{\Omega_i} g_i(x) v(x)\, dx, \quad i = 1,2. \end{aligned} \tag{1.9}$$

Then it follows from (1.6) and (1.7) that the solution $u(x) \in H$ of (1.3) satisfies the integral identity

$$(u,v) = (u,v)_1 + g_2(v) \quad \forall\, v \in H. \tag{1.10}$$

Now, using (1.10), the following iterative process can be suggested for (1.3):

$$\begin{aligned} u^0 \in H:\ (u^0,v) &= g_1(v) + g_2(v) \quad \forall\, v \in H, \\ u^k \in H:\ (u^k,v) &= (u^{k-1},v)_1 + g_2(v) \quad \forall\, v \in H,\ k = 1,2,\ldots \end{aligned} \tag{1.11}$$

Theorem 1. *If for any $v \in H$ there exists $v_i^* \in H$ such that*

$$\begin{aligned} v_i^*(x) &= v(x), \quad x \in \Omega_i, \\ \alpha(v_i^*,v_i^*) &\le (v,v)_i, \quad i = 1,2, \end{aligned} \tag{1.12}$$

where $\alpha > 0$ is independent of v and v_i^*, then the sequence u^k, $k = 0,1,\ldots$, of the method of fictitious components (1.11) *converges to $u^* \in H$ satisfying the integral identity* (1.10) *and the identity*

$$(u^*,v) = g_1(v) \quad \forall\, v \in H, \quad v = 0 \text{ in } \Omega_2. \tag{1.13}$$

The validity of this theorem readily follows from Theorem 2.

The integral identity (1.10) can be written as

$$(u,v) = (u,v) - \tau[(u,v)_2 - g_2(v)],$$

so that the iterative process (1.11) coincides with the following method of fictitious components:

$$\begin{aligned} w^0 \in H: \quad (w^0,v) &= g_1(v) + g_2(v) \quad \forall\, v \in H\,, \\ w^k \in H: \quad (w^k,v) &= (w^{k-1},v) - \tau_k\,[(w^{k-1},v)_2 - g_2(v)]\,, \\ &\quad \forall\, v \in H, \quad k = 1,2,\ldots\,, \end{aligned} \tag{1.14}$$

where $\tau_k = 1$, $k = 1,2,\ldots$.

Theorem 2. *If* (1.12) *is valid then the sequence* $\{w^k\}$ *of the method of fictitious components* (1.14) *with* $\tau_k = \tau$ *for any* $\tau \in (0,2)$ *converges to* $u^* \in H$ *satisfying integral identities* (1.10) *and* (1.13).

The proof of this theorem will be given in the next section.

We note that it is necessary to solve the boundary value problem for the domain Ω_0 at every step of the method of fictitious components. Also, if the latter is applied to solving (1.1), then Dirichlet boundary conditions can be imposed on $\Gamma = \partial\Omega_0$. Similarly, if it is necessary to solve the problem with natural boundary conditions for the domain Ω_1, then both forced and natural boundary conditions can be imposed on $\Gamma = \partial\Omega_0$ in constructing the method of fictitious components.

2. Convergence of the method of fictitious components

Before investigating the convergence of the method of fictitious components (1.11) or (1.14), let us formally define the problem in Hilbert space H, to the solution of which the sequence $\{w^k\}$ of this method converges when $k \to \infty$. Let H_0, H_1 and H_{0i}, $i = 1,2$, be closed subspaces of H mutually orthogonal in scalar product (u,v) in H, and such that

$$H = H_0 + H_1\,, \qquad H_0 = H_{01} + H_{02}\,. \tag{2.1}$$

For the examples considered in section 1 these subspaces can be defined by

$$\begin{aligned} H &= W_2^1(\Omega_0)\,, \\ H_0 &= \{u \in H:\ u(x) = 0,\ x \in S\}\,, \\ H_1 &= \{u \in H:\ (u,v) = 0,\ \forall\, v \in H\}\,, \\ H_{0i} &= \{u \in H_0:\ u(x) = 0,\ x \in \Omega_{3-i}\}\,,\ i = 1,2\,. \end{aligned} \tag{2.2}$$

Here H_{0i} is a set of functions of $\overset{\circ}{W}{}_2^1(\Omega_i)$ continued by zero outside the domain Ω_i, $i = 1,2$, and in this case the validity of conditions (2.1) depends on the smoothness of the boundaries of domains Ω_0, Ω_1 and Ω_2.

Let us assume that continuous bilinear forms $(u,v)_i$ and linear functionals $g_i(v)$, $i = 1,2$, are given in H and satisfy the conditions:

$$\left|\begin{array}{lll} (u,u)_i & \geq 0 & \forall\, u \in H\,, \\ (u,v)_i & = \overline{(v,u)}_i & \forall\, u,v \in H\,, \\ (u,v)_i & = 0 & \forall\, u,v \in H_{0\,3-i}\,; \quad \forall\, u \in H_0,\, v \in H_1\,; \\ & & \forall\, u \in H_{0i},\, v \in H_{0\,3-i}\,; \end{array}\right. \tag{2.3}$$

$$\left|\begin{array}{l} (u,v) = (u,v)_1 + (u,v)_2\,, \quad \forall\, u,v \in H\,, \\ \alpha_i(u,u) \leq (u,u)_i \leq \beta_i(u,u) \quad \forall\, u \in H_1\,, \end{array}\right. \tag{2.4}$$

$$g_i(v) = 0 \quad \forall\, v \in H_{0\;3-i}\,, \quad i = 1,2\,, \tag{2.5}$$

where α_i and β_i are positive constants and $\beta_i \leq 1$.

It is easy to see that the bilinear forms and linear functionals (1.9) satisfy (2.3)–(2.5) if Hilbert space H and its subspaces H_0, H_1 and H_{0i}, $i = 1,2$, are defined by (2.2).

Projections of any element $v \in H$ onto subspaces H_0, H_{01}, H_{02} and H_1 will be denoted by v_0, v_{01}, v_{02} and v_1, so that:

$$\begin{array}{l} v = v_0 + v_1\,, \quad v_0 \in H_0,\; v_1 \in H_1\,, \\ v_0 = v_{01} + v_{02}\,, \quad v_{01} \in H_{01},\; v_{02} \in H_{02}\,. \end{array} \tag{2.6}$$

Let us consider the following problem for $u^* \in H$:

$$(u^*,v)_2 = g_2(v) \quad \forall\, v \in H\,, \tag{2.7}$$

$$(u^*,v)_1 = g_1(v) \quad \forall\, v \in H_{01}\,. \tag{2.8}$$

For the examples considered in the previous section, (2.7) is the weak form of (1.2) with natural boundary conditions, and (2.8) is the weak form of (1.1), the forced boundary conditions of which are defined by the solution of (2.7).

Lemma 1. *If the conditions* (2.1), (2.3)–(2.5) *are valid, then there exists a unique element* $w_1 \in H_1$ *and a unique element* $w_{02} \in H_{02}$, *such that* $w \in H$,

$$w = w_1 + w_{02} + w_{01}\,, \tag{2.9}$$

is the solution of (2.7) *for every* $w_{01} \in H_{01}$. *There are no other solutions of* (2.7).

P r o o f. Using (2.6) and conditions (2.3)–(2.5), it is easy to show that

$$(u,v)_2 = (u_1,v_1)_2 + (u_{02},v_{02})_2 \quad \forall\, u,v \in H\,,$$

$$\alpha_2(u,u) \leq (u,u)_2 \leq (u,u) \quad \forall\, u \in H_1 + H_{02}\,,$$

$$g_2(v) = g_2(v_1+v_{02}) \quad \forall\, v \in H.$$

Therefore the problem

$$u \in H_1 + H_{02}\colon\ (u,v)_2 = g_2(v) \quad \forall\, v \in H_1 + H_{02}$$

has the unique solution

$$u = w_1 + w_{02}\,, \quad w_1 \in H_1,\ w_{02} \in H_{02}\,, \tag{2.10}$$

which is also the solution of (2.7). Since the decomposition (2.10) of the element $u \in H_1+H_{02}$ is unique and

$$(w_{01},v)_2 = 0\,, \quad \forall\, w_{01} \in H_{01},\ v \in H\,,$$

the first proposition of the lemma is proved.

Let z and y be any solutions of (2.7). Then their difference $v = z-y$ satisfies

$$0 = (v,v)_2 \geq \alpha_2[(v_1,v_1)+(v_{02},v_{02})] \geq 0\,.$$

Hence $z_1 = y_1$, $z_{02} = y_{02}$, and the projections of the solutions of (2.7) onto subspaces H_1 and H_{02} are unique and are defined by (2.9).

The lemma is proved.

Lemma 2. *If the conditions* (2.1), (2.3)–(2.5) *are valid, then there exists a unique element* $z_{01} \in H_{01}$ *such that* $z \in H$,

$$z = z_{01} + z_{02} + z_1\,, \tag{2.11}$$

is the solution of (2.8) *for every* $z_{02} \in H_{02}$ *and* $z_1 \in H_1$. *There are no other solutions of* (2.8).

The proof is similar to that of Lemma 1.

Theorem 3. *If the conditions* (2.1), (2.3)–(2.5) *are valid, then there exists the unique solution* u^* *of* (2.7)–(2.8),

$$u^* = \overset{*}{u}_{01} + \overset{*}{u}_{02} + \overset{*}{u}_1 = z_{01} + w_{02} + w_1 , \tag{2.12}$$

where $\overset{*}{u}_{01} = z_{01} \in H_{01}$ *is the component of the decomposition* (2.11) *and* $\overset{*}{u}_{02} = w_{02} \in H_{02}$, $\overset{*}{u}_1 = w_1 \in H_1$ *are components of the decomposition* (2.9).

The validity of Theorem 3 follows directly from Lemmas 1 and 2 since the intersection of sets of solutions of (2.7)–(2.8) is the single point defined by (2.12). Note that in order to solve (2.7)–(2.8) it is sufficient to find the element $u^* \in H$ satisfying the identities (1.10) and (1.13). Hence, if the solution of (1.3), $u(x) = (v_1(x),v_2(x))$, belongs to the Sobolev space $H = W_2^1(\Omega_0)$, then it is the solution of (2.7)–(2.8).

Theorem 4. *If the conditions* (2.1), (2.3)–(2.5) *are valid, the sequence* $\{w^k\}$ *of the method of fictitious components* (1.14),

$$\begin{aligned} w^0 \in H:\ (w^0,v) &= g_1(v) + g_2(v) \quad \forall\, v \in H , \\ w^k \in H:\ (w^k,v) &= (w^{k-1},v) - \tau[(w^{k-1},v)_2 - g_2(v)] \\ &\qquad \forall\, v \in H,\ k = 1,2,\dots , \end{aligned} \tag{2.13}$$

converges to the solution $u^* \in H$ *of the problem* (2.7)–(2.8) *for every* $\tau \in (0,2)$, *the error* $\psi^k = u^k - u^*$ *belongs to the subspace* H_1, *and the following estimate holds*:

$$\|\psi^k\|^2 = (\psi^k,\psi^k) \le q^{2k}\ \|\psi^0\|^2, \quad k = 1,2,\dots , \tag{2.14}$$

where $q = \max\{|1-\tau\alpha_2|,\ |1-\tau|\} < 1$, *and the constant* $\alpha_2 \in (0,1]$ *is that from inequalities* (2.4).

P r o o f. First we need to prove that $\psi^k \in H_1$ for $k = 0,1,2,\dots$. Indeed, it follows from (2.13) and 2.3 that

$$(w^0_{0i},v) = (w^0_{0i},v)_i = g_i(v) \quad \forall\, v \in H_{0i},\ i = 1,2 ,$$

and using Lemmas 1–3 we obtain

$$w^0_{0i} = w_{0i} = u^*_{0i} ,\ i = 1,2 .$$

Suppose that $w^k_{0i} = u^*_{0i}$, $i = 1,2$ for all $k \ge m$ and let $k = m + 1$. From (2.13), (2.3) and the previous assumption we have that

$$(w^{m+1}_{0\,i},v) = (w^m_{0\,i},v) = (\overset{*}{u}_{0i},v) \quad \forall\, v \in H_{0i} ,\quad i = 1,2 ,$$

so that $w^{m+1}_{0\,i} = \overset{*}{u}_{0i}$, $i = 1,2$, for every m, and $\psi^k = w^k - u^* = (w_1^k - \overset{*}{u}_1) \in H_1$. It is obvious that the sequence $\{\psi^k\}$ is defined:

$$(\psi^k,v) = (\psi^{k-1},v) - \tau(\psi^{k-1},v)_2 \quad \forall\, v \in H_1,\ k = 1,2,\dots . \tag{2.15}$$

It follows from (2.4) that the bilinear form $(\psi,v)_2$ defines the self–adjoint linear operator A_2 from H_1 in H_1:

$$\begin{aligned} (\psi,v)_2 &= (A_2\psi,v) \quad \forall\, \psi, v \in H_1 , \\ \alpha_2(\psi,\psi) \le (A_2\psi,\psi) &\le (\psi,\psi) \quad \forall\, \psi \in H_1 . \end{aligned} \tag{2.16}$$

Then the iterative process (2.15) can be written as

$$\psi^k = (E-\tau A_2)\psi^{k-1} = T\psi^{k-1} .$$

Here E is the identity operator in H_1, the operator $T = E-\tau A_2$ is linear self–adjoint, and

$$(1-\tau)(\psi,\psi) \le (T\psi,\psi) \le (1-\tau\alpha_2)(\psi,\psi) \quad \forall\, \psi \in H_1 .$$

Hence [11]

$$\|T\| = \sup_{\psi \in H_1} \frac{\|T\psi\|}{\|\psi\|} \le \max\{|1-\tau|, |1-\tau\cdot\alpha_2|\} = q .$$

It is clear that if $\tau \in (0,2)$, then $q < 1$ so that the method of fictitious components converges and

$$\|\psi^k\| \le \|T\| \cdot \|\psi^{k-1}\| \le q^k \|\psi^0\|, \qquad k = 1,2,\dots .$$

Theorem 4 is proved.

Since the operator A_2 which is defined by the identity (2.16) is self–adjoint and strictly positive definite in H_1, the convergence of the method of fictitious components can be improved by the proper choice of the parameter $\tau = \tau_k$ at every step of the process (2.13).

Theorem 5. *If the conditions* (2.1), (2.3)–(2.5) *are valid, then the sequence* u^k, $k = 0,1,2,\dots$, *of the method of fictitious components*

$$\left\{ \begin{aligned} & u^0 \in H\colon\ (u^0,v) = g_1(v) + g_2(v) \quad \forall\, v \in H , \\ & u^k \in H\colon\ (u^k,v) = (u^{k-1},v) - \tau_k[(u^{k-1},v)_2 - g_2(v)] \quad \forall\, v \in H , \end{aligned} \right. \tag{2.17}$$

$$\left\{ \begin{aligned} & \tau_k = \frac{(\psi^{k-1},\xi^{k-1})_2}{(\xi^{k-1},\xi^{k-1})_2} = \frac{(\xi^{k-1},\xi^{k-1})}{(\xi^{k-1},\xi^{k-1})_2} , \\ & \xi^k = A_2\psi^k \in H_1 , \quad k = 1,2,\dots , \end{aligned} \right. \tag{2.18}$$

converges to the solution $u^* \in H$ *of the problem* (2.7)–(2.8).

Theorems 1 and 2 formulated in the previous section follow from Theorem 4 if the conditions (2.1), (2.3)–(2.5) hold for the spaces H, H_{i-1} and H_{0i}, $i = 1,2$, defined by (2.2). In order to prove this, it suffices to show that from (1.12), i.e., from

$$\forall\, v \in H \;\exists\, v_i^* \in H\colon\; (v - v_i^*, z) = 0 \quad \forall\, z \in H_1 + H_{0i}\,,$$

$$(v,v)_i \geq \alpha\cdot(v_i^*, v_i^*)\,, \quad i = 1,2\,,$$

we have (2.4). If

$$v = v_{01} + v_{02} + v_1,$$

then v_i^* can be defined by

$$v_i^* = v_1 + v_{0i}\,, \quad i = 1,2\,,$$

and (2.4) follows with $\alpha_1 = \alpha_2 = \alpha$, $\beta_1 = \beta_2 = 1$.

3. Alternating-subdomains method

The Schwarz alternating–subdomains method is dual to the method of fictitious components. It consists in construction of an iterative process for solution of boundary value problems in the domain Ω_0, at every step of which it is necessary to solve boundary value problems (2.7) and (2.8) for the nonintersecting subdomains Ω_2 and Ω_1 such that $\overline{\Omega}_0 = \overline{\Omega}_1 \cup \overline{\Omega}_2$. Let us formulate this method, assuming that conditions (2.1), (2.3)–(2.5) are valid, and using the notation of the previous section.

Let $g(v)$ be some linear functional in H. Consider the following problem:

$$u^* \in H\colon\; (u^*, v) = g(v) \quad \forall\, v \in H \tag{3.1}$$

and the iterative process

$$u^0 \in H_0\colon\; (u^0, v)_i = g(v) \quad \forall\, v \in H_{0i},\; i = 1,2\,, \tag{3.2}$$

$$u^k \in H\colon\; (u^k, v)_2 = g_2^{(k)}(v) \quad \forall\, v \in H\,, \tag{3.3}$$

$$(u^k, v)_1 = g_1^{(k)}(v) \quad \forall\, v \in H_{01}\,, \tag{3.4}$$

$$\left\{\begin{aligned} g_2^{(k)}(v) &= (u^{k-1}, v)_2 - \tau[(u^{k-1}, v) - g(v)]\,,\\ g_1^{(k)}(v) &= (u^{k-1}, v)_1\,, \quad k = 1,2,\ldots\,. \end{aligned}\right. \tag{3.5}$$

Lemma 3. *If the conditions* (2.1), (2.3)–(2.5) *are valid, then there exists a unique sequence* u^k, $k = 0,1,\dots$, *of the alternating–subdomains method* (3.2)–(3.5).

Proof. Since $g(v)$ is a linear functional and

$$(u,v)_i = (u,v) \quad \forall\, u,v \in H_{0i}, \quad i = 1,2 ,$$

there exists a unique solution u^0 of (3.2). Hence the linear functionals $g_2^{(k)}(v)$ and $g_1^{(k)}(v)$ are defined in H and H_{01}, and

$$g_1^{(k)}(v) = g(v) \quad \forall\, v \in H_{01} , \quad k = 1 . \tag{3.6}$$

Furthermore, it follows from (2.3) that

$$g_2^{(k)}(v) = -\tau[(u^{k-1},v)_1 - g(v)] = 0 \quad \forall\, v \in H_{01}, \quad k = 1. \tag{3.7}$$

Theorem 3 implies that (3.3)–(3.4) has the unique solution $u^k \in H$ for k=1. Assuming that the properties which hold for k=1 hold also for $k \le m$ and repeating the preceding considerations, we obtain that for every $k \ge 1$, (3.6) and (3.7) are valid and (3.3)–(3.4) has a unique solution. The lemma is proved.

Theorem 6. *If the conditions* (2.1), (2.3)–(2.5) *are valid, then the sequence* u^k, $k = 0,1,\dots$, *of the alternating–subdomains method converges to the solution* $u^* \in H$ *of* (3.1) *for any* $\tau \in (0,2\alpha_2)$, *where* α_2 *is defined by* (2.4) *and the error* $\psi^k = u^k - u^*$ *belongs to subspace* H_1. *Moreover, the following estimate holds*

$$(\psi^k,\psi^k) \le cq^{2k}(\psi^0,\psi^0) , \quad k = 1,2,\dots ;$$

where constant c *is independent of* τ, *and* $q = q(\tau) < 1$.

Proof. Existence and uniqueness of the sequence $\{u^k\}$ follows from Lemma 3. It is easy to see that for $i = 1, 2$

$$(u^0,v)_i = (u^k,v)_i = (u^*,v)_i = g(v) \quad \forall\, v \in H_{0i} ,$$

hence

$$\begin{aligned} u^0_{0i} &= u^k_{0i} = \overset{*}{u}_{0i} \in H_{0i} , \quad i = 1, 2 , \\ u^0 &= \overset{*}{u}_{01} + \overset{*}{u}_{02} , \\ \psi^k &= u^k - u^* = (\overset{k}{u}_1 - \overset{*}{u}_1) \in H_1 , \\ (\psi^k,v)_2 &= (\psi^{k-1},v)_2 - \tau(\psi^k,v) \quad \forall\, v \in H_1 , \; k = 1,2,\dots . \end{aligned} \tag{3.8}$$

By the definition (2.16) of the operator A_2, (3.8) can be written as

$$A_2\psi^k = A_2\psi^{k-1} - \tau\psi^{k-1} = T\psi^{k-1}, \quad k \geq 1,$$

or

$$\psi^k = A_2^{-1}T\psi^{k-1} = \tilde{T}\psi^{k-1}, \quad k \geq 1. \tag{3.9}$$

Define the following inner product and the norm in H_1:

$$(\psi,v)_2 = (A_2\psi,v) \quad \forall\, \psi,v \in H_1,$$

$$\|\psi\|_2 = ((\psi,\psi)_2)^{1/2} \quad \forall\, \psi \in H_1.$$

Then the operator $\tilde{T}$ is self-adjoint in H_1 with respect to this inner product, and from (2.4) we have

$$(1 - \frac{\tau}{\alpha_2}) \cdot (\psi,\psi)_2 \leq (\tilde{T}\psi,\psi)_2 \leq (1 - \tau) \cdot (\psi,\psi)_2 \quad \forall\, \psi \in H_1.$$

Therefore

$$\|\tilde{T}\|_2 \leq \max\,\{|1 - \tau|, |1 - \frac{\tau}{\alpha_2}|\} = q$$

and $q < 1$, if $\tau \in (0,2\alpha_2)$, for $0 < \alpha_2 \leq 1$. Then from (3.9) and (2.4) it is easy to obtain the following estimates:

$$\sqrt{\alpha_2}\ \|\psi^k\| \leq \|\psi^k\|_2 \leq q^k\|\psi^0\|_2 \leq q^k\|\psi^0\|, \quad k \geq 1, \tag{3.10}$$

and since $q < 1$, we have $\psi^k \to 0$ or $u^k \to u^*$ i+ H as $k \to \infty$.

The theorem is proved.

In fact, solution of the problem (3.3)–(3.4) is equivalent to solution of the following two problems:

$$z \in H_1 + H_{02}:\ (z,v)_2 = g_2^{(k)}(v) \quad \forall\, v \in H_1 + H_{02},$$

$$y \in H_{01}:\ (y,v)_1 = g_1^{(k)}(v) - (z,v)_1 \quad \forall\, v \in H_{01},$$

$$u^k = z + y, \quad k = 1,2,\ldots.$$

Hence the alternating–subdomains method can also be called the alternating–subspaces method with respect to subspaces $V_1 = H_{01}$ and $V_2 = H_1 + H_{02}$.

The alternating–subspaces method can be formulated for the case when the subspaces are not orthogonal complements of each other. Let V_i, $i = 1,\ldots,m$, be some closed subspaces of the Hilbert space H:

$$H = V_1 + V_2 + \ldots + V_m. \tag{3.11}$$

Let us assume that for every element $v \in H$ there exist $\overline{v}_i \in V_i$ such that

$$v = \overline{v}_1 + \overline{v}_2 + \dots + \overline{v}_m\ , \quad (\overline{v}_i,\overline{v}_i) \le \gamma\cdot(v,v)\ , \quad i = 1,\dots,m\ , \tag{3.12}$$

with constant γ independent of v. Assume in addition that some continuous bilinear forms $(u,v)_i$ are given:

$$\begin{gathered}(u,v)_i = \overline{(v,u)}_i \quad \forall\, u,v \in V_i\ ,\\ \alpha\cdot(u,u) \le (u,u)_i \le \beta(u,u) \quad \forall\, u \in V_i\ ,\ i = 1,\dots,m,\end{gathered} \tag{3.13}$$

where α and β are some positive constants. Consider the iterative process:

$$\begin{gathered}u^k \in H:\ u^k = u^{k-1} - \tau\sum_{i=1}^{m} z_i^k\ ,\\ z_i^k \in V_i:\ (z_i^k,v)_i = (u^{k-1},v) - g(v) \quad \forall\, v \in V_i\ ,\\ i = 1,\dots,m\ , \quad k = 1,2,\dots\ ,\end{gathered} \tag{3.14}$$

where $u^0 \in H$ is given and $g(v)$ is some linear functional.

Denote by $V_i^{\perp}$ the orthogonal supplement of the subspace V_i to H:

$$\forall\, v \in H\ \exists\, v_i \in V_i,\ v_i^{\perp} \in V_i^{\perp}:\ v = v_i + v_i^{\perp}\ , \quad i = 1,\dots,m\ . \tag{3.15}$$

Define the operators R_i and B_i:

$$\begin{gathered}(R_iu,v) = (u_i,v_i) \quad \forall\, u,v \in H\ ,\\ (B_iu,v) = (u,v)_i \quad \forall\, u,v \in V_i\ ,\ i = 1,\dots,m\ .\end{gathered} \tag{3.16}$$

It is easy to see that R_i is the operator of orthogonal projection on V_i, and B_i is a linear self–adjoint continuous operator from V_i into V_i, $i = 1,\dots,m$. Also, it follows from (3.13) [11] that the norm of the operator B_i^{-1} is estimated by $1/\alpha$. Let us define the operators B_i^{+} and B:

$$\begin{gathered}B_i^{+} = B_i^{-1}R_i = R_iB_i^{-1}R_i\ , \quad i = 1,\dots,m\ ,\\ B = B_1^{+} + B_2^{+} + \dots + B_m^{+}\ .\end{gathered} \tag{3.17}$$

From properties of R_i and B_i, it follows that B_i^{+} is a linear continuous and self–adjoint operator from H into H and its norm is less than or equal to $1/\alpha$. Furthermore, the elements z_i^k from (3.14) are given by

$$z_i^k = B_i^{+}(u^{k-1} - g)\ ,$$

where $g \in H$ satisfies $g(v) = (g,v)$. Hence, the alternating–subspaces method (3.14) can be written as

$$u^k = u^{k-1} - \tau B(u^{k-1} - g) , \quad u^0 \in H , \quad k = 1,2,\ldots . \tag{3.18}$$

Theorem 7. *If the conditions* (3.11)–(3.13) *are valid the alternating–subspaces method* (3.14) or (3.18) *converges to the solution of the problem* (3.1) *for every* $\tau \in (0, 2\alpha/m)$, *and the error* $\psi^k = u^k - u^*$ *is estimated by*

$$(\psi^k,\psi^k) \leq q^{2k}(\psi^0,\psi^0) , \quad k \geq 1 \quad (u^* = g) ,$$

with $q = q(\tau,\alpha,\gamma,\beta,m) < 1$.

P r o o f. First let us estimate the supremum and infimum of the quadratic functional (Bv,v). It follows from (3.13) and (3.17) that for every $v \in H$

$$\frac{m}{\alpha}(v,v) \geq (Bv,v) = \sum_{i=1}^{m} (B_i^{-1}R_iv,R_iv) \geq \frac{1}{\beta}\sum_{i=1}^{m} (R_iv,v) . \tag{3.19}$$

Let u be an arbitrary element of H, let $\ell(v) = (u,v)$ be some linear functional in H, and let

$$\ell_i(v) = (R_iu,v) = (R_iu,R_iv) = (u,v) = \ell(v) \ \forall\ v \in V_i,\ i = 1,\ldots,m$$

be linear functionals in V_i. The norms of these functionals as elements of dual spaces are defined by

$$\|\ell\|_{H'} = \sqrt{(u,u)} , \qquad \|\ell_i\|_{V_i'} = \sqrt{(R_iu,R_iu)} ,\ i = 1,\ldots,m .$$

Let us estimate the norm of the functional ℓ. For any v, by (3.12) we have for $\ell(v)$:

$$\begin{aligned} |\ell(v)| &= |\ell(\overline{v}_1) + \ldots + \ell(\overline{v}_m)| = |\ell_1(\overline{v}_1) + \ldots + \ell_m(\overline{v}_m)| \\ &\leq [\|\ell_1\|_{V_1'} \cdot \|\overline{v}_m\| + \ldots + \|\ell_m\|_{V_m'} \cdot \|\overline{v}_m\|] \\ &\leq \sqrt{\gamma}\cdot(\|\ell_1\|_{V_m'} + \ldots + \|\ell_m\|_{V_m'}) \cdot \|v\| . \end{aligned}$$

Therefore

$$\|\ell\|_{H'} \leq \sqrt{\gamma}\cdot(\|\ell_1\|_{V_1'} + \ldots + \|\ell_m\|_{V_m'}) ,$$

i.e.,

$$(u,u) \leq \gamma\,[\sum_{i=1}^{m}(R_iu,R_iu)^{1/2}]^2 \leq \gamma \cdot m^2 \sum_{i=1}^{m}(R_iu,R_iu) . \tag{3.20}$$

By (3.20) and (3.19) we now obtain

$$(Bv,v) \geq (m^2\gamma\beta)^{-1} \cdot (v,v) \quad \forall\, v \in H\,. \tag{3.21}$$

Since the solution of (3.1) satisfies

$$u^* = u^* - \tau B(u^*-g),$$

we have

$$\psi^k = \psi^{k-1} - \tau B\psi^{k-1} = T\psi^{k-1}\,, \quad k \geq 1\,.$$

Since the operator T is self–adjoint and inequalities (3.19), (3.21) hold, we have

$$\|T\| \leq \max\{|1 - \frac{\tau m}{\alpha}|, |1 - \frac{\tau}{m^2\gamma\beta}|\} = q < 1$$

for $\tau \in (0,2\alpha/m)$. Hence,

$$\|\psi^k\| \leq \|T\| \cdot \|\psi^{k-1}\| \leq q^k \|\psi^0\| \to 0\,, \quad k \to \infty\,.$$

The theorem is proved.

4. Examples

Let us consider some simple examples illustrating the convergence of the fictitious–components method and the alternating–subspaces method.

Let H be equal to $\overset{\circ}{W}{}^1_2(0,2)$, H_{0i} be the set of functions belonging to H, which are equal to zero at $(2-i,3-i)$, $i = 1,2$, and H_1 be the set of functions $c(1-|1-x|)$, where c is an arbitrary constant. It is clear that these subspaces satisfy (2.1), (2.3)–(2.4) if we define

$$(u,v) = \int_0^2 u'(x)\cdot v'(x)\,dx\,,$$

$$(u,v)_i = \int_{i-2}^{i} u'(x)\cdot v'(x)\,dx \quad \forall\, u,v \in H,\ i = 1,2$$

and set $\alpha_1=\alpha_2=0.5$, $\beta_1=\beta_2=1$.

Example 1. Consider the Dirichlet problem

$$u''(x) = -2\,, \quad x \in (0,1)\,, \quad u(0) = u(1) = 0\,. \tag{4.1}$$

The solution of (4.1) is equal to $u^*(x) = x(1-x)$, and the sequence $\{w^k\}$ of the fictitious–components method (2.13) is defined by

$$w^k(x) \;=\; u^*(x) - [(1-\tau)^k \cdot 2(1-|1-x|)]\,, \quad k = 0,1,\ldots\,; \tag{4.2}$$

if we set $u^*(x) = 0$ for $x \in (1,2)$,

$$g_1(v) \;=\; \int_0^1 2 \cdot v(x)\,dx\,, \quad g_2(v) = 0 \quad \forall\, v \in H\,.$$

It is easy to see that for any $\tau \in (0,2)$ the sequence $\{w^k\}$ converges to u^* and the error $w^k - u^*$ belongs to the subspace H_1, which agrees with Theorem 4.

Example 2. Consider the problem

$$u''(x) = -2\,, \quad x \in (1,2)\,, \quad u'(1) = u(2) = 0\,. \tag{4.3}$$

The solution of (4.3) is equal to $u^*(x) = x(2-x)$, and we set $u^*(x) = x$ on $(0,1)$. Then the sequence $\{w^k\}$ of fictitious–components method (2.13) is defined by

$$w^k(x) \;=\; u^*(x) - [(1-\tau)^k \cdot (1-|1-x|)]\,, \quad k = 0,1,\ldots\,, \tag{4.4}$$

if $g_1(v) = 0$, $g_2(v) = \int_1^2 2\cdot v(x)\,dx$. It is obvious that for any $\tau \in (0,2)$, w^k converges to u^* as $k \to \infty$, and the error $\psi^k = w^k - u^*$ belongs to subspace H_1.

Example 3. Consider the problem

$$u''(x) = -2\,, \quad x \in (0,2)\,, \quad u(0) = u(2) = 0\,. \tag{4.5}$$

The solution of (4.5) is equal to $u^*(x) = x(2-x)$, and it is easy to see that the sequence $\{u^k\}$ of the alternating–subdomains method (3.2)– (3.5) is defined by the following formula:

$$u^k(x) \;=\; u^*(x) - [(1-2\tau)^k \cdot (1-|1-x|)]\,, \quad k = 0,1,\ldots\,, \tag{4.6}$$

if we set $g(v) = \int_0^2 2\cdot v(x)\,dx$.

It follows from (4.6) that u^k converges to u^* for any $\tau \in (0,2\alpha_2) = (0,1)$ and the error $\psi^k = u^k - u^*$ belongs to the subspace H_1.

Example 4. Consider the problem

$$-(pu'(x))' \;=\; g(x)\,, \quad x \in (0,2), \;\; u(0) = u(2) = 0\,,$$

$$g(x) \in L_2(0,2)\,, \quad p(x) \;=\; \begin{cases} 1\,, & x < 1\,, \\ 2\,, & x > 1\,. \end{cases} \tag{4.7}$$

Define in H the inner product (u,v) and bilinear forms $(u,v)_i$ by

$$(u,v) = \int_0^2 p(x)\cdot u'(x)\cdot v'(x)\, dx ,$$

$$(u,v)_1 = \int_0^{1+t} u'(x)\cdot v'(x) dx , \quad (u,v)_2 = \int_{1-t}^{2} u'(x) v'(x) dx ,$$

where $t \in (0,1)$ is fixed. Let

$$V_1 = \{v \in H:\ v(x) = 0,\ x \in (1+t,2)\} ,$$

$$V_2 = \{v \in H:\ v(x) = 0,\ x \in (0,1-t)\} .$$

It is easy to show that $H = V_1+V_2$ and conditions (3.12)–(3.13) are valid for $\gamma = (2+0.75/t)$, $\alpha = 0.5$ and $\beta = 1$. Hence the alternating–subspaces method (3.14) with respect to subspaces V_1 and V_2 can be used for solving (4.7). The initial approximation u^0 of the method (3.14) is selected in special form [12]: $u^0 = z^0 + y^0$, where

$$z^0 \in V_1:\ (z^0,v)_1 = \int_0^{1-t} gv\, dx + \frac{1}{2}\int_{1-t}^{1} gv\, dx + \frac{1}{4}\int_1^{1+t} gv\, dx \quad \forall\, v \in V_1 ,$$

$$y^0 \in V_2:\ (y^0,v)_2 = \frac{1}{2}\int_{1-t}^{1} gv\, dx + \frac{1}{4}\int_1^{1+t} gv\, dx + \frac{1}{2}\int_{1+t}^{2} gv\, dx \quad \forall\, v \in V_2 .$$

Then it is easy to show that the error $\psi^k = u^k - u^*$ of (3.14) is the linear function at segments $(0,1-t)$, $(1-t,1)$, $(1,1+t)$ and $(1+t,2)$, i.e., is defined by the vector $\overline{\psi^k} = (\psi^k(1-t,\psi^k(1),\psi^k(1+t))^{\mathrm{T}}$. Moreover,

$$\overline{\psi^k} = (E-\tau\Lambda)\overline{\psi^{k-1}} , \quad k = 1,2,\ldots ,$$

$$\Lambda = \frac{1}{1+t}\begin{bmatrix} 1+t & 1-t & -2(1-t) \\ -1 & 3(1+t) & -2 \\ -(1-t) & -(1-t) & 2(1+t) \end{bmatrix}$$

and for $t \in (0,1)$ the eigenvalues of the matrix Λ are real and positive. Figure 1 shows the behavior of maximal (solid line) and minimal (broken line) eigenvalues of the matrix Λ as a function of t:

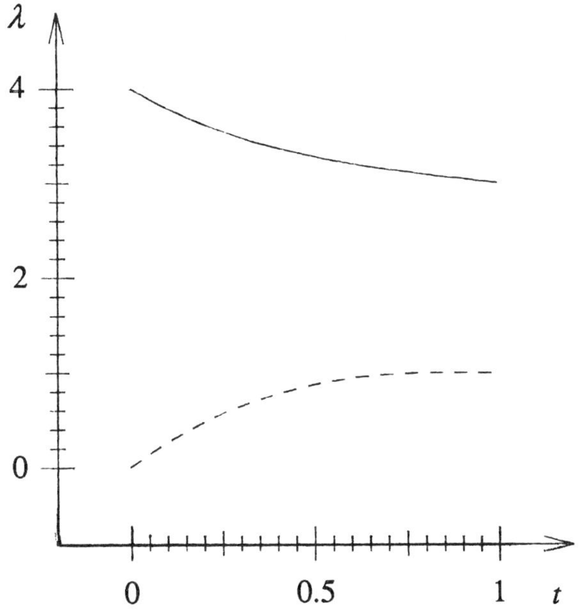

Fig. 1. Bounds of the spectrum

Since for any $t \in (0,1)$ the maximal eigenvalue of the matrix Λ is less than 4, the alternating method converges for any $\tau \in (0,0.5) = (0,2\alpha/m)$. On the other hand, for $t \to 0$ the minimal eigenvalue of Λ tends to zero, so that the convergence rate decreases. But in this case, $\gamma(t) \to \infty$ and therefore this follows also from the proof of Theorem 7.

5. Remarks.

A. The results formulated in sections 2 and 3 are valid also for finite-dimensional problems corresponding to elliptic boundary value problems [5], [6], [8], [9].

B. This method can also be used for investigation of the so-called bordering method [13], the capacitance matrix method [14], both for continuous and discrete cases.

REFERENCES

[1] Marchuk, G.I., and Yu.A. Kuznetsov. 1972. Some problems involving iterative methods (in Russian). In *Vychislitel'nye Metody Linejnoj Algebry*, 4–20. Computing Center of the USSR Academy of Sciences, Siberian Branch, Novosibirsk.

[2] Astrakhantsev, G.P. 1972. Iterative methods for solving variate–difference schemes for two–dimensional second–order elliptic equations (in Russian). Ph.D. diss., LOMI Akademii Nauk SSSR, Leningrad.
[3] Kuznetsov, Yu.A., and A.M. Matsokin. 1974. A matrix analog of the fictitious–domains method (in Russian). Preprint, Computing Center of the USSR Academy of Sciences, Siberian Branch, Novosibirsk.
[4] ————. 1977. On optimization of the method of fictitious components (in Russian). In *Vychislitel'nye Metody Linejnoj Algebry*, 79–86. Computing Center of the USSR Academy of Sciences, Siberian Branch, Novosibirsk.
[5] Matsokin, A.M. 1980. The method of fictitious components and a modified difference analog of the Schwarz method. In *Vychislitel'nye Metody Linejnoj Algebry*, 66–77. Computing Center of the USSR Academy of Sciences, Siberian Branch, Novosibirsk.
[6] Kaporin, I.E., and E.S. Nikolaev. 1980. The method of fictitious unknowns for solving the finite–difference elliptic boundary value problems in irregular domains. *Differential Equations* 16, no. 7: 1211–25.
[7] Saul'ev, B.K. 1963. On the solution of some boundary value problems on high–speed computers by the method of fictitious domains (in Russian). *Sibirskij Matem. Zh.* 4, no. 4: 333–33.
[8] Matsokin, A.M. Forthcoming. On relation between the bordering method, fictitious–component method, and alternating–subdomains method. Paper read at the International Conference on Partial Differential Equations, Novosibirsk, October 1983.
[9] Matsokin, A.M., and S.V. Nepomnyashchikh. 1981. On the convergence of alternating Schwarz method for nonintersecting subdomains (in Russian). In *Metody Interpolyatsii i Approksimatsii*, 85–97. Computing Center of the USSR Academy of Sciences, Siberian Branch, Novosibirsk.
[10] Kuznetsov, Yu.A. 1984. Computational methods in subspaces (in Russian). In *Vychislitel'nye Protsessy i Sistemy*, ed. G.I. Marchuk, vol. 2. Moscow: Nauka.
[11] Riesz, F., and B. Sz–Nady. *Lectures on Functional Analysis*. Budapest: Akad. Kiado, 1952.
[12] Kuznetsov, Yu.A., A.M. Matsokin, and V.V. Shajdurov. Forthcoming. A high–speed iterative method for solving systems of mesh equations (in Russian). In *Dejstvitel'nye Problemy Vychislitel'noj Matematiki*.
[13] Nepomnyashchikh, S.V. On the application of the bordering method to mixed boundary value problems for elliptic equations and on mesh norms in $W_2^{1/2}(S)$. Preprint no. 106. Computing Center of the USSR Academy of Sciences, Siberian Branch, Novosibirsk.
[14] Dryja, M. August 1983. Finite–element–capacitance matrix method for the elliptic problem. *SIAM J. Numer. Anal.* 20, no. 4: 671–80.

OBSTACLE PROBLEMS: DO CONTINUOUS SOLUTIONS EXIST UNDER WILDLY IRREGULAR CONSTRAINTS?

Umberto Mosco
Dipartimento di Matematica
Universita di Roma
Rome, Italy

Introduction

An *obstacle problem* can be formulated in simplest terms as follows: we minimize an "energy" functional of the Dirichlet type

$$E(u) = \int_{\Omega} |Du|^2 \, dx ,$$

Ω being some open region of $\mathbf{R}^n$, under a unilateral constraint

$$u \geq \psi \quad \text{in } \Omega$$

on the solution u and possibly additional boundary conditions on Ω.

Here ψ is a given function, called the *obstacle*; Du denotes the gradient of the function u.

A minimizing u can be seen as a locally optimal configuration of some distributed system in $\mathbf{R}^n$ subject in the region Ω to the constraint $u \geq \psi$, the optimality criterion being of the integral type $E(u)$.

Models of this kind, and more generally the so–called *variational inequalities* (v.i.), of which obstacle problems represent a fundamental example, have been studied in recent years and have a wide range of application, from several free–boundary problems in physics and engineering to optimal control and game theory, to mathematical programming, inventory management and so on. As general references see, for instance [1], [2], [4], [6], [7], [9], [12].

In the present paper we shall be concerned with a particular aspect of the theory: the *regularity*, i.e., smoothness, of minimizing functions, namely their continuity at a given point of the domain.

For the corresponding unconstrained minimization problems, regularity properties and estimates, however technical, are indeed of crucial importance in the applications, as well as in numerical approximation procedures.

With respect to regularity, the obstacle problem has a peculiar feature: the solutions cannot be too regular; for instance, they have no continuous second–order derivatives no matter how smooth the obstacle might be. For simple one–dimensional examples see [9].

Hence, the Euler condition satisfied by a minimizing u, which is the v.i.

$$\min \{u-\psi, -\Delta u\} = 0 \quad \text{in } \Omega ,$$

$\Delta = \Sigma_{i=1}^{m} \partial^2/\partial x_i^2$ being the Laplace operator in $\mathbf{R}^n$, cannot be given a classical pointwise meaning; u can only be a weak solution of the above v.i. in a suitable Sobolev space and $-\Delta u$ a measure in Ω.

It is therefore remarkable that such weak solutions nevertheless possess the weaker regularity property—continuity—for large classes of possibly wildly irregular obstacles ψ. This "regularizing" effect is due to the elliptic nature of our integral–optimality condition $E(u)$.

Special examples of discontinuous obstacles have been known from the classical potential theory. However, our main interest in irregular constraints is of a different nature. It comes from the study of certain quasivariational inequalities (q.v.i.) arising in the dynamic programming approach to some stochastic optimal impulse–control problems; see, for instance, [2], [3], [8], [10].

These q.v.i. have the form of an implicit obstacle problem: the obstacle ψ is not known *ex ante*, as the datum of the problem, but it can only be identified *ex post* once the solution u itself is known, via some mapping $\psi = M(u)$. Furthermore, in the control problems mentioned above this map M converts the weak solution u in an *a priori* discontinuous ψ.

It is worthwhile also to mention, incidentally, that similar "circularities" between solution and constraints occur in many other cases of implicit optimization, for example, Nash equilibria, implicit complementarity systems, and so on.

It is remarkable that a vast class of problems of this type can be dealt with in a unified abstract framework by combining variational and fixed–point techniques. We refer to [4], [5], [13] for more details.

In section 1 below we formulate our problem more precisely. In section 2 we state a qualitative continuity result at the so–called Wiener points of the obstacle, and in section 3 we give an estimate of the modulus of continuity of u in terms of the Wiener modulus of the obstacle. For application to impulse control we refer to [3], [8].

More general results of this type have been presented in [14], which are based on an analogue of the Saint–Venant principle of elasticity theory; see, for instance [15].

1. The local minimizing functions

We are given a function

$$\psi\colon\ \mathbf{R}^n \to [-\infty,\infty) \tag{1}$$

which is assumed to be defined up to sets of capacity zero in $\mathbf{R}^n$ (c.a.e.).

We fix a point

$$x_0 \in \mathbf{R}^n \tag{2}$$

and a set

$$\Omega, \text{ an open subset of } \mathbf{R}^n \text{ containing } x_0\ . \tag{3}$$

Also, we consider an arbitrary solution u of the problem

$$\left\{\begin{array}{c} u \in H^1(\Omega)\ ,\quad u \geq \psi \quad \text{c.a.e. in } \Omega\ , \\ E(u) \leq E(v) \quad \forall\ v \in H^1(\Omega),\ v-u \in C_0^1(\Omega)\ , \\ \text{such that } v \geq \psi \quad \text{c.a.e. in } \Omega\ . \end{array}\right. \tag{4}$$

Our objective is to find out under what general assumptions on ψ will u be continuous at x_0, as well as to estimate the modulus of continuity of u.

First we make some remarks on the above assumptions and notation.

The value $-\infty$ is extended to ψ in order to include the case where the constraint $u \geq \psi$ is prescribed only on some given subset E of $\mathbf{R}^n$ (then ψ will be $\equiv -\infty$ on $\mathbf{R}^n-E$). Moreover, in order to allow *thin sets* E to be carriers of constraints, we assume that both ψ and u have been defined to be sets of capacity zero; see, e.g. [11]. Accordingly, the condition $u \geq \psi$ is required to hold in Ω, perhaps only with the exception of sets of capacity zero.

The capacity considered here is the usual Newtonian (or harmonic) external capacity in $\mathbf{R}^n$, $n \geq 3$. For simplicity, we keep this restriction on the dimension n throughout the paper. For an arbitrary set F of $\mathbf{R}^n$ and an arbitrary open subset A of $\mathbf{R}^n$ containing $\overline{F}$, the capacity, cap(F,A), is defined by the usual extension procedure from the cap(K,A), K being a compact subset of A,

$$\operatorname{cap}(K,A) = \inf\left\{\int_A |Dv|^2\, dx : v \in C_0^1(A),\ v \geq 1 \text{ on } K\right\} ;$$

see, for instance, [11]. If the property holds everywhere in some $A \subset \mathbf{R}^n$ with the possible exception of a subset of points of capacity zero, then we say it holds c.a.e. in A.

The space $H^1(\Omega)$ is the Sobolev space of all (real) functions v in Ω which are Lebesgue square integrable in Ω together with their first-order distribution derivatives $D_i v = v_{x_i}$, $i = 1,\ldots,n$. The functions of $H^1(\Omega)$ are assumed to be defined in the c.a.e. sense in Ω; see, for instance, [11].

2. Continuity at a Wiener point

As formulated in section 1, our basic question is the following: Given a function ψ as in (1), which points $x_0 \in \mathbf{R}^n$ are points of continuity for every solution u of the local obstacle problems (3), (4)? We will answer this question, using the notion of a *Wiener point* of ψ.

We need some preliminary notation. For arbitrary $\omega > 0$ and $\rho > 0$, we consider the following "level sets" of ψ:

$$E(\omega,\rho) = \{x \in B(x_0,\rho) \colon \psi(x) \geq \operatorname*{c-sup}_{B(x_0,\rho)} \psi - \omega\} ,$$

where $B(x_0,\rho)$ denotes the open ball of radius ρ centered at x_0 and the supremum of ψ in $B(x_0,\rho)$ is taken in the c.a.e. sense (see section 1).

Next we consider the following *relative capacities* of the sets $E(\omega,\rho)$:

$$\delta(\omega,\rho) = \frac{\operatorname{cap}(E(\omega,\rho), B(x_0, 2\rho))}{\operatorname{cap}(B(x_0,\rho), B(x_0, 2\rho))} .$$

Note that $0 \leq \delta(\omega,\rho) \leq 1$ for all ω and ρ and that $\operatorname{cap}(B(x_0,\rho),B(x_0,2\rho)) = c\rho^{n-2}$, $c = \operatorname{cap}(B(0,1),B(0,2))$ being a constant depending only on n.

We say that $x_0 \in \mathbf{R}^n$ is a *Wiener point* of ψ if for every $\varepsilon > 0$

$$\int_0^1 \delta(\varepsilon,\rho) \frac{d\rho}{\rho} = +\infty .$$

The meaning of this condition is clear: the level sets $E(\omega,\rho)$ of ψ in balls $B(x_0,\rho)$ shrinking to x_0 must not become too "thin" as $\rho \to 0$, when "measured" by their relative capacities $\delta(\omega,\rho)$ in $B(x_0,\rho)$.

The following theorem clarifies our point.

Theorem. *Under assumptions* (1)–(4), u *is continuous at every Wiener point* x_0 *of* ψ.

By saying that u is continuous at x_0 we mean that

$$\operatorname*{osc}_{B(x_0,r)} u := \sup_{B(x_0,r)} u - \inf_{B(x_0,r)} u \to 0 \quad \text{as } r \to 0 ,$$

where the supremum and infimum of u are taken in the essential a.e. sense.

In particular,

Corollary. *u is continuous at every point of continuity of ψ.*

In fact, it is easy to show that every point x_0 at which ψ is continuous is a Wiener point of ψ. By saying that ψ is continuous at x_0 we mean that

$$\underset{B(x_0,r)}{\text{c–osc}}\ \psi := \underset{B(x_0,r)}{\text{c–osc}}\ \psi - \underset{B(x_0,r)}{\text{c–osc}}\ \psi \to 0 \ \text{ as } r \to 0\ ,$$

the supremum and infimum being taken now in the c.a.e. essential sense.

This theorem is, however, general since there exist Wiener points which are not continuity points. As a simple example, assume ψ to be the characteristic function of the nonnegative orthant in $\mathbf{R}^n$, i.e., $\psi(x) = 1$ if $x \geq 0$, $\psi(x) = 0$ if $x \ngeq 0$, and $x_0 = 0$.

On the other hand, it can be shown that the condition that x_0 be a Wiener point of ψ is also *necessary* in order that every local solution of u of (3) and (4) be continuous at x_0; see [15].

Thus, we conclude that a *Wiener criterion* holds for the obstacle problem that generalizes the classical Wiener criterion of potential theory.

3. The Wiener modulus

We now define the *Wiener modulus of ψ at the point* x_0 as the function

$$\omega_\sigma(r,R)$$

of the variables $0 \leq r \leq R$ and $\sigma > 0$ given by

$$\omega_\sigma(r,R) = \inf\{\omega > 0 \colon \omega \exp \int_r^R \delta(\sigma\omega,\rho)\, \frac{d\rho}{\rho} \geq 1\}\ ,$$

where $\delta(\omega,\rho)$ are the relative capacities associated with ψ at x_0 as in section 2.

Note that $\delta(\omega,\rho)$ is nondecreasing in ω, making thus the above definition consistent. Roughly speaking, $\omega_\sigma(r,R)$ is implicitly defined by

$$\omega_\sigma(r,R) \sim \exp\Big(-\int_r^R \delta(\sigma\omega_\sigma(r,R),\rho)\, \frac{d\rho}{\rho}\Big)\ .$$

We can then prove the following

Theorem. *Under assumptions* (1)–(4), *there exist constants C, k and $\beta > 0$ such that*

$$\underset{B(x_0,r)}{\text{osc}}\ u \leq C\omega_\sigma(r,R)^\beta + k\sigma\omega_\sigma(r,R)$$

for all $0 \leq r \leq R$ with $B(x_0,2R) \subset \Omega$ and all $\sigma > 0$. The constants k and β depend only on n, the constant C depends only on n, on the c.a.e. essential supremum of ψ on $B(x_0,2R)$ and on the L^2–norm of u on $B(x_0,2R)$.

This theorem includes the qualitative theorem of section 2. However, it is a much more powerful result for it provides an estimate of the modulus of continuity of u at an arbitrary Wiener point of ψ.

For a better understanding of this estimate, let us write ψ in the form

$$\psi(x) = \phi(x) \text{ if } x \in E, \quad \psi(x) = -\infty \text{ if } x \in \mathbf{R}^n - E\,,$$

where the set $E \subset \mathbf{R}^n$ and the c.a.e. defined function $\phi: E \to \mathbf{R}$ are given. The theorem implies then, in particular,

Corollary. *Under* the *assumptions of the theorem, we have*

$$\operatorname*{osc}_{B(x_0,r)} u \le C \exp\left(-\beta \int_r^R \operatorname{cap}(E \cap B(x_0,\rho), B(x_0,2\rho))\rho^{1-n}\, d\rho\right)$$
$$+\, k \operatorname*{c\text{-}osc}_{E \cap B(x_0,R)} \phi$$

for all $0 < r \le R$, $B(x_0,2R) \subset \Omega$, *the constants* C, k *and* β *being given as in the theorem.*

In the latter estimate we can distinguish in the second member two different terms: the first one takes into account the possibly irregular "geometry" of the set E where the constraint is actually imposed; the second one takes into account the "analytical" behavior of ψ on that set E.

In the case of an everywhere finite constraint ψ: $\mathbf{R}^n \to \mathbf{R}$, hence $E = \mathbf{R}^n$, the above estimate takes the form

$$\operatorname*{osc}_{B(x_0,r)} u \le C\left(\frac{r}{R}\right)^{\beta} + k \operatorname*{c\text{-}osc}_{B(x_0,r)} \psi\,,$$

which in particular implies that if ψ is Hölder continuous at x_0, then u too is Hölder continuous at x_0.

For the application to the discontinuous implicit obstacles arising in impulse control we refer the reader to [8]. Let us only mention here that a slightly more general version of this theorem yields the following somewhat surprising result: if ψ is an arbitrary *monotone* function, i.e., $\psi(x) \le \psi(x)$ for all $x \le y$ in $\mathbf{R}^n$, then u is everywhere Hölder continuous in Ω.

Conclusion

Locally "energy"–optimal distributed systems remain continuous in $\mathbf{R}^n$ even if they are subject to wildly distributed unilateral constraints. What matters for continuity is that the constraint, where it is active, be "thick" enough in capacity to support the local "energy" of the system. Situations of this type are encountered, for example, in stochastic impulse control.

REFERENCES

[1] Baiocchi, C., and A. Capelo. *Disuguaglianze variazionali*, ed. Pitagora, Roma.

[2] Bensoussan, A., and J.L. Lions. *Applications des inequations variationnelles en controle stochastique*. Paris: Dunod, 1978.

[3] Bensoussan, A., J. Frehse, and U. Mosco. 1982. A stochastic impulse control problem with quadratic growth Hamiltonian and the corresponding quasi–variational inequality. *Jour. für die reine und ang. Math.* (1982): 125–145.

[4] Cottle, R., F. Giannessi, and J.L. Lions, eds. *Variational Inequalities*. New York: John Wiley & Sons Publ. Co., 1980.

[5] Capuzzo–Dolcetta, I., and U. Mosco. Implicit complementarity problems and quasi–variational inequalities. Ibid.

[6] Duvaut, G., and J.L. Lions. *Application des inequations variationnelles en mechanique*. Paris: Dunod, 1972.

[7] Friedman, A. *Variational Principles and Free Boundary Problems*. New York: John Wiley & Sons Publ. Co., 1982.

[8] Frehse, J., and U. Mosco. 1982. Irregular obstacles and quasi–variational inequalities of stochastic impulse control. *Ann. Sc. Normale Sup. Pisa*, Serie IV, IX, 1:105–97.

[9] Kinderlehrer, D., and G. Stampacchia. *An Introduction to Variational Inequalities and Their Application*. New York: Academic Press, 1982.

[10] Matzeu, M., U. Mosco, and M.A. Vivaldi. 1983. Optimal impulse and continuous control with Hamiltonian of quadratic growth. *The Proc. Conf. Oper. Res.*(Karlsruhe), ed. Pallaschke.

[11] Maz'ja, V.G., and V.P. Khavin. 1972. Nonlinear potential theory. *Russian Math. Surveys* 27:71–148.

[12] Mosco, U. 1973. An introduction to the approximate solution of variational inequalities. *CIME Erice* 1971. Rome: Cremonese.

[13] Mosco, U. Implicit variational problems and quasi–variational inequalities. Lecture Notes in Mathematics 534. Berlin New York Heidelberg Tokyo: Springer–Verlag, 1976.

[14] Mosco, U. 1982. Module de Wiener et estimation du potential pour le probleme d'obstacle. *C.R. Acad. Sci. Paris*, t. 299, Serie I, no. 17:851–54.

[15] Mosco, U. 1985. Wiener criterion and potential estimates for the obstacle problem. IMA Preprint Series no. 135. *Indiana Univers. Math. J.* Forthcoming.

THE THEORETICAL ASPECTS OF MULTIGRID METHODS

V.V. Shajdurov
Department of Computational Mathematics
The USSR Academy of Sciences
Moscow, USSR

In this article the application of multigrid methods is discussed with respect to the solution of second–order elliptic equations. For discretization of differential problems, the Bubnov–Galerkin method with piecewise–linear trial functions on triangles is used. The algebraic system thus obtained is solved by means of a multigrid algorithm which is based on the notion of reducing the dimension of the subspace in projection methods [1]. It is similar to the methods of Fedorenko [2] and Bakhvalov [3], which were realized for finite differences. Modifications of this algorithm for algebraic systems of the finite–element method are suggested and proved by many authors (see bibliography in [4]); in particular, in the articles of Hackbusch [5], [6] quoted in this paper.

We will consider possible ways of increasing the efficiency of these algorithms by appropriately choosing smoothing iterative procedures. In section 1 we carry out the discretization of the differential problem and formulate multigrid algorithms which will be used later. In section 2 we consider the problem of optimizing the convergence rate of W–cycles, using the Chebyshev polynomials. In section 3 a similar problem for V–cycles is solved by choosing the iterative parameters and changing the number of iterations. In sections 4 and 5 we consider W–cycles with special smoothing iterative procedures which allow one to solve systems of the Bubnov–Galerkin method for problems with non–self–adjoint operators and differential similarities. In section 6 we extend these construction techniques to two–dimensional and three–dimensional problems in regions with curvilinear boundaries.

1. Discretization of the problem and formulation of algorithms

Consider the Dirichlet problem for a convex polygon Ω with boundary Γ:

$$Lu \equiv -\sum_{i,j=1}^{2} \frac{\partial}{\partial x_i}\left(a_{ij}\frac{\partial u}{\partial x_j}\right) + au = f \text{ in } \Omega, \tag{1}$$

$$u = 0 \quad \text{on } \Gamma. \tag{2}$$

The coefficients and the right–hand side satisfy the conditions

$$\mu\sum_{i=1}^{2} \xi_i^2 \le \sum_{i,j=1}^{2} a_{ij}\xi_i\xi_j \le \nu\sum_{i=1}^{2} \xi_i^2 \quad \text{on } \overline{\Omega} \tag{3}$$

$$\forall\ \xi_i \in \mathbf{R} \quad \text{with the constants } \nu \ge \mu > 0\ ;$$

$$a_{12} = a_{21} \quad \text{and} \quad 0 \le a \le c_1 \quad \text{on } \overline{\Omega}\ ; \tag{4}$$

$$f \in L_2(\Omega)\ . \tag{5}$$

Here and in the sequel the following notation is used:

$$\mathcal{L}(u,v) = \int_\Omega \left(\sum_{i,j=1}^{2} a_{ij}\frac{\partial u}{\partial x_i}\frac{\partial v}{\partial x_j} + auv\right) dx\ , \tag{6}$$

$$(u,v) = \int_\Omega uv\, dx\ , \quad \|u\|_{L_2} = (u,u)^{1/2}\ ,$$

$$\|u\|^2_{\mathring{W}^1_2} = \int_\Omega \left\{\left(\frac{\partial u}{\partial x_1}\right)^2 + \left(\frac{\partial u}{\partial x_2}\right)^2\right\} dx\ ,$$

$$\|u\|^2_{W^2_2} = \int_\Omega \left\{u^2 + \sum_{i,j=1}^{2}\left(\frac{\partial^2 u}{\partial x_i \partial x_j}\right)^2\right\} dx\ .$$

L_2, $\mathring{W}^1_2$, W^2_2 are usual Sobolev spaces of functions which are measured on Ω, having the corresponding bounded norms, and vanish on Γ in the case of $\mathring{W}^1_2$.

To discretize the problem we break $\overline{\Omega}$ into a small number of closed triangles, so that each two triangles neither intersect nor have a common side or vertex. We denote the maximum length of the sides of all the triangles by ℓ_0. Let $n_i = 2^i$, $h_i = \ell_0/n_i$ and for all $i = 0,1,\dots,p$ we break each original triangle into n_i^2 equal elementary triangles. Let $\overline{\Omega}_{h_i}$ denote the union of all vertices of the obtained triangles, $\Omega_{h_i} = \overline{\Omega}_{h_i} \cap \Omega$, and N_i the number of vertices in Ω_{h_i}. At each vertex $y \in \Omega_{h_i}$ we introduce the trial function $\varphi_y^{h_i}$. It is equal to 1 at the vertex y, to zero at all other vertices of $\overline{\Omega}_{h_i}$ and is linear on each elementary triangle. Let H^{h_i} denote the linear subspace whose basis consists of these functions. Note that each trial function $\varphi_y^{h_{i-1}}$, $y \in \Omega_{h_{i-1}}$, is a linear combination of few (in most cases it is equal to 7) trial functions of the coarser grid Ω_{h_i}

$$\varphi_y^{h_{i-1}}(x) = \sum_{z \in \Omega_{h_i}} \beta_z^y \, \varphi_z^{h_i}(x) \quad \forall\, y \in \Omega_{h_{i-1}} . \tag{7}$$

Here $\beta_y^y = 1$, several weights β_z^y are equal to 1/2, and the remaining weights are equal to zero.

In accordance with the Bubnov–Galerkin method, the approximate solution $u^{h_i} \in H^{h_i}$ is sought in the form of a sum

$$u^{h_i}(x) = \sum_{y \in \Omega_{h_i}} \alpha_y^{h_i} \, \varphi_y^{h_i}(x) \quad \text{on } \overline{\Omega} ,$$

where $\{\alpha_y^{h_i}\}$ is the set of parameters defined from the system of linear equations

$$\sum_{y \in \Omega_{h_i}} \alpha_y^{h_i} \, \mathcal{L}(\varphi_y^{h_i}, \varphi_z^{h_i}) = (f, \varphi_z^{h_i}) , \quad z \in \Omega_{h_i} . \tag{8}$$

This system has a unique solution and the estimates

$$\| u - u^{h_i} \|_{L_2} \le c_2 h_i^2 \, \| f \|_{L_2} , \tag{9}$$

$$\| u - u^{h_i} \|_{\overset{\circ}{W}{}_2^1} \le c_3 h_i \| f \|_{L_2} \tag{10}$$

hold. In these inequalities, C_i denote the constants not depending on h_i, N_i and functions on both sides of these inequalities.

For each vector W^{h_i} with the components $W_y^{h_i}$, $y \in \Omega_{h_i}$, we set into correspondence the piecewise–linear interpolant from H^{h_i}

$$w^{h_i}(x) = \sum_{y \in \Omega_{h_i}} W_y^{h_i} \varphi_y^{h_i}(x) .$$

Now we introduce the vector norms

$$\| W^{h_i} \|_{h_i} = \| w^{h_i} \|_{L_2} , \quad \| W^{h_i} \|_{h_i}^{(1)} = \mathcal{L}^{1/2}(w^{h_i}, w^{h_i}) .$$

Let us assign the number 1 to N_i the knots of Ω_{h_i} arbitrarily and write down the system (8) in matrix form:

$$L^{h_i} V^{h_i} = F^{h_i} , \tag{11}$$

where L^{h_i} is the square symmetric $N_i \times N_i$ matrix and V^{h_i}, F^{h_i} are the vectors with components $V_y^{h_i} = \alpha_y^{h_i}$, $F_y^{h_i} = (f, \varphi_y^{h_i})$, $y \in \Omega_{h_i}$.

We will assume next that any system with the matrix L^{h_0} is solvable by a direct method involving a small number M_0 of arithmetic operations. Then the solution V^{h_0} is also sought with M_0 operations and the algorithm of computing the V^{h_1}, V^{h_2},... is formulated recurrently in the form of two procedures. Indeed, let the approximate solution $\widetilde{V}^{h_{i-1}}$ of system (11) with index $i-1$ be found. Then the procedure A for finding the approximate solution of (11) consists of two stages.

A_1. To the vector $\widetilde{V}^{h_{i-1}}$ we set into correspondence the piecewise–linear interpolant $\widetilde{v}^{h_{i-1}} \in H^{h_{i-1}}$ and construct the vector $\overline{V}^{h_i}$ with components $\overline{V}_y^{h_i} = \widetilde{v}^{h_{i-1}}(y)$ $\forall\, y \in \Omega_{h_i}$.

A_2. Using this initial approximation, we find the approximate solution $\widetilde{V}^{h_i}$ of (11) using the procedure $B(i)$ described below.

Next we will describe the procedure $B(i)$ on the grid Ω_{h_i} for the solution of (11). On the coarse grid Ω_{h_0} the procedure $B(0)$ is realized, as above, by direct methods. Now let $i \geq 1$ and there is some approximation $V_0^{h_i}$ to the solution V^{h_i}. Then $B(i)$ consists of four stages.

B_1. We make m iterations using the formula

$$U_{\ell+1} = U_\ell - \tau_\ell (L^{h_i} U_\ell - F^{h_i}) \,, \quad \ell = 0,1,...,m-1 \,, \tag{12}$$

with the initial approximation $V_0^{h_i}$ and parameters τ_ℓ which we choose later. Finally we get the vector U_m and the residual

$$G^{h_i} = L^{h_i} U_m - F^{h_i} \,. \tag{13}$$

B_2. We project G^{h_i} with components $G_z^{h_i}$, $z \in \Omega_{h_i}$, in the vector space of dimension N_{i-1} by the rule

$$G_y^{h_{i-1}} = \sum_{z \in \Omega_{h_i}} \beta_z^y G_z^{h_i} \quad \forall\, y \in \Omega_{h_{i-1}} \,, \tag{14}$$

where the coefficients β_z^y are the same as in (7). We obtain the vector $G^{h_{i-1}}$.

B_3. We take the vector $G^{h_{i-1}}$ as the right–hand side of the system

$$L^{h_{i-1}} W^{h_{i-1}} = G^{h_{i-1}} \tag{15}$$

and for its approximate solution we use twice the procedure $B(i-1)$ on the grid $\Omega_{h_{i-1}}$ with the zero vector and next with the obtained vector as an initial approximation. This yields the vector $\widetilde{W}^{h_{i-1}}$.

B_4. The vector $\widetilde{W}^{h_{i-1}}$ corresponds to the piecewise–linear interpolant $\widetilde{w}^{h_{i-1}} \in H^{h_{i-1}}$. Using the values of this function at the knots $z \in \Omega_{h_i}$ we construct the vector $\widetilde{W}^{h_i}$ and take the vector

$$V_2^{h_i} = U_m - \widetilde{W}^h \qquad (16)$$

as a new approximation to the solution of system (11).

The procedure B is called a *W–cycle,* due to the transition from the upper to the lower segment of the Ω. In contrast, the procedure C is called a *V–cycle,* which we shall refer to later.

$C(0)$ coincides with $B(0)$, and $C(i)$ consists of the stages B_1, B_2, C_3, B_4, C_5.

C_3. We take the vector $G^{h_{i-1}}$ as the right–hand side of the system (15) and for its approximate solution we use the procedure $C(i–1)$ on the grid $\Omega_{h_{i-1}}$ with the initial zero vector. Let $\widetilde{W}^{h_{i-1}}$ denote the vector thus obtained.

C_5. We use the vector $V_1^{h_i}$ as the initial approximation of the iterative process (12). Let $V_2^{h_i}$ denote the vector obtained after m iterations. We take it as the outcome of the procedure $C(i)$.

2. Optimization of convergence of W-cycles

Now we consider different choices of the parameters τ_ℓ. To do this, we re–call that eigenvalues of the algebraic spectral problem

$$L^{h_i}U = \lambda U \qquad (17)$$

lie on the interval $(0,d]$ for all h_i and we may choose constant d not depending on h_i. For practical purposes, it can be done with Gershgorin circles.

For the stationary choice of τ_ℓ it is usually assumed that

$$\tau_\ell = 1/d \quad \forall\, \ell = 0,\ldots,m-1 \,. \qquad (18)$$

This leads to the following estimate of convergence of the procedure B in the mean square norm:

$$\|V^{h_i} - V_1^{h_i}\|_{h_i} \le \frac{C_4}{m+1} \|V^{h_i} - V_0^{h_i}\|_{h_i} \,. \qquad (19)$$

Consider the nonstationary choice of parameters τ_ℓ based on the following notion. A solution of the system

$$L^{h_i}W^{h_i} = G^{h_i} \qquad (20)$$

is the vector yielding the correction for U_m up to the exact solution:

$$V^{h_i} = U_m - W^{h_i} \,.$$

But system (20) coincides with the Bubnov–Galerkin method for the problem (1)–(2) with a given right–hand side $g \in H^{h_i}$. Without defining this function, we may convince ourselves that to the differential problem obtained on the more sparse grid $\Omega_{h_{i-1}}$ there corresponds the system of the Bubnov–Galerkin method

$$L^{h_{i-1}} W^{h_{i-1}} = G^{h_{i-1}} \tag{21}$$

in which the vector $G^{h_{i-1}}$ is the same as in (14). For the piecewise–linear interpolants $w^{h_i} \in H^{h_i}$ and $w^{h_{i-1}} \in H^{h_{i-1}}$, we have

$$\|w^{h_i} - w^{h_{i-1}}\|_{L_2} \leq 5C_2 h_i^2 \|g\|_{L_2} .$$

Passing to the vector norms implies that the error

$$\|V^{h_i} - V_1\|_{h_i} = \|W^{h_i} - \widetilde{W}^{h_i}\|_{h_i}$$

decreases as the Euclidean norm of vector G^{h_i} decreases. Therefore, we arrive at the problem of minimizing the Euclidean norm of the residual in the iterative process (12) provided m and the initial error $\|V^{h_i} - V_0^{h_i}\|_{h_i}$ are fixed by the choice of parameters τ_ℓ. Using spectral analysis, this problem becomes the following: to find the polynomial $P_{m+1}(\lambda)$ of the form

$$\lambda \prod_{\ell=0}^{m-1} (1-\tau_\ell \lambda) ,$$

which deviates minimally from zero on the interval $[0,d]$. Such a polynomial is unique [7]:

$$P_{m+1}(\lambda) = -q \cos\{(m+1)\arccos(\cos\alpha - \frac{\lambda}{d}(1 + \cos\alpha))\} , \tag{22}$$

where

$$\alpha = \frac{\pi}{2(m+1)} , \quad q = \frac{\alpha}{m+1} tg \frac{\alpha}{2} .$$

All roots of this polynomial

$$\omega_k = \frac{d(\cos\alpha - \cos(2k+1)\alpha)}{1 + \cos\alpha} , \quad k = 0,\dots,m ,$$

are different and lie on the interval $[0,d]$, and $\omega_0 = 0$. Therefore, to achieve our objective, we need to choose the iterative parameters in (12) by the formula

$$\tau_\ell = 1/\omega_{\ell+1} , \quad \ell = 0,\dots,m-1 . \tag{23}$$

Under these conditions the following estimate is valid [8]:

$$\|V^{h_i} - V_1^{h_i}\|_{h_i} \leq \frac{\pi C_4}{2(m+1)^2} \|V^{h_i} - V_0^{h_i}\|_{h_i} . \tag{24}$$

Finally, this leads to an essentially decreased number of iterations at stage B_1 with the same accuracy; this has been proved by numerical experiments.

For the algorithm A, in this case the following result holds.

Theorem 1. *For each $\rho > 0$ we may choose $M > 0$ independent of h_i and such that for every $m \geq M$ the algorithm A gives an approximate solution $\tilde{V}^{h_p}$ with the interpolant $\tilde{v}^{h_p} \in H^{h_p}$ satisfying the estimate*

$$\|u - \tilde{v}^{h_p}\|_{L_2} \leq (C_2+\rho)h^2 p \|f\|_{L_2} \,. \tag{25}$$

Also, the number of arithmetic operations is estimated by the quantity $C_5 mN_p$.

Spectral analysis of convergence of the procedure B in energy norm leads to the search of a function $Q_{m+1/2}(\lambda)$ of the form

$$\lambda^{1/2} \prod_{\ell=0}^{m-1} (1-\tau_\ell \lambda) \,, \tag{26}$$

which deviates minimally from zero on the interval $[0,d]$. The solution of this problem has the form [9]:

$$Q_{m+1/2}(\lambda) = \frac{\sqrt{a}}{2m+1} \cos\{(2m+1)\arccos(\lambda/d)^{1/2}\} \,. \tag{27}$$

This function has the following roots:

$$\sigma_\ell = d \cos \frac{\pi(2\ell+1)}{2(2m+1)} \,, \; \ell = 0,\ldots,m \,. \tag{28}$$

Then iterative parameters are chosen by the rule

$$\tau_\ell = 1/\sigma_\ell \,. \tag{29}$$

For the procedure B in this case the following estimate of decreasing error in energy norm is obtained [8]:

$$\|V^{h_i} - V_1^{h_i}\|_{h_i}^{(1)} \leq \frac{C_6}{2m+1} \|V^{h_i} - V_0^{h_i}\|_{h_i}^{(1)} \,. \tag{30}$$

For the stationary choice of parameters (18), the analogous proof gives the worst multiplier on the right-hand side: $C_6/\sqrt{2m+1}$. The numerical experiments confirm this ratio between the rates of convergence.

Thus, for the choice of iterative parameters by the rule (29) for the procedure A we have the result similar to Theorem 1 if we replace inequality (25) with

$$\|u - \tilde{v}^{h_p}\|_{\mathring{W}_2^1} \leq (C_3+\rho)h_p \|f\|_{L_2} \,. \tag{31}$$

Note that by appropriately choosing τ_ℓ we may not only increase the convergence rate but expand the field of application of the method as well. Consider, for example, the case of a nonsingular operator with an alternating spectrum, when the function $a \in L_2(\Omega)$ may be negative. Then the eigenvalues of (17) lie on the interval $[-bh_i^2, d]$. For a sufficiently small h_i the inequality

$$bh_i^2 \le d\,tg^2\alpha/2 \tag{32}$$

holds. It guarantees the optimality of the polynomial $P_{m+1}(\lambda)$ on the interval $[-bh_i^2, d]$ and the validity of (24).

For a large mesh h_i, (32) may not hold. Then the roots of another polynomial should be used:

$$P^k_{m'+1}(\lambda) = q^k \cos\{(m'+1)\arccos(\cos\alpha_k - \frac{\lambda}{d}(1+\cos\alpha_k))\} \tag{33}$$

with parameters

$$\alpha_k = \frac{\pi(2k-1)}{2(m'+1)}, \quad q^k = \frac{d}{m'+1}\,tg\,\frac{\alpha_k}{2}$$

and roots

$$\omega_i^k = \frac{d(\cos\alpha_k - \cos\alpha_i)}{1 + \cos\alpha_k}.$$

The number k of this polynomial is chosen as to satisfy the condition

$$k = [8(m+1)^2 bh_i^2/d\pi^2] + 1 .$$

It ensures the optimality of $P^k_{m'+1}(\lambda)$ on the interval $[-bh_i^2, d]$. As it gives a smaller rate of decreasing residual, the number of iterations m' should be increased by the following rule:

$$m' = [\sqrt{2k-1}(m+1)] .$$

Finally, the iterative process (12) is carried out on the grid Ω_{h_i} at the unrealized inequality (32) with parameters

$$\tau_\ell \in \{1/\omega_i^k,\ i = 0,\ldots,m';\ i \ne k\} .$$

Note that in this case the result of Theorem 1 is fully valid. To ensure the computational stability for large m', it is necessary to mix parameters τ_ℓ by a special rule [1].

An application of this technique to the operators with an alternating spectrum allowed us to construct the effective multigrid algorithm for solving spectral problems [10].

3. Optimization of convergence for V-cycles

We use spectral analysis for the investigation of the coefficient ε_i of the error suppression by the procedure C:

$$\|V^{h_i} - V_2^{h_i}\|_{h_i} \le \varepsilon_i \|V^{h_i} - V_0^{h_i}\|_{h_i} . \tag{34}$$

Using the computations from [1], we get the inequality

$$\varepsilon_i \le \max_{(0,d]} |C_7(1-\varepsilon_{i-1})\lambda R_m(\lambda) + \varepsilon_{i-1} R_m(\lambda)| , \tag{35}$$

where $R_m(\lambda)$ is a polynomial of the form

$$\prod_{\ell=0}^{m-1} (1 - \tau_\ell \lambda) .$$

As a rule, the static regime $\varepsilon_i = \varepsilon_{i-1}$ is considered. This, however, complicates solution of the optimization problem for the right–hand side of (35). Moreover, the constant C_7 may be estimated only roughly for each concrete problem. Therefore this solution of the minimization problem for the right–hand side of (35) with such a constant may not be the best solution at all.

We study a dynamic regime where ε_i and m_i are different on each level. This is due to the fact that $\varepsilon_0 = 0$, for example. Furthermore, we also make a simplification, based on a real situation, that the value $\max_{\lambda \in (0,d]} |R_m(\lambda)|$ is close to 1. Then we obtain

$$\varepsilon_i \le C_7(1-\varepsilon_{i-1}) \max_{\lambda \in (0,d]} |P_{m_{i+1}}(\lambda)| + \varepsilon_{i-1} . \tag{36}$$

At first we optimize the choice of parameters τ_ℓ to decrease the first term on the right–hand side of (36). The solution of this problem was given in the preceding section. It yields the estimates

$$\varepsilon_i \le \frac{C_8(1-\varepsilon_{i-1})}{(m_i+1)^2} + \varepsilon_{i-1}, \quad i = 1,2,\dots ; \quad \varepsilon_0 = 0 .$$

Summing up and taking into consideration the smallness of ε_i, we get the inequality

$$\varepsilon_i \le \sum_{j=1}^{i} \frac{C_8}{(m_j+1)^2} . \tag{37}$$

The number of arithmetic operations needed for the realization of the V–cycle is

$$C_g N_i \sum_{j=1}^{i} (m_j+1) 4^{j-i} + O(N_i) , \tag{38}$$

where C_g is a constant not depending on m_j and the number of knots N_i of the grid Ω_{h_i}. Fixing the main term in (38), we find the minimum on the right–hand side of (37) by choosing the m_j. Using the method of Lagrange multipliers, we arrive at the following relation for m_j:

$$\frac{m_{j-1}+1}{m_j+1} = 4^{1/3} .$$

Hence

$$m_{j-1} = [4^{1/3}(m_j+1)] . \tag{39}$$

Thus the number of iterations m_j increases from a dense grid to a sparse one.

Now, the dynamic procedure C with the algorithm A consists in the following. Fix a certain integer $m > 0$. Let the approximate solution $\tilde{V}^{h_{i-1}}$ of system (11) exist. Make a step A_1. Then, using the obtained vector $\overline{V}^{h_i}$ as the initial approximation, apply the procedure $C(i)$ with $m_i = m$ iterations and parameters τ_ℓ defined by formula (23) at stages B_1 and C_5. For the procedure $C(j)$ with index $j < i$ the number of iterations m_j is given by the recurrence formula (39) and the parameters τ_ℓ are computed by (23), replacing m by m_j. The parameters τ_ℓ should be mixed between stages B_1 or C_5 to ensure the computational stability.

In spite of the rapidly decreasing number of iterations, the total number of arithmetic operations remains proportional to the number of unknowns N_i, and the method on the whole is more economical than the static regime m = const. and τ_ℓ = const.

Theorem 2. *For each $\rho > 0$ we may choose $M > 0$ independently of h_i and such that for every $m \geq M$ the constructed algorithm with a dynamic choice of the number of iterations gives the approximate solution $\tilde{V}^{h_p}$ for the interpolant of which $\tilde{v}^{h_p} \in H^{h_p}$ the estimate (25) is valid. The number of arithmetic operations in this algorithm is estimated by the quantity $C_{10}mN_p$.*

4. The solution of the problem with a non–self–adjoint operator

Now consider a more general case of the Dirichlet problem with the operator

$$L_1 u \equiv Lu + \sum_{i=1}^{2} b_i \frac{\partial u}{\partial x_i}.$$

We require a unique solution in $W_2^1(\Omega)$ for the new problem. Introduce a new bilinear form

$$\mathcal{L}(u,v) = \int_\Omega \Big(\sum_{i,j=1}^{2} a_{ij} \frac{\partial u}{\partial x_i}\frac{\partial v}{\partial x_j} + \sum_{i=1}^{2} b_i \frac{\partial u}{\partial x_i} v + auv \Big)\, dx$$

and keep the notation of sections 1 and 2 for this norm as well as the subsequent vectors and matrices. Then for sufficiently small h_i the system (8) of Bubnov–Galerkin method has a unique solution and the estimate (9) holds.

We retain without change the algorithm A for the solution of (11) with a square asymmetric matrix, and in the procedure B we replace the smoothing iterative process (12) by the following:

$$U_{\ell+1} = U_\ell - \tau_\ell (L^{h_i})^{\mathrm{T}} (L^{h_i} U_\ell - F^{h_i}), \quad \ell = 0,1,\ldots,m-1 \,, \tag{40}$$

where $(\cdot)^{\mathrm{T}}$ denotes transposition. Using the notions of spectral analysis, the optimization problem of the parameters τ_ℓ for the mean square norm coincides with (26)–(28), where d is equal to the spectral radius of the symmetric matrix $(L^{h_i})^{\mathrm{T}} L^{h_i}$. Therefore, τ_ℓ are chosen by the rule (28)–(29) with a new d.

Then for the algorithm A with this modified procedure B for a non–self–adjoint Dirichlet problem with the operator L_1 the statement of Theorem 1 is fully valid [8].

5. The problem with differential singularity

Returning to the problem (1)–(2) on the polygon Ω, one of the interior angles is greater than π, for example, with the vertex in the origin. It leads to a decreasing smoothness of the solution U in the neighborhood of the point (0,0) and U does not, in general, belong to $W_2^2(\Omega)$. In turn, it decreases the order of accuracy of the Bubnov–Galerkin method formulated above.

To provide the necessary order of accuracy, one may use various techniques: additive separation of singularity, norms with singular weight, condensation of [11]. We will consider the triangulation condensation to a singular point.

Let us introduce the condensation index $\rho \geq 1$ and consider the situation after initially dividing $\overline{\Omega}$ into a small number of closed triangles. We shall call this partition a zero partition. We continue partitioning. If a triangle of the ith division does not touch the origin, then it is divided into 4 equal triangles of the $(i+1)^{\text{th}}$ division if the midpoints of its sides are connected. Now consider the triangle ABC of the ith division with the vertex A = (0,0). First we cut off from it the triangle $A'B'C'$ which is similar to ABC with the coefficient $2^{-\rho}$ by drawing a segment $B'C'$ parallel to BC (see figure 1). Next we divide the left part into 3 triangles, connecting points B' and C' with the midpoint of the side BC. Sequentially dividing the triangles for i = $1,2,\ldots,\rho$, we get the necessary condensation of triangulation near the singular point. Within the bounds of one initial triangle we get only 4 types of triangles similar to the triangles of the first division. Therefore, the triangles obtained recurrently do not have degeneration of angles.

As above, let Ω_{h_i} denote the union of all vertices of the ith division and preserve the notation of section 1. Following the lines of [10], one may choose the condensation index ρ so that for the solution U^h of (8) the estimates (9), (10) hold. The maximal edges of triangulation at any ρ is related to the number of knots N_i by $N_i \leq C_{11} h_i^{-2}$ as for uniform division.

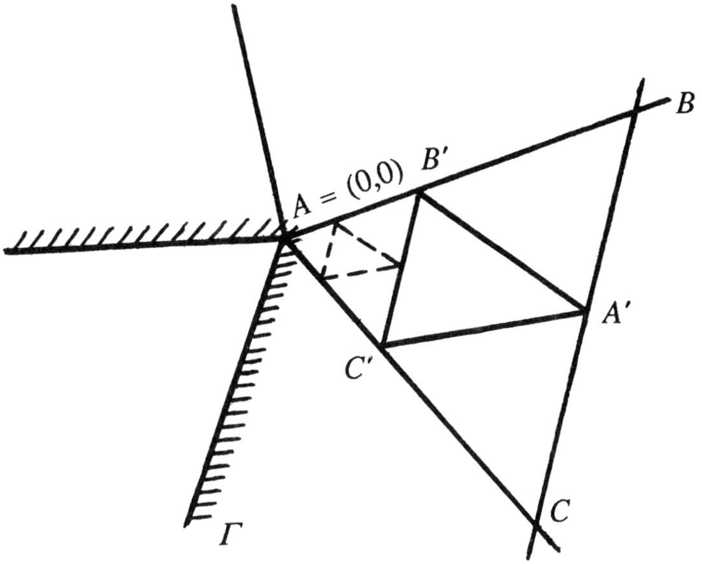

Fig. 1. The condensation of a grid

Note that condensation of the grid essentially worsens the conditionality of the matrix L^{h_i}. It results in a poor convergence of B. To improve the conditionality, it is convenient to normalize L^{h_i} directly in (12). We restrict ourselves to W–cycles.

We introduce the normalization in the following way. To each knot $y \in \Omega_{h_i}$ we set into correspondence the number $d_y^{h_i}$ equal to the summation area of the triangles of the ith division with the vertex at y. Next, we introduce the diagonal matrix $\mathscr{D}^{h_i}$ with elements $\mathscr{D}_{yy}^{h_i} = d_y^{h_i}$ and replace (12) by

$$U_{\ell+1} = U_\ell - \tau_\ell(\mathscr{D}^{h_i})^{-1}(L^{h_i}U_\ell^{h_i} - F^{h_i}), \quad \ell = 0,1,\ldots,m-1 .$$

The quantity d in (22) for the construction of τ_ℓ is equal to the spectral radius of the matrix $(\mathscr{D}^{h_i})^{-1}L^{h_i}$. We leave without change the other stages of B. Let B' denote the procedure thus constructed.

Theorem 3. *Let for the solution of* (1)–(5) *on polygon* Ω *with an interior angle being greater than* π, *the Bubnov–Galerkin method be used with the condensation index* $\rho > 1$ *of triangulation* Ω_{h_i}. *Then one may choose* $M > 0$ *so that for any integer* $m \geq M$ *the algorithm* A *with procedure* B' *gives an approximate solution* $\tilde{V}^{h_p}$ *with the interpolant* $\tilde{v}^{h_p} \in H^{h_p}$ *satisfying* (25). *The number of arithmetic operations is estimated by the quantity* $C_{12}mN_p = C_{13}mh_p^{-2}$.

6. The solution of two–dimensional and three–dimensional problems in the region with curvilinear boundary

At first we consider a two–dimensional case of the region Ω with a piecewise–smooth boundary. First we devide the Ω into a small number of triangles, perhaps, with one or two curvilinear sides being a smooth segment of the boundary Γ. Each triangle is then divided into four triangles by connecting the midpoints of three sides, including curvilinear ones, by the segments of straight lines. This procedure of dividing is repeated p times and on the last grid $\overline{\Omega}_{h_p}$ the knots of the boundary are sequentially connected by chords [12]. On the triangulation thus constructed the piecewise–linear trial functions $\varphi_y^{h_p}$ $\forall\ y \in \Omega_{h_p}$ are introduced, as was done earlier.

Near the convex section of the boundary, a further construction of the Bubnov–Galerkin method does not cause any difficulty. Near the concave section the variational principle is violated because of the main boundary conditions (2). Nevertheless, following [12], the estimate (9) for the approximate solution U^{h_i} is found in the same way as before if for calculating the elements of the matrix L^{h_i} and the vector F^{h_i} the coefficients and right–hand side of the problem are extended with the same smoothness class to small holes $0(h_i^2)$ wide near the boundary. This assumption is however unnecessary in practical problems where quadrature formulas with knots inside triangles and in these vertices are used.

Note that in this case it is enough to construct the matrix L^{h_p} on the smallest grid, and all auxiliary matrices L^{h_s} with indices $s < p$ are to be obtained from it by summing the rows and columns, since by (7) the elements of $L^{h_{i-1}}$ are represented as linear combinations of the elements of L^{h_i}:

$$L^{h_{i-1}}_{y_1,y_2} = \mathcal{L}(\varphi^{h_{i-1}}_{y_1},\varphi^{h_{i-1}}_{y_2}) = \sum_{z_1,z_2\in\Omega_{h_i}} \beta^{y_1}_{z_1}\beta^{y_2}_{z_2}\,\mathcal{L}(\varphi^{h_i}_{y_1},\varphi^{h_i}_{y_2})$$

$$= \sum_{z_1,z_2\in\Omega_{h_i}} \beta^{y_1}_{z_1}\beta^{y_2}_{z_2}\,L^{h_i}_{z_1,z_2} \qquad \forall\ y_1,y_2 \in \Omega_{h_{i-1}}\,.$$

The elements of the right–hand side can be calculated in a similar manner:

$$F^{h_{i-1}}_y = \sum_{z\in\Omega_{h_i}} \beta^y_z F^{h_i}_z \qquad \forall\ y \in \Omega_{h_{i-1}}\,.$$

With this formulation of the intermediate systems (11) for $i = 0,\dots,p-1$, the algorithm A and the procedures B,C remain unchanged. The results of Theorems 1,2 are valid for them, too. However, the proof is different and consists in proving the approximation properties (9), (10) for the composite trial functions $\varphi_y^{h_i}$ obtained for $i = 0,\dots,p-1$ from $\varphi_y^{h_p}$ by the recurrence formula (7).

The methods constructed extend to three–dimensional problems when the region Ω is a polyhedron, perhaps with curvilinear smooth faces. The initial closed region $\overline{\Omega}$ is divided first into a set of k closed tetrahedrons, perhaps, with curvilinear faces being smooth segments of the boundary Γ. We call this division coordinated if any two tetrahedrons either have no common points or have only a common vertex, or have one common rib, or have one common face. We call the initial division zero division. The tetrahedrons obtained are then subdivided. Take one tetrahedron of the ith division. For each four vertices we draw a plane passing over the midpoint of the three ribs coming out of this vertex (fig. 2(a)). These planes cut off four tetrahedrons, perhaps, with curvilinear faces, too. In the left octahedron we join by a straight line two vertices from different faces. There are three possible steps: take the one which gives the shortest segment (fig. 2(b)), which is the rib of four tetrahedrons of the $(i+1)^{\text{th}}$ division. Note that the obtained division will be coordinated, again.

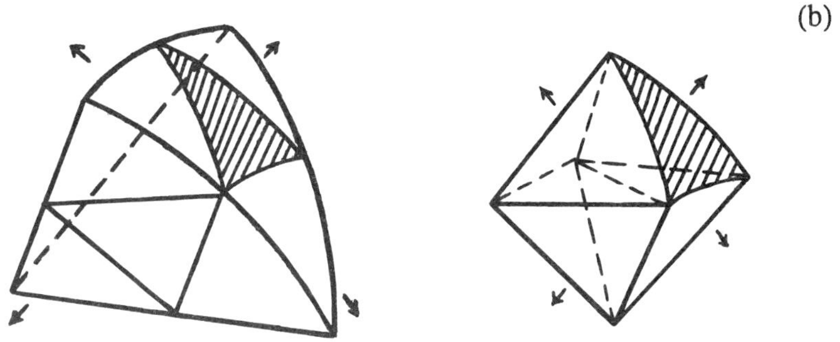

Fig. 2. The stages of dividing a tetrahedron into 8 parts

We repeat such division p times and on the last grid $\overline{\Omega}_{h_p}$, instead of curvilinear faces on Γ of an elementary tetrahedron we draw the plane faces being triangles with vertices on Γ. Then on the obtained spatial triangulation the piecewise–linear trial functions $\varphi_y^{h_p}$ $\forall\ y \in \Omega_{h_p}$ and the Bubnov–Galerkin system is constructed in the usual way.

The other results are formulated for a three–dimensional case in the obvious manner. Note only that the weights β_z^y in (7) are defined in the following way. Suppose from the point $y \in \Omega_{h_{i-1}}$ there come out k_1 ribs of spatial triangulation. Then $\beta_y^y = 1$, once more k_1 weights β_z^y are equal to 1/2 for $z \in \Omega_{h_i}$ lying at the midpoints of these ribs. The left weights are equal to zero.

Finally the algorithm yields the approximate solution $\tilde{v}^{h_p}$ of the Bubnov–Galerkin method with the accuracy $\|\tilde{v}^{h_p} - U\|_{L_2} = 0(h_p^2)$, where h_p is the maximal length of the ribs of spatial triangulation. The number of arithmetic operations in these algorithms is $0(h_p^{-3})$ and is proportional to the number of unknowns.

REFERENCES

[1] Marchuk, G.I., and V.I. Lebedev. *Numerical Methods in the Theory of Neutron Transport* (in Russian). Moscow: Izdatel'svo "Atomnaya Fizika," 1981.

[2] Fedorenko, R.P. 1962. A relaxation method for solving elliptic difference equations. *U.S.S.R. Computat. Math. and Math. Physics* 1, no. 4:1092–96. (English transl.)

[3] Bakhvalov, N.S. 1966. On the convergence of a relaxation method with natural constraints on the elliptic operator. *U.S.S.R. Comput. Math. and Math. Physics* 6, no. 5:101–35. (English transl.)

[4] Hackbusch, W., and U. Trottenberg, eds. *Multigrid Methods.* Proceedings of the Conference on multigrid methods in Koln–Porz, November 1981. Lecture Notes in Mathematics, vol. 960. Berlin New York Heidelberg Tokyo: Springer–Verlag, 1982.

[5] Braess, D., and W. Hackbusch. 1983. A new convergence proof for the multigrid method including the *V*–cycle. *SIAM J. Numer. Anal.* 20, no. 5:967–75.

[6] Hackbusch, W. 1979. On the fast solutions of nonlinear elliptic equations. *Numer. Math.* 32, no. 1:83–95.

[7] Saff, E.B., and R.S. Varga. 1981. On incomplete polynomials. II. *Pacif. J. Math.* 1:161–72.

[8] Shajdurov, V.V. 1983. Projection–grid schemes on a sequence of grids (in Russian). In *Vychislitel'nye Metody Linejnoj Algebry,* 238–46. Department of Numerical Mathematics of the USSR Academy of Sciences, Moscow.

[9] Marchuk, G.I. *Methods of Computational Mathematics.* Berlin New York Heidelberg Tokyo: Springer–Verlag, 1981.

[10] Shajdurov, V.V. 1984. Solution of a spectral variate–difference problem on a sequence of grids (in Russian). In *Variatsionno–raznostnye Metody Matematicheskoj Fiziki,* 149–60. Department of Numerical Mathematics of the USSR Academy of Sciences, Moscow.

[11] ———————. 1982. Numerical solution of Dirichlet problem in the domain with angles (in Russian). In *Vychislitel'nye Metody Prikladnoj Matematiki,* 173–88. Novosibirsk: Nauka.

[12] Korneev, V.G. 1977. *Finite–element schemes for accuracy of higher order* (in Russian). Leningrad: Izdatel'stvo LGU.

ON THE REALIZATION OF THE QUADRATIC PROGRAMMING ALGORITHM OF GOLDFARB AND IDNANI

Josef Stoer

Institut für Angewandte Mathematik und Statistik
Universitat Würzburg
Würzburg, The Federal Republic of Germany

Abstract

The paper describes a realization of the dual method of Goldfarb and Idnani [1] for solving strictly convex quadratic programs, $\min\{\frac{1}{2}\mathbf{x}^T\mathbf{D}\mathbf{x} + \mathbf{d}^T\mathbf{x} \mid \mathbf{A}^T\mathbf{x} \le \mathbf{b}\}$. The techniques proposed avoid the numerical difficulties to be expected with the algorithm of [1], if $\mathbf{D}$ is badly conditioned.

The method can also be used to solve constrained least squares problems, $\min\{\|\mathbf{C}\mathbf{x} - \mathbf{x}\|_2 \mid \mathbf{A}^T\mathbf{x} \le \mathbf{b}\}$.

1. Introduction

Recently, Goldfarb and Idnani [1] proposed a method for solving quadratic programs of the form

$$\begin{aligned} &\min \frac{1}{2}\mathbf{x}^T\mathbf{D}\mathbf{x} + \mathbf{d}^T\mathbf{x} \\ &\mathbf{x}:\ \mathbf{a}_i^T\mathbf{x} \le b_i\ ,\ i \in M := \{1,2,\ldots,m\}\ , \end{aligned} \qquad (1.1)$$

where $\mathbf{D}$ is a positive definite $n \times n$ matrix, $\mathbf{a}_i$, $\mathbf{d} \in \mathbf{R}^n$. Let

$$\mathbf{A} := (\mathbf{a}_1,\ldots,\mathbf{a}_m)\ , \quad \mathbf{b} := (b_1,\ldots,b_n)^T\ ,$$

so that $\mathbf{x}$ is feasible for (1.1) iff $\mathbf{A}^T\mathbf{x} \le \mathbf{b}$. For ease of presentation only we assume that there are only inequality and no equality constraints in (1.1).

Instead of (1.1) we prefer to consider a linearly constrained least squares problem, as in [4]:

$$\min \frac{1}{2} \|\mathbf{Cx} - \mathbf{c}\|^2 \; := \; \mathbf{f}(\mathbf{x}) \tag{P}$$

$$\mathbf{x}: \; \mathbf{A}^\mathsf{T}\mathbf{x} \le \mathbf{b}$$

where $\mathbf{C}$ is a $p \times n$ matrix of rank n.

Clearly, using the Cholesky decomposition $\mathbf{D} = \mathbf{LL}^\mathsf{T}$ of $\mathbf{D}$ and setting $\mathbf{C} := \mathbf{L}^\mathsf{T}$, $\mathbf{c} := -\mathbf{L}^{-1}\mathbf{d}$, (1.1) is reduced to (P).

Let us use the following handy notation: if $\mathbf{J} = (j_1,\dots,j_l) \in M$, we write briefly $\mathbf{J} \subset M$ and

$$\mathbf{A_J} := (\mathbf{a}_{j_1},\dots,\mathbf{a}_{j_l}) \,, \quad \mathbf{b_J} := (b_{j_1},\dots,b_{j_l})^\mathsf{T} \,.$$

Following [1], let us call a pair $(\mathbf{x},\mathbf{J})$ consisting of a vector $\mathbf{x} \in \mathbf{R}^n$ and an index vector $\mathbf{J} \subset M$ an S–pair for (P) if $\mathbf{A_J}$ has linearly independent columns and $\mathbf{x}$ is an optimal solution of

$$\min \mathbf{f}(\mathbf{y}) \tag{P_J}$$

$$\mathbf{y}: \; \mathbf{A_J}^\mathsf{T}\mathbf{x} \; \le \; \mathbf{b_J}$$

with $\mathbf{A_J}^\mathsf{T}\mathbf{x} = \mathbf{b_J}$. The method of [1] is a dual method, giving a finite sequence $(\mathbf{x}_k,\mathbf{J}_k)$ of S–pairs, beginning with $(\mathbf{x}_0,\mathbf{J}_0)$, $\mathbf{J}_0 := \emptyset$ and the unconstrained minimum $\mathbf{x}_0$ of (P), according to the following scheme:

0. Start: Set $\mathbf{J}_0 := \emptyset$ and compute

$$\mathbf{x}_0 := \arg\min \{\mathbf{f}(\mathbf{x}) \mid \mathbf{x} \in \mathbf{R}^n\}$$

For $k = 0,1,\dots$ (1.2)
Given an S–pair $(\mathbf{x}_k,\mathbf{J}_k)$, construct $(\mathbf{x}_{k+1},\mathbf{J}_{k+1})$ as follows:

1. If $\mathbf{A}^\mathsf{T}\mathbf{x}_k \le \mathbf{b}$, stop: $\mathbf{x}_k$ is optimal for (P). Otherwise,

2. find a constraint violated by $\mathbf{x}_k$, say $\mathbf{a}_r^\mathsf{T}\mathbf{x}_k > \mathbf{b}_r$, and set $\mathbf{J}' := (j_1,\dots,j_l,r) = \mathbf{J}_k \cup \{r\}$, if $\mathbf{J} = (j_1,\dots,j_l)$.

3. Stop, if $(P_{\mathbf{J}'})$ has no feasible solutions. Otherwise find an S–pair $(\mathbf{x}_{k+1},\mathbf{J}_{k+1})$ with

$$r \in \mathbf{J}_{k+1} \subset \mathbf{J}_k \cup \{r\} \; = \; \mathbf{J}'$$

$$\mathbf{f}(\mathbf{x}_{k+1}) \; > \; \mathbf{f}(\mathbf{x}_k) \,.$$

Clearly, the algorithm terminates, as there is no repetition of index vectors $\mathbf{J}_k$ because of $\mathbf{f}(\mathbf{x}_{k+1}) > \mathbf{f}(\mathbf{x}_k)$, and it gives the optimal solution of (P) after finitely many steps, if (P) has feasible solutions.

The practical importance of this algorithm stems from the fact that, unlike the more usual primal algorithms, (1.2) has no "phase 1"; it can be started with the unconstrained minimum $\mathbf{x}_0$, which need not be feasible for (P). Moreover, Goldfarb and Idnani [1] and Powell [2] have described a very elegant numerical realization which is much more efficient than other dual methods. However, one may doubt the suitability of their realizations for very ill–conditioned matrices $\mathbf{D}$ for the following reasons: a basic tool for efficiently performing the arithmetics in step k of (1.2), are an $n\times n$ matrix $\mathbf{Z}_k$ and an upper triangular $|\mathbf{J}_k| \times |\mathbf{J}_k|$ matrix $\mathbf{R}_k$ with

$$\mathbf{Z}_k\mathbf{Z}_k^{\top} = \mathbf{D}^{-1}, \quad \mathbf{Z}_k^{\top}\mathbf{A}_{\mathbf{J}_k} = \begin{bmatrix}\mathbf{R}_k\\ \mathbf{0}\end{bmatrix}. \tag{1.3}$$

Initially, one starts with the Cholesky decomposition $\mathbf{D} = \mathbf{L}\mathbf{L}^{\top}$ of $\mathbf{D}$, and sets $\mathbf{Z}_0 := \mathbf{L}^{-\top}$ ($\mathbf{R}_0$:= the empty 0×0 matrix, since $\mathbf{J}_0 = \emptyset$). The matrices $\mathbf{Z}_k$, $\mathbf{R}_k$, $k \geq 0$, are updated recursively to give $\mathbf{Z}_{k+1}$, $\mathbf{R}_{k+1}$, using essentially only numerically stable pre/postmultiplications of $\mathbf{Z}_k$, $\mathbf{R}_k$ by suitable orthogonal matrices. Since Cholesky factorization is numerically stable, the computed Cholesky factor $\overline{\mathbf{L}} = \mathrm{fl}(\mathbf{L})$ is such that $\overline{\mathbf{D}} := \overline{\mathbf{L}} \cdot \overline{\mathbf{L}}^{\top}$ is very close to $\mathbf{D}$, so that $\overline{\mathbf{L}}$ can be interpreted as the exact Cholesky factor of a close–by matrix $\overline{\mathbf{D}}$, even if $\mathbf{D}$ is very ill–conditioned. However, the computed $\overline{\mathbf{Z}}_0 = \mathrm{fl}(\overline{\mathbf{L}}^{-\top})$ is not such that

$$(\overline{\mathbf{Z}}_0)^{-\top} \cdot (\overline{\mathbf{Z}}_0)^{-1}$$

is close to $\overline{\mathbf{D}}$, if $\mathbf{D}$ is ill conditioned. The same holds for the recursively computed $\overline{\mathbf{Z}}_k = \mathrm{fl}(\mathbf{Z}_k)$; for ill–conditioned $\mathbf{D}$, $(\overline{\mathbf{Z}}_k)^{-\top}(\overline{\mathbf{Z}}_k)^{-1}$ may not at all be close to $\overline{\mathbf{D}}$. The numerically stable transformations leading from (the computed) $\overline{\mathbf{Z}}_k$ to (the computed) $\overline{\mathbf{Z}}_{k+1}$ guarantee only

$$\overline{\mathbf{Z}}_0\overline{\mathbf{Z}}_0^{\top} \simeq \overline{\mathbf{Z}}_k\overline{\mathbf{Z}}_k^{\top} \simeq \overline{\mathbf{Z}}_{k+1}\overline{\mathbf{Z}}_{k+1}^{\top} \simeq \ldots$$

but not $\overline{\mathbf{Z}}_i^{-\top}\overline{\mathbf{Z}}_i^{-1} \simeq \mathbf{D}$.

This possible instability of the Goldfarb–Idnani algorithm (GI–algorithm) was already noted by Powell [3]; as an alternative he also discussed a QR–type algorithm, which uses instead of (1.3) decompositions of the form

$$\mathbf{A}_{\mathbf{J}_k} = (\overline{\mathbf{Q}}_k^{(c)}, \overline{\mathbf{Q}}_k^{(u)})\begin{bmatrix}\overline{\mathbf{R}}_k\\ \mathbf{0}\end{bmatrix}, \quad \mathbf{U}_k\mathbf{U}_k^{\top} = \overline{\mathbf{Q}}_k^{(u)\top}\mathbf{D}\overline{\mathbf{Q}}_k^{(u)}, \tag{1.4}$$

where $\mathbf{Q}_k = (\overline{\mathbf{Q}}_k^{(c)}, \overline{\mathbf{Q}}_k^{(u)})$ is orthogonal $n\times n$, and $\overline{\mathbf{R}}_k$, $\mathbf{U}_k$ are upper triangular $l\times l$ and $(n-l)\times(n-l)$ matrices, respectively, where $l := |\mathbf{J}_k|$. Powell compared the QR–type algorithm with a carefully coded version of the GI–algorithm (ZQPCVX, see [2]), which contains repeated iterative refinement steps in order to overcome the numerical instabilities mentioned above. On the basis of test results, he finally recommended the GI–method over the QR–method, because of the greater efficiency. However, by using other QR–type decomposi–

tions than (1.4) one may improve the efficiency of these methods. It is the purpose of this paper to describe such techniques; they are essentially based on decompositions (see (2.2))

$$A_J^T Q = (0,L) , \quad UCQ = R , \tag{1.5}$$

where $\mathbf{Q}$ is nonsingular (not necessarily unitary) $\mathbf{L}$ = is triangular $l \times l$, $\mathbf{R}$ is upper triangular $p \times n$, and $\mathbf{U}$ is unitary. Here, however, only $\mathbf{Q},\mathbf{L},\mathbf{R}$ need be stored, not $\mathbf{U}$. Also, in distinction to the QR–method of [3] based on (1.4), the matrix $\mathbf{D}(\mathbf{C})$ need not be retained; the corresponding information is kept in $\mathbf{R}$. Also, some of the updating mechanisms simplify. This holds in particular for the so–called dropping step (see section 3), where the use of the decomposition (1.5) leads to some savings over (1.4).

Before we describe the algorithm in detail in sections 2 and 3, it is useful to outline how the crucial step 3 of (1.2) is performed:

Given an S–pair $(\mathbf{x}_k,\mathbf{J}_k)$, and a constraint r violated by $\mathbf{x}_k$, $\overline{\alpha} := \mathbf{a}_r^T\mathbf{x}_k - \mathbf{b}_r > \mathbf{0}$, one constructs for $\mathbf{0} \le \alpha \le \overline{\alpha}$ a continuous piecewise linear curve $\mathbf{x}(\alpha)$, with $\mathbf{x}(\mathbf{0}) = \mathbf{x}_k$, and a family of index vectors $\mathbf{J}(\alpha)$, with $\mathbf{J}(\mathbf{0}) = \mathbf{J}_k$, $\mathbf{J}(\alpha) \subset \mathbf{J}_k$, such that $\mathbf{x}(\alpha)$ is the optimal solution of

$$\begin{aligned} &\min \frac{1}{2} \|\mathbf{Cx} - \mathbf{c}\| \\ &\mathbf{x}:\ \mathbf{A}_{\mathbf{J}(\alpha)}^T \mathbf{x} \le \mathbf{b}_{\mathbf{J}(\alpha)} \\ &\mathbf{a}_r^T\mathbf{x} \le \mathbf{b}_r + \overline{\alpha} - \alpha = \mathbf{a}_r^T\mathbf{x}_k - \alpha \end{aligned} \tag{1.6}$$

with $\mathbf{A}_{\mathbf{J}(\alpha)}^T\mathbf{x}(\alpha) = \mathbf{b}_{\mathbf{J}(\alpha)}$, $\mathbf{a}_r^T\mathbf{x}(\alpha) = \mathbf{a}_r^T\mathbf{x}_k - \alpha$, $\mathbf{0} \le \alpha \le \overline{\alpha}$. The optimality of $\mathbf{x}(\mathbf{a})$ is equivalent to the existence of Lagrange multipliers $\mathbf{u}(\alpha)$, $\lambda_r(\alpha)$ such that for $\mathbf{0} \le \alpha \le \overline{\alpha}$

$$\nabla \mathbf{f}(\mathbf{x}(\alpha)) + \mathbf{A}_{\mathbf{J}(\alpha)}\mathbf{u}(\alpha) + \mathbf{a}_r \cdot \lambda_r(\alpha) = \mathbf{0} ,$$

$$\mathbf{u}_{\mathbf{J}(\alpha)} \ge \mathbf{0} , \quad \lambda_r(\alpha) \ge \mathbf{0} .$$

The vectors $\mathbf{u}(\alpha)$ and $\lambda_r(\alpha)$ are again piecewise linear functions in α, which can be explicitly computed together with $\mathbf{x}(\alpha)$. Starting with $\alpha = \mathbf{0}$, $\mathbf{x}(\mathbf{0}) = \mathbf{x}_k$, $\mathbf{J}(\mathbf{0}) = \mathbf{J}_k$, $\lambda_r(\mathbf{0}) = \mathbf{0}$, one increases α in $[\mathbf{0},\overline{\alpha}]$ and observes the function $\mathbf{u}(\alpha)$. Everytime a component of $\mathbf{u}(\alpha)$ becomes 0, say $\mathbf{u}_i(\alpha_0) = 0$, $\mathbf{u}(\alpha) \ge \mathbf{0}$, for $\alpha \le \alpha_0$, then the corresponding component j_i of $\mathbf{J}(\alpha)$ is dropped:

$$\mathbf{J}(\alpha_0) := \mathbf{J}(\alpha_0 -) \setminus \{j_i\} ,$$

so that $\mathbf{x}(\alpha_0)$ is still optimal for (1.3) ($\lambda_r(\alpha) > \mathbf{0}$ holds for $\alpha > \mathbf{0}$). Clearly for $\alpha = \overline{\alpha}$, $(\mathbf{x}_{k+1},\mathbf{J}_{k+1}) := (\mathbf{x}_k(\overline{\alpha}),\mathbf{J}_k(\overline{\alpha}) \cup \{r\})$ then is an S–pair for (P) with $\mathbf{f}(\mathbf{x}_{k+1}) > \mathbf{f}(\mathbf{x})$, $r \in \mathbf{J}_{k+1} \subset \mathbf{J}_k$.

For the realization of this algorithm, it is therefore important to have efficient methods for the computation of $\mathbf{x}(\alpha)$ and $\mathbf{u}(\alpha)$. Such methods, which are closely related to the technique employed in [1]–[3], are described in the following sections.

2. The computation of a new *S*–pair

Let us suppose that we are at the beginning of step 3 of (1.2) and we are given an S–pair $(\mathbf{x},\mathbf{J}) := (\mathbf{x}_k,\mathbf{J}_k)$ and a violated constraint r, that is $\overline{\alpha} := \mathbf{a}_r^T\mathbf{x} - \mathbf{b}_r > 0$. Moreover, assume that in addition to $(\mathbf{x},\mathbf{J})$, we are given a 7–tuple

$$\mathcal{M} \equiv (\mathbf{x},\mathbf{J},\mathbf{Q},\mathbf{R},\mathbf{L},\mathbf{h},\mathbf{u}) \tag{2.1}$$

with the following meaning:

(a) $\mathbf{Q}$ is a nonsingular $n\times n$ matrix, with (2.2)

$$\mathbf{A}_\mathbf{J}^T\mathbf{Q} = (\mathbf{0},\mathbf{L}) ,$$

where the lower triangular $l\times l$ matrix $\mathbf{L} := |\mathbf{J}|$ is of the form (called lower pseudotriangular)

$$\mathbf{L} = \begin{bmatrix} 0 & & . x \\ & . \cdot^{\cdot} & \vdots \\ x & \cdots & x \end{bmatrix}$$

(b) $\mathbf{R}$ is an upper triangular $p\times n$ matrix

$$\mathbf{R} = \begin{bmatrix} \mathbf{R}_{11} & \mathbf{R}_{12} \\ \mathbf{0} & \mathbf{R}_{22} \end{bmatrix} = \begin{bmatrix} x & \cdots & x \\ 0 & \ddots & x \\ \vdots & & 0 \\ \vdots & & \vdots \\ 0 & \cdots & 0 \end{bmatrix}$$

where the partitioning is such that $\mathbf{R}_{11}$ has $n-l$ columns, and there is a unitary $p\times p$ matrix $\mathbf{U}$ (which need not be stored) such that

$$\mathbf{UCQ} = \mathbf{R} , \quad \mathbf{U}(\mathbf{c} - \mathbf{Cx}) = \mathbf{h} .$$

If necessary, $\mathbf{h}$ is partitioned similarly to $\mathbf{R}$,

$$\mathbf{h} = \begin{bmatrix} \mathbf{h}_1 \\ \mathbf{h}_2 \end{bmatrix}, \qquad \mathbf{h}_1 \in \mathbf{R}^{n-l} .$$

(c) $\mathbf{u} \in \mathbf{R}^l$ is a vector of Lagrange multipliers such that

$$\nabla \mathbf{f}(\mathbf{x}) + \mathbf{A_J u} = 0 .$$

Note that $\mathbf{u} \geq \mathbf{0}$ and $\mathbf{A_J^T x} = \mathbf{b_J}$, since $(\mathbf{x},\mathbf{J})$ is an S–pair. It is easy to find such an $\mathcal{M}$ for the initial S–pair $(\mathbf{x},\mathbf{J})$ with $\mathbf{J} := \emptyset$: Set $l := 0$, $\mathbf{u}$ and $\mathbf{L}$ are empty, $\mathbf{Q} := \mathbf{I}$; the usual orthogonalization method for finding $\mathbf{x}$ with $\|\mathbf{Cx} - \mathbf{c}\| = \min \|\mathbf{Cy} - \mathbf{c}\|$ gives an orthogonal $\mathbf{U}$, an upper $p{\times}n$ triangle $\mathbf{R}$, and a vector $\mathbf{h}$ with

$$\mathbf{UC} = \mathbf{R}\,,\quad \mathbf{U}(\mathbf{c}-\mathbf{Cx}) = \mathbf{h} = \begin{bmatrix}\mathbf{h}_1\\ \mathbf{h}_2\end{bmatrix} \quad \text{with } \mathbf{h}_1 = \mathbf{0}\,.$$

Now let $(\mathbf{x},\mathbf{J})$ be an S–pair, r a constraint violated by $\mathbf{x}$, $\alpha := \mathbf{a}_r^T\mathbf{x} - \mathbf{b}_r > 0$, and $\mathcal{M}$ a 7–tuple (2.1) associated with $(\mathbf{x},\mathbf{J})$ which satisfies (2.2). Our aim is to construct a new S–pair $(\overline{\mathbf{x}},\overline{\mathbf{J}})$, and an associated $\overline{\mathcal{M}}$ with (2.2) such that

$$r \in \overline{\mathbf{J}} \subseteq \mathbf{J} \cup \{r\}\ ,\ \mathbf{f}(\overline{\mathbf{x}}) > \mathbf{f}(\mathbf{x})\ .$$

Since $(\mathbf{x},\mathbf{J})$ is an S–pair, $\mathbf{s} := \mathbf{0}$ is the optimal solution of

$$\min_{\mathbf{s}:\ \mathbf{A_J^T s} \leq \mathbf{0}} \|\mathbf{C}(\mathbf{x}+\mathbf{s}) - \mathbf{c}\| \equiv \|\mathbf{UCs} - \mathbf{h}\|\ ,$$

that is, using the transformed variables $\mathbf{y}$, $\mathbf{s} = \mathbf{Qy}$, the vector $\mathbf{y} = \mathbf{0}$ is also the optimal solution of

$$\min_{\mathbf{y}:\ \mathbf{A_J^T Q y} \leq \mathbf{0}} \|\mathbf{Ry} - \mathbf{h}\| \equiv \min \left\| \begin{bmatrix}\mathbf{R}_{11} & \mathbf{R}_{12}\\ \mathbf{0} & \mathbf{R}_{22}\end{bmatrix} \cdot \begin{bmatrix}\mathbf{y}_1\\ \mathbf{y}_2\end{bmatrix} - \begin{bmatrix}\mathbf{h}_1\\ \mathbf{h}_2\end{bmatrix} \right\|$$

$$\mathbf{y}:\ (\mathbf{0},\mathbf{L}) \begin{bmatrix}\mathbf{y}_1\\ \mathbf{y}_2\end{bmatrix} \equiv \mathbf{L}\mathbf{y}_2 \leq \mathbf{0}$$

so that $\mathbf{h}_1 = \mathbf{0}$, $\mathbf{h} = \begin{bmatrix}\mathbf{0}\\ \mathbf{h}_2\end{bmatrix}$.

Following the ideas explained at the end of section 1, we first try to find the optimal solution $\mathbf{s}(\alpha)$ for $\alpha \geq 0$ of

$$\min \|\mathbf{C}(\mathbf{x}+\mathbf{s}) - \mathbf{c}\| \qquad (\mathrm{P}_\alpha)$$

$$\mathbf{s}:\ \mathbf{A_J^T s} = \mathbf{0}$$

$$\mathbf{a}_r^T\mathbf{s} = -\alpha\ .$$

We then try to find those $\alpha \geq 0$, for which $s(\alpha)$ is also optimal for

$$\min \|\mathbf{C}(\mathbf{x}+\mathbf{s}) - \mathbf{c}\| \qquad (P_\alpha^{\leq})$$

$$\mathbf{s}:\ \mathbf{A}_\mathbf{J}^\mathsf{T}\mathbf{s} \leq \mathbf{0}$$

$$\mathbf{a}_r^\mathsf{T}\mathbf{s} \leq -\alpha\ .$$

Note that for $\alpha = 0$, $s(0) = 0$ is optimal for $P_0^{\leq}$.

It is easy to compute $s(\alpha)$ by means of $\mathcal{M}$. One sets

$$\mathbf{J}' := (j_1,\ldots,j_l,r) = \mathbf{J} \cup \{r\}\ ,\ \text{if } \mathbf{J} = (j_1,\ldots,j_l)$$

and, using the updating techniques of section 3, one easily finds a modified 7–tuple

$$\mathcal{M}' = (\mathbf{x},\mathbf{J}',\mathbf{Q}',\mathbf{R}',\mathbf{L}',\mathbf{h}',\mathbf{u}')\ ,$$

satisfying (2.2), $\mathbf{u}' = \begin{bmatrix}\mathbf{u}\\ \mathbf{0}\end{bmatrix}$ and

$$\mathbf{A}_{\mathbf{J}'}^\mathsf{T}\mathbf{Q} = \begin{bmatrix}\mathbf{A}_\mathbf{J}^\mathsf{T}\\ \mathbf{a}_r^\mathsf{T}\end{bmatrix} \cdot \mathbf{Q}' = (0,\mathbf{L}') = \left[\begin{array}{c|c|c}\mathbf{0} & 0 & \mathbf{L}\\ \mathbf{0} & \delta & \mathbf{a}^\mathsf{T}\end{array}\right]$$

We partition the matrix $\mathbf{R}'$ similarly:

$$\mathbf{R}' = \left[\begin{array}{c|c|c}\mathbf{R}_{11}' & r & \mathbf{R}_{12}\\ \hline \mathbf{0} & \rho & \mathbf{s}^\mathsf{T}\\ \hline \mathbf{0} & 0 & \mathbf{R}_{22}'\end{array}\right]$$

Let $\mathbf{U}'$ be the unitary matrix with the properties (2.2) with respect to $\mathcal{M}'$.

Then in terms of the transformed variables $\mathbf{y} = (\mathbf{Q}')^{-1}\mathbf{s}$, (P_α) is equivalent to

$$\min \|\mathbf{R}'\mathbf{y} - \mathbf{h}'\| \qquad (P_\alpha')$$

$$\mathbf{y}:\mathbf{A}_{\mathbf{J}'}^\mathsf{T}\mathbf{Q}'\mathbf{y} = \begin{bmatrix}0\\ -\alpha\end{bmatrix}$$

that is

$$\min \left\| \begin{bmatrix}\mathbf{R}_{11}' & r & \mathbf{R}_{12}'\\ \mathbf{0} & \rho & \mathbf{s}^\mathsf{T}\\ \mathbf{0} & 0 & \mathbf{R}_{22}'\end{bmatrix} \cdot \begin{bmatrix}\mathbf{y}_1\\ \eta\\ \mathbf{y}_2\end{bmatrix} - \begin{bmatrix}\mathbf{0}\\ \mathbf{0}\\ \mathbf{h}_2'\end{bmatrix} \right\|$$

$$\mathbf{y}: \begin{bmatrix}\mathbf{0} & 0 & \mathbf{L}\\ \mathbf{0} & \delta & \mathbf{a}^\mathsf{T}\end{bmatrix} \cdot \begin{bmatrix}\mathbf{y}_1\\ \eta\\ \mathbf{y}_2\end{bmatrix} = \begin{bmatrix}\mathbf{0}\\ \alpha\end{bmatrix}$$

We distinguish two cases:

I. $\delta \neq 0$, that is, $rk(\mathbf{A}_{\mathbf{J}'}) = |\mathbf{J}'|$, $\mathbf{L}' = \begin{bmatrix} 0 & \mathbf{L} \\ \delta & \mathbf{a}^{\mathrm{T}} \end{bmatrix}$ is nonsingular. (2.3)

II. $\delta = 0$, that is, $\mathbf{a}^r$ depends linearly on the columns of $\mathbf{A}_{\mathbf{J}}$,

$$\mathbf{a}_r = \mathbf{A}_{\mathbf{J}}\mathbf{v}, \quad \mathbf{a} = \mathbf{L}^{\mathrm{T}}\mathbf{v}, \quad \mathbf{v} := \mathbf{L}^{-\mathrm{T}}\mathbf{a} .$$

We consider case I first.

In this case, the optimal solution of (P'_α), which is linear in α, is given by

$$\mathbf{y}(\alpha) = \begin{bmatrix} \mathbf{y}_1(\alpha) \\ \eta(\alpha) \\ \mathbf{y}_2(\alpha) \end{bmatrix}, \quad \mathbf{y}_2(\alpha) := 0 , \quad \eta(\alpha) := -\frac{\alpha}{\delta},$$

$$\mathbf{y}_1(\alpha) := \frac{\alpha}{\delta}\mathbf{R}'^{-1}_{11} r. \tag{2.4}$$

It is easy to compute the Lagrange multipliers $\mathbf{u}'(\alpha) = \begin{bmatrix} \mathbf{u}(\alpha) \\ \lambda_r(\alpha) \end{bmatrix}$ for the optimal solution $\mathbf{s}(\alpha) := \mathbf{Q}'\mathbf{y}(\alpha)$ of (P_α)

$$\mathbf{0} = \nabla \mathbf{f}(\mathbf{x}+\mathbf{s}(\alpha)) + \mathbf{A}_{\mathbf{J}'}\mathbf{u}'(\alpha) = \nabla \mathbf{f}(\mathbf{x}+\mathbf{s}(\alpha)) + \mathbf{A}_{\mathbf{J}}\mathbf{u}(\alpha) + \mathbf{a}_r\lambda_r(\alpha) . \tag{2.5}$$

$\mathbf{u}'(\alpha)$ is given by

$$\mathbf{u}'(\alpha) = \begin{bmatrix} \mathbf{u}(\alpha) \\ \lambda_r(\alpha) \end{bmatrix} = (\mathbf{L}')^{-\mathrm{T}} \begin{bmatrix} \rho & \mathbf{s}^{\mathrm{T}} \\ 0 & \mathbf{R}'_{22} \end{bmatrix}^{\mathrm{T}} \left[\begin{bmatrix} \mathbf{0} \\ \mathbf{h}'_2 \end{bmatrix} - \eta(\alpha) \cdot \begin{bmatrix} \rho \\ 0 \end{bmatrix} \right]$$

$$= \mathbf{u}'(0) + \frac{\alpha\rho}{\delta} \begin{bmatrix} 0 & \delta \\ \mathbf{L}^{\mathrm{T}} & \mathbf{a} \end{bmatrix}^{-1} \cdot \begin{bmatrix} \rho \\ \mathbf{s} \end{bmatrix} , \tag{2.6}$$

where $\mathbf{u}'(0) \geq \mathbf{0}$, since $\mathbf{s}(0)$ is optimal for $(\mathrm{P}_0^{\leq})$.

In particular,

$$\lambda_r(\alpha) = \lambda_r(0) + \alpha\frac{\rho^2}{\delta^2} \geq \mathbf{0} \quad \text{for all } \alpha \geq \mathbf{0} . \tag{2.7}$$

Note that

$$\mathbf{f}(\mathbf{x}+\mathbf{s}(\alpha)) = \frac{1}{2}\|\mathbf{R}'\mathbf{y}(\alpha) - \mathbf{h}'\|^2 = \|\mathbf{h}'_2\|^2 + \rho^2\eta(\alpha)^2$$

$$= \|\mathbf{h}'_2\|^2 + \rho^2 \cdot \frac{\alpha^2}{\delta^2}$$

increases strictly with α.

The vector $s(\alpha) := Qy(\alpha)$ will be optimal for

$$\begin{aligned} &\min \|C(x+s) - c\| && (P_{\alpha}^{\leq}) \\ &s: A_J^T s \leq 0 \\ &a_r^T s \leq -\alpha , \end{aligned}$$

for all $0 \leq \alpha$ with $u(\alpha) \geq 0$. Let $\hat{\alpha}$ be the maximal $\alpha \geq 0$ for which $u(\alpha) \geq 0$, which can easily be computed from (2.6) (note that $\hat{\alpha} = 0, \infty$ is possible).

Let $\overline{\alpha} := \min(\hat{\alpha}, a_r^T x - b_r)$ and define

$$\begin{aligned} \overline{x} &:= x + s(\overline{\alpha}) , \quad s(\overline{\alpha}) := Q'y(\alpha) \\ \overline{h} &:= U'(c - C\overline{x}) = U'(c - Cx - CQ'y(\alpha)) \\ &= h' - R'y(\overline{\alpha}) \\ &= \begin{bmatrix} 0 \\ 0 \\ h_2' \end{bmatrix} - \eta(\overline{\alpha}) \begin{bmatrix} 0 \\ \rho \\ 0 \end{bmatrix} = \begin{bmatrix} 0 \\ \rho\overline{\alpha}/\delta \\ h_2' \end{bmatrix} \end{aligned} \tag{2.8}$$

We distinguish two cases: 1. $\overline{\alpha} = a_r^T x - b_r$, and 2. $\overline{\alpha} = \hat{\alpha} < a_r^T x - b_r$. In case 1, $(\overline{x}, \overline{J})$, $\overline{J} := J' = J \cup \{r\}$ is a new S–pair with the properties required in step 3) of (1.2), and a corresponding 7–tuple with (2.2)

$$\overline{\mathcal{M}} := (\overline{x}, \overline{J}, \overline{Q}, \overline{R}, \overline{L}, \overline{h}, \overline{u})$$

is given by (2.8) and

$$\overline{J} := J' = J \cup \{r\} , \quad \overline{Q} := Q' , \quad \overline{R} := R' , \quad \overline{L} := L', \quad \overline{u} := u'(\alpha) .$$

In case 2, $\overline{\alpha} = \hat{\alpha} < a_r^T x - b_r$, there is an index $i \neq r$ with $u(\overline{\alpha})_i = 0$.

We now set

$$\overline{J} := J \setminus \{j_i\} , \quad \overline{J}' := \overline{J} \cup \{r\} = J' \setminus \{j_i\}$$

and $\overline{u}'$ is obtained from $u'(\overline{\alpha})$ by removing its ith component $u'(\overline{\alpha})_i$. By applying the dropping step of the update algorithms in section 3, the 7–tuple $\mathcal{M}' = (x, J', Q', R', L', h', u')$ is transformed into a new 7–tuple $\overline{\mathcal{M}}' = (\overline{x}, \overline{J}', \overline{Q}', \overline{R}', \overline{L}', \overline{h}', \overline{u}')$ again satisfying (2.2). We then replace $\mathcal{M}'$ by $\overline{\mathcal{M}}'$ and repeat the algorithm starting with (2.4).

Now consider case II, $\delta = 0$.

In this case, $\mathbf{a}_r$ is linearly dependent on the columns of $\mathbf{A_J}$, $\mathbf{a}_r = \mathbf{A_J v}$, where $\mathbf{v}$ can be computed as the solution of

$$\mathbf{L}^T\mathbf{v} = \mathbf{a} .$$

If $\mathbf{v} \leq \mathbf{0}$ then $\mathbf{A_J^T s} \leq \mathbf{0}$ implies $\mathbf{a}_r^T\mathbf{s} \geq \mathbf{0}$, that is, for $\alpha > 0$, $(P_\alpha^{\leq})$ and therefore (P) has no feasible solutions, and we may stop. Suppose therefore $\mathbf{v} \not\leq \mathbf{0}$. Then one can find an index i such that

$$\frac{\mathbf{u}_i}{\mathbf{v}_i} = \min \left\{\frac{\mathbf{u}_j}{\mathbf{v}_j} \mid \mathbf{v}_j > 0\right\}$$

Then $\mathbf{a}_r = \mathbf{A_J v}$ implies

$$\mathbf{a}_{j_i} = \frac{1}{\mathbf{v}_i}\mathbf{a}_r - \sum_{k \neq i} \frac{\mathbf{v}_k}{\mathbf{v}_i}\mathbf{a}_{j_k}$$

Since $(\mathbf{x},\mathbf{J})$ is an S–pair, we therefore get, by elimination of $\mathbf{a}_{j_i}$,

$$\mathbf{0} = \nabla \mathbf{f}(\mathbf{x}) + \mathbf{A_J u} = \nabla \mathbf{f}(\mathbf{x}) + \sum_{\substack{k=1 \\ k \neq i}}^{l} \mathbf{a}_{j_k}\left(\mathbf{u}_k - \frac{\mathbf{u}_i \mathbf{v}_k}{\mathbf{v}_i}\right) + \mathbf{a}_r \frac{\mathbf{u}_i}{\mathbf{v}_i} \tag{2.9}$$

Since

$$\mathbf{u}_k - \mathbf{u}_i\mathbf{v}_k/\mathbf{v}_i \geq \mathbf{0} \qquad \text{for } k \neq i$$

and $\mathbf{u}_i \geq \mathbf{0}$, $\mathbf{s} = \mathbf{0}$ is optimal for $P_0^{\leq}$, if we replace $\mathbf{J}$ by $\mathbf{J} \setminus \{j_i\}$ in the definition of $P_0^{\leq}$. By means of the dropping step of section 3, we may compute a new 7–tuple

$$\overline{\mathcal{M}}' = (\overline{\mathbf{x}},\overline{\mathbf{J}}',\overline{\mathbf{R}}',\overline{\mathbf{L}}',\overline{\mathbf{h}}',\overline{\mathbf{u}})$$

which satisfies (2.2) for $\overline{\mathbf{J}} := \mathbf{J}' \setminus \{j_i\} = (j_1,\ldots,j_{i-1},j_{i+1},\ldots,j_l,r)$. Note that in (2.9) $\overline{\mathbf{u}}'$ is given by

$$\overline{\mathbf{u}}_k' = \begin{cases} \mathbf{u}_k - \mathbf{u}_i\mathbf{v}_k/\mathbf{v}_i , & \text{for } k \leq i-1 \\ \mathbf{u}_{k+1} - \mathbf{u}_i\mathbf{v}_{k+1}/\mathbf{v}_i , & \text{for } i \leq k \leq l-1 \\ \mathbf{u}_i/\mathbf{v}_i , & \text{for } k := l . \end{cases} \tag{2.10}$$

One now replaces $\mathcal{M}'$ by $\overline{\mathcal{M}}'$ and returns to (2.3).

3. Update techniques

Let $\mathcal{M} = (\mathbf{x},\mathbf{J},\mathbf{Q},\mathbf{R},\mathbf{L},\mathbf{h},\mathbf{u})$ satisfy (2.2). In the course of the algorithm of section 2, one has to compute new 7–tuples $\mathcal{M}'$ satisfying (2.2), if $\mathbf{J}$ is changed by one index i: $\mathbf{J}' = \mathbf{J} \cup \{i\}$ (adding step), or $\mathbf{J}' = \mathbf{J} \setminus \{j_i\}$ (dropping step).

Let us consider the *adding step* first and let $i \in \{1,...,m\}$ be an index with $i \notin \mathbf{J}$, and set

$$\mathbf{J}' := (j_1,...,j_l,i) \quad \text{if } \mathbf{J} = (j_1,...,j_l)\ .$$

The problem is to compute an $\mathcal{M}' = (\mathbf{x},\mathbf{J}',\mathbf{Q}',\mathbf{R}',\mathbf{L}',\mathbf{h}',\mathbf{u}')$ with (2.2). By the definition of $\mathcal{M}$ we have

$$\mathbf{A}_{\mathbf{J}'}^{\top}\mathbf{Q} = \begin{bmatrix} \mathbf{A}_{\mathbf{J}}^{\top}\mathbf{Q} \\ \mathbf{a}_i^{\top}\mathbf{Q} \end{bmatrix} = \begin{bmatrix} \mathbf{0} & \mathbf{L} \\ \mathbf{b}^{\top} & \mathbf{a}^{\top} \end{bmatrix}, \qquad (\mathbf{b}^{\top},\mathbf{a}^{\top}) = \mathbf{a}_i^{\top}\mathbf{Q}\ .$$

Let us sketch the further transformations for the special case $l = |\mathbf{J}| = 2$, $n = 5$, $p = 6$. Then there is a unitary $\mathbf{U}$ such that

$$\mathbf{B} := \mathbf{A}_{\mathbf{J}}^{\top}\mathbf{Q} = \begin{bmatrix} O & & & & x \\ & & & x & x \\ x & x & x & x & x \end{bmatrix}$$

$$\mathbf{UCQ} = \mathbf{R} = \begin{bmatrix} x & x & x & x & x \\ & x & x & x & x \\ & & x & x & x \\ O & & & x & x \\ & & & & x \\ 0 & 0 & 0 & 0 & 0 \end{bmatrix}$$

By postmultiplying $\mathbf{B} := \mathbf{A}_{\mathbf{J}}^{\top}\mathbf{Q}$ by a suitable Givens rotation operating on the columns 1 and 2 one can annihilate $\mathbf{B}_{31}$. (Instead of a Givens rotation one could also use Gaussian elimination operating on columns 1 and 2 with pivot $\mathbf{B}_{32}$ in order to annihilate $\mathbf{B}_{31}$; if necessary, an interchange of columns 1 and 2 can guarantee $0 \neq |\mathbf{B}_{32}| \geq |\mathbf{B}_{31}|$. This would reduce the number of operations by a factor of 3, without losing numerical stability.)

Applying the same operation also to $\mathbf{R} = \mathbf{UCQ}$, transforming $\mathbf{R}$ to $\mathbf{R}_1$, generates a subdiagonal element in position (2,1) of $\mathbf{R}_1$. This in turn is annihilated by premultiplying $\mathbf{R}_1$ by a suitable Givens rotation operating on rows 1 and 2 of $\mathbf{R}_1$. The same premultiplication is also applied to $\mathbf{U}(\mathbf{c}-\mathbf{C}\mathbf{x}) = \mathbf{h}$. (See the following sketch where changing elements are denoted by *.)

$$\mathbf{A}_{\mathbf{J}}^{\top}\mathbf{Q} \to \mathbf{A}_{\mathbf{J}'}^{\top}\mathbf{Q}_1 = \begin{bmatrix} & & & & x \\ & & & x & x \\ 0 & * & x & x & x \end{bmatrix}$$

$$\mathbf{UCQ} = \mathbf{R} \to \mathbf{UCQ}_1 = \mathbf{R}_1 = \begin{bmatrix} * & * & x & x & x \\ * & * & x & x & x \\ & & x & x & x \\ & & & x & x \\ & & & & x \\ 0 & & & & 0 \end{bmatrix} \to \mathbf{U}_1\mathbf{CQ}_1 = \begin{bmatrix} * & * & * & * & * \\ & * & * & * & * \\ & & x & x & x \\ & & & x & x \\ & & & & x \\ 0 & & & & 0 \end{bmatrix}$$

$$U(c-Cx) = h = \begin{bmatrix} x \\ x \\ x \\ x \\ x \\ x \end{bmatrix} \rightarrow U_1(c-Cx) = \begin{bmatrix} * \\ * \\ x \\ x \\ x \\ x \end{bmatrix}$$

In the same way, all elements in the last row of $A_J^T \cdot Q$ are annihilated one by one until $A_J^T \cdot Q$ is transformed into a lower triangular matrix

$$A_J^T \cdot Q' = (0,L'),L' = \begin{bmatrix} 0 & L \\ \delta & a^T \end{bmatrix} = \begin{bmatrix} 0 & & & x \\ & & \cdot & \vdots \\ x & \cdots & & x \end{bmatrix}$$

of the required shape. Likewise $UCQ = R$ is transformed into a new upper triangular

$$U'CQ' = R',$$

where U' is unitary and $h = U(c-Cx)$ into $h' = U'(c-Cx)$.

Since

$$\nabla f(x) + A_J u = 0,$$

$u' := \begin{bmatrix} u \\ 0 \end{bmatrix}$ satisfies

$$\nabla f(x) + A_{J'} u' = 0,$$

and the construction of $\mathcal{M}' = (x,J',Q',R',L',h',u')$ is complete. Note that the computation of $\mathcal{M}'$ from $\mathcal{M}$ requires only $0(n^2)$ operations.

For the *dropping step* we have the following situation: we are given $\mathcal{M} = (x,J,Q,R,L,h,u)$ satisfying (2.2), and an index $j_i \in J$ to be removed from J. Now,

$$J' := J \setminus \{j_i\} = (j_1,\ldots,j_{i-1},j_{i+1},\ldots,j_l),$$

where i is such that $u_i = 0$.

A 7–tuple $\mathcal{M}' = (x,J',Q',R',L',h',u')$ satisfying (2.2) is obtained as follows: $A_J^T \cdot Q$ has the form (sketched for $n = 5$, $i = 2$, $p = 6$, $l = |J| = 4$)

$$A_J^T \cdot Q = \begin{bmatrix} 0 & 0 & 0 & 0 & x \\ 0 & 0 & x & x & x \\ 0 & x & x & x & x \end{bmatrix}$$

By postmultiplying $A_J^T \cdot Q$ by a suitable Givens rotation (or Gaussian elimination matrices) operating on columns (3,4), one annihilates the (2,3) element and finds a nonsingular Q_1 such that

$$A_J^T \cdot Q_1 = \begin{bmatrix} O & & & & x \\ & & & 0 & * & x \\ 0 & x & * & * & x \end{bmatrix}$$

$$UCQ_1 = \begin{bmatrix} x & x & * & * & x \\ & x & * & * & x \\ & & * & * & x \\ & & * & * & x \\ & & & & x \\ 0 & & & & 0 \end{bmatrix} \rightarrow U_1CQ_1 = \begin{bmatrix} x & x & x & x & x \\ & x & x & x & x \\ & & * & * & * \\ & & & * & * \\ & & & & x \\ 0 & & & & 0 \end{bmatrix}$$

and we can again restore the triangular structure of UCQ_1 by removing the newly introduced subdiagonal (4,3)–element by premultiplying UCQ_1 by a suitable Givens rotation operating on the rows (3,4). $A_J^T \cdot Q$ and U_1CQ_1 are then treated in the same way as $A_J^T \cdot Q$ and $UCQ = R$. In this way one finally finds a nonsingular Q', a unitary U', so that $A_J^T \cdot Q'$ and $U'CQ'$ have the required shapes

$$A_J^T \cdot Q' = (0, L'), \quad L' = \begin{bmatrix} 0 & & x \\ & \cdot^{\cdot^{\cdot}} & \vdots \\ x & \cdots & x \end{bmatrix}$$

$$U'CQ' = R' = \begin{bmatrix} x & \cdots & & x \\ 0 & \ddots & & \vdots \\ \vdots & & & x \\ \vdots & & & 0 \\ \vdots & & & \vdots \\ 0 & \cdots & \cdot & 0 \end{bmatrix}$$

Clearly, by applying the successive left multiplications of UCQ by orthogonal matrices also to $h = U(c-Cx)$, one obtains the vector

$$h' = U'(c-Cx) .$$

If we finally set $u' := (u_1, \ldots, u_{i-1}, u_{i+1}, \ldots, u_l)^T$, (note that $u_i = 0$), then the 7–tuple $\mathcal{M}' = (x, J', Q', R', L', h', u')$ again satisfies (2.2).

4. Concluding remarks

The above algorithm easily extends to the case where (P) involves equality constraints. Also, it is possible but more difficult to extend the method to quadratic programs (1.1), where D is only positive semidefinite, or the matrix C in (P) does not have full column rank. In this case, the finiteness of the method is much harder to prove.

The storage requirement for the algorithm is somewhat higher than for the rival methods in [1], [2], since one has to store the matrix **R**. On the other hand, it is not necessary to retain **C**, which may be overwritten by **R**. The code of Powell [2] for the GI method needs the storage of **C** for the periodic iterative refinement of the current matrix partitionings (1.3) of the GI method [1], [2] in order to limit the loss of accuracy connected with a badly conditioned **D**/**C**. The QR method discussed by Powell [3] needs the storage of **D**/**C** for the realization of the dropping step. If in (1.4) $\mathbf{J}_k$ is replaced by $\mathbf{J}_k' := \mathbf{J}_k \setminus \{i\}$, then the computation of $\mathbf{U}_k'$ requires the computation of a product $\mathbf{q}^{\mathrm{T}}\mathbf{D}\mathbf{Q}_k^{(u)}$ for a $\mathbf{q} \in \mathbf{R}^n$ and the solution of a triangular system of linear equations with the $(n-|\mathbf{J}_k|) \times (n-|\mathbf{J}_k|)$ matrix $\mathbf{U}_k$ (1.4). On the average this requires more work than the corresponding dropping step of this paper (unless $|\mathbf{J}_k|$ is quite large, say $|\mathbf{J}_k| \geq 0.8n$).

Naturally, this difference is felt only if many dropping steps occur in the course of the algorithm.

The coding of the algorithm is under way. Test results will be reported separately.

REFERENCES

[1] Goldfarb, G., and A. Idnani. 1983. A numerically stable dual method for solving strictly convex quadratic programs. *Math. Programming* 2, no. 7: 1–33.

[2] Powell, M.J.D. 1983. ZQPCVX A Fortran subroutine for convex quadratic programming. Technical Report DAMTP/1983/NA17, Dept. of Applied Mathematics and Theoretical Physics, University of Cambridge, England.

[3] ——————. 1983. On the quadratic programming algorithm of Goldfarb and Idnani. Technical Report DAMTP/1983/NA19, Dept. of Applied Mathematics and Theoretical Physics, University of Cambridge, England.

[4] Stoer, J. 1971. On the numerical solution of constrained least squares problems. *SIAM J. Numer. Anal.* 8: 382–411.

THE FINITE ELEMENT APPROXIMATION OF MINIMAL SURFACES

V.A. Vasilenko

Computing Center
Siberian branch of the USSR Academy of Sciences
Novosibirsk, USSR

Introduction

Let Ω be some bounded domain in R^n, and W_2^m be the Sobolev space of functions with m^{th} partial derivatives in $L_2(\Omega)$. Let us define the operator of the generalized gradients by the formula

$$D^m u = \left[\left(\frac{m!}{\alpha!}\right)^{1/2} D^\alpha u, |\alpha| = m\right], \tag{1}$$

where $\alpha = (\alpha_1,...,\alpha_n)$ is multi-index, $\alpha_i \geq 0$, $\alpha! = \alpha_1!\cdots\alpha_n!$, $|\alpha| = \Sigma_{i=1}^n \alpha_i$. The operator D^m is the mapping from W_2^m to the space $Y = \otimes_{i=1}^R L_2(\Omega)$, where $R = (n+m-1)!/n!/(m-1)!$ is the number of all indices α with $|\alpha| = m$. The norm in Y is introduced by

$$\|v\|_Y = \|v\|_{L_2} = \left(\sum_{k=1}^R \|v_k\|_{L_2(\Omega)}\right)^{1/2}, \quad v = (v_1,...,v_n) . \tag{2}$$

The range of operator D^m is closed in Y under some natural conditions [1].

Let $m > n/2$, so that the embedding of the space W_2^m to the space $C(\Omega)$ of continuous functions occurs. Consider in Ω an arbitrary subset ω_h which forms some h-net in Ω,

$$h = \sup_{p\in\Omega}\ \inf_{Q\in\omega_h} \|P - Q\|_2 , \tag{3}$$

where $\|\cdot\|$ is the usual Euclidean norm. The problem is to find the interpolant $\sigma_h \in W_2^m(\Omega)$ of the given function $\varphi_* \in W_2^m(\Omega)$ from the conditions

$$\sigma_h = \varphi_* \quad \text{in } \omega_h ,$$
$$\|D^m \sigma_h\|^2_{L_2} = \sum_{|\alpha| = m} \frac{\alpha!}{m!} \int_\Omega (D^\alpha \sigma_h)^2 \, d\Omega = \min . \tag{4}$$

The solution of this problem is known as *D^m–spline*, or surface with minimal energy. Spline–interpolation of this type was studied by this author in [1], [2], [3], and by others in [4], [5], [6], [9].

Denote by Π_{m-1} the space of polynomials of n variables with order not greater than m–1. The dimension of this space is $R = (n+m-1)!/n!/(m-1)!$. The set of points $p_1,...,p_R$ is called *L*–solvable if the Lagrange problem for the polynomial $L_{m-1} \in \Pi_{m-1}$, determined by the condition

$$L_{m-1}(p_k) = z_k , \quad k = \overline{1,R} \tag{5}$$

has a unique solution. Then the general existence and uniqueness theorem for splines [1] leads to the following

Theorem 1. *The problem* (4) *is uniquely solvable if the subset ω_h contains some L–solvable set.*

The general convergence theorem for splines [1] shows that $\sigma_h \to \varphi_*$ in W_2^m–norm. Moreover, for the case $\Omega = \mathrm{R}^n$ [4] and for the bounded domain Ω [6] the following error estimate holds:

$$\|D^k(\sigma_h - \varphi_*)\|_{L_q(\Omega_\delta)} \le C h^{m-k-n/2+n/q} \|D^m(\sigma_h - \varphi_*)\|_{L_2(\Omega)} . \tag{6}$$

Here Ω_δ is the δ–interior of the bounded domain Ω, and $m > n/2$, $2 \le q \le \infty$, $k - n/q \le m - n/2$, excluding the case $k = m - n/2$, $q = \infty$. To prove this error estimate we have to assume that the domain satisfies the following "cone condition": it is possible to touch any point of the boundary (from the inside and from the outside) by the top of the n–dimensional sector of any radius $R > 0$ and with angle $\theta > 0$.

To construct the D^m spline we need to know the explicit representation of Green's function (see [5], [1]) for the polyharmonic operator Δ^m in the domain Ω. But, in general, for bounded domains the explicit representation of Green's function is unknown. For $\Omega = \mathrm{R}^n$ we have the necessary formula (see [4], [5]), but computation of splines σ_h requires the solution of a linear algebraic system with a dense matrix; the analytic representation of spline σ_h includes logarithms (in even–dimensional domain Ω) and square roots, and the number of these functions grows if the number of points in ω_h increases. But the main (and important for practical implementation) property of piecewise–polynomial splines is the simplicity of computation of the spline in every point of the domain. This leads to a natural solution technique: approximate the nonpolynomial splines by finite elements, which, in turn, leads to sparse matrices and simplest polynomial representations (see [1], [2]). The general convergence theorems proved show the convergence of these approximations in the W_2^m-norm. The objective of this paper is to obtain the error estimate in L_q-norms which are similar to (6). But first we need to make some preliminary assumptions, which are, in fact, of independent interest.

1. D^m-approximation as the orthogonal projection

Let ω_h be some finite h-net in the domain Ω containing some L-solvable set $p_1,\dots,p_R$. Let us define in the space W_2^m the scalar product and the norm in the following way:

$$(u,v)_* = \sum_{i=1}^{R} u(p_i)v(p_i) + (D^m u, D^m v)_{L_2}, \qquad \|u\|_* = (u,u)_*^{1/2}. \tag{7}$$

This special norm is equivalent to the conventional norm in W_2^m (see [7]),

$$C_1\|u\|_* \leq \|u\|_{W_2^m} \leq C_2\|u\|_* . \tag{8}$$

Denote by $\Pi_{m-1}^{\perp}$ the set of functions from W_2^m orthogonal to the space of polynomials Π_{m-1} in the scalar product $(,)_*$. Let $u \in \Pi_{m-1}^{\perp}$. Then for every monomial $t^\alpha = t_1^{\alpha_1}\cdots t_n^{\alpha_n}$, $|\alpha| \leq m-1$ we have

$$(u,t^\alpha)_* = \sum_{i=1}^{R} u(p_i)p_i^\alpha = 0 . \tag{9}$$

Equalities (9) form the linear algebraic system for $u(p_i)$, and the matrix of this system is transformed to the matrix corresponding to the Lagrange polynomial. This matrix is nonsingular, so that $u(p_i) = 0$, $i = \overline{1,R}$. Therefore the subspace $\Pi_{m-1}^{\perp}$ consists of the functions from $W_2^m(\Omega)$, vanishing on the L-solvable set. In the subspace $\Pi_{m-1}^{\perp}$ the expressions $\|D^m u\|_{L_2}$, $(D^m u, D^m v)_{L_2}$ are exactly the norm and scalar product.

If $\varphi_* \in W_2^m$, the unique representation in the form

$$\varphi_* = Q_{m-1} + \varphi_*^{\perp}, \quad Q_{m-1} \in \Pi_{m-1}, \quad \varphi_*^{\perp} \in \Pi_{m-1}^{\perp} \tag{10}$$

is valid. If we construct the D^m splines σ_h in the set of meshes ω_h, and the intersection of ω_h includes some L-solvable set $p_1,p_2,\dots,p_R$, then the polynomial part Q_{m-1} will be reproduced exactly,

$$\sigma_h = Q_{m-1} + \sigma_h^{\perp},$$

and $\varphi_*^{\perp}$ will be interpolated by D^m spline $\sigma_h^{\perp}$, which vanishes at the points $p_1,\dots,p_R$. In the subspace $\Pi_{m-1}^{\perp}$ the structure of D^m splines becomes simpler. Let D^m: $\Pi_{m-1}^{\perp} \to D^m(\Pi_{m-1}^{\perp})$. Then the conjugate operator $(D^m)^*$: $D^m(\Pi_{m-1}^{\perp}) \to \Pi_{m-1}^{\perp}$, defined by the Lagrange identity

$$(D^m u,v)_{L_2} = (u,(D^m)^*v)_* , \tag{11}$$

has the property $(D^m)^* = (D^m)^{-1}$. Indeed,

$$(D^m u,v)_{L_2} = (u,(D^m)^*v)_* = (D^m u,D^m(D^m)^*v)_{L_2}$$

for every $u \in \Pi_{m-1}^{\perp}$, $v \in D^m(\Pi_{m-1}^{\perp})$.

Denote by k_p the functionals in $\Pi_{m-1}^{\perp}$ given by

$$\forall\, u \in \Pi_{m-1}^{\perp} \quad (k_p,u)_* = u(P) . \tag{12}$$

Then using the well-known fact [1] from spline theory that $T^*T\sigma = \sum \lambda_i k_i$, we have in this case

$$\sigma_h^{\perp} = \sum_{p\in \omega_h'} \lambda_p k_p , \tag{13}$$

where ω_h' is the mesh ω_h without a L–solvable set $p_1,\dots,p_R$. The constants λ_p are found in the interpolation conditions

$$\sigma_h^{\perp} = (k_Q,\sigma_h^{\perp})_* = \sum_{p\in \omega_h'} (k_p,k_Q)_*\lambda_p = (k_Q,\varphi_*^{\perp}) = \varphi_*^{\perp}(Q) .$$
$$\forall\, Q \in \omega_h' . \tag{14}$$

It is obvious that (14) is equivalent to the condition

$$\|\varphi_*^{\perp} - \sum_{p\in \omega_h'} \lambda_p k_p \|_* = \min_{\lambda p} , \tag{15}$$

and linear algebraic system (14) has a nonsingular matrix, if the mesh ω_h' does not include any equal points. Thus we no longer need the variational principle $\|D^m\sigma_h^{\perp}\|_{L_2} = \|\sigma_h^{\perp}\|_* = \min$.

So, the D^m spline $\sigma_h^{\perp}$ is the orthogonal projection in the scalar product $(u,v)_*$ of the function $\varphi_*^{\perp}$ to the linear finite–dimensional space with basis k_p, $p \in \omega_h'$.

2. Finite element approximations of D^m splines

Let us consider in the space $\Pi_{m-1}^{\perp}$ some system of the finite–dimensional subspaces E_τ, $\tau > 0$, any of them having the finite basis $v_1,v_2,\dots,v_{N(t)}$. For example, E_τ can be the finite element subspace with elements of size $\tau > 0$. In general, E_τ is a Hilbert space with scalar product defined by

$$(u^\tau,v^\tau)_* = (D^m u^\tau,D^m v^\tau)_{L_2} .$$

Let us fix the element $\varphi_*^\perp \in \Pi_{m-1}^\perp$ and the family of condensing meshes ω_h'. Then the spline σ_h^τ in the subspace E_τ ([1],[2]) is the solution of

$$\sigma_h^\tau = \varphi_*^\perp \quad \text{in } \omega_h' , \tag{16}$$

$$\|D^m \sigma_h^\tau\|_{L_2} = \min_{E_\tau} . \tag{17}$$

The interpolation condition (16) for given E_τ seems contradictory. But it is natural to assume that subspaces E_τ are dense in $\Pi_{m-1}^\perp$, $\tau \to 0$, so that for $\tau < \tau(h)$, (16) becomes correct (for sufficiently small τ the finite–element interpolation in E_τ of the given values in the given nodes of the ω_h' does exist). Then the solution of (16)–(17) exists and is unique.

Denote by k_p^τ the elements of E_τ with the property

$$(k_p^\tau, u^\tau)_* = u^\tau(P) , \quad \forall\, u^\tau \in E_\tau . \tag{18}$$

Then the functionals k_p^τ, $\tau < \tau(h)$, are linearly independent, $p \in \omega_h'$ (the existence of k_p^τ follows from the Riesz theorem in E_τ). In the same way as before, we can obtain the analogue of (13) in the subspace

$$\sigma_h^\tau = \sum_{p \in \omega_h'} \lambda_p^\tau k_p^\tau , \tag{19}$$

where coefficients λ_p^τ are determined from (16):

$$\sum_{p \in \omega_h'} \lambda_p^\tau (k_p^\tau, k_Q^\tau)_* = (\varphi_*^\perp, k_Q)_* , \quad Q \in \omega_h' . \tag{20}$$

Then for $\tau < \tau(h)$ (20) is uniquely solvable, and we do not need the variational principle $\|D^m \sigma_h^\perp\|_{L_2} = \min$.

Let us clarify the structure of the functional $k_p^\tau \in E^\tau$, which can be represented in the form

$$k_p^\tau = \sum_{i=1}^{N(\tau)} c_i v_i . \tag{21}$$

It is clear that $(k_p^\tau, v_j)_* = v_j(p) = (k_p, v_j)_*$, so that the following system of algebraic equations obtains:

$$\sum_{i=1}^{N(\tau)} c_i (v_i, v_j)_* = (k_p, v_j)_* , \quad j = \overline{1, N(\tau)} . \tag{22}$$

In other words, k_p^τ is the orthogonal projection of k_p on the subspace E_τ. Let us define the projector B_τ of the element $\varphi_* \in \Pi_{m-1}^\perp$ to E^τ by the condition

$$\|\varphi - B_\tau \varphi\|_* = \min_{u^\tau \in E_\tau} \|\varphi - u^\tau\|_* , \tag{23}$$

for which $k_p^\tau = B^\tau k_p$.

Denote by A_h: $\Pi_{m-1}^\perp \to R^{N(h)}$ the trace operator to the mesh ω_h'. Then the operator A^*: $R^{N(h)} \to \Pi_{m-1}^\perp$, i.e., the conjugate to A_h, satisfies the Lagrange identity

$$(A_h\varphi,\overline{\lambda})_{R^{N(h)}} = \sum_{p\in\omega'_h} \lambda_p(k_p,\varphi)_* = (\varphi,A_h^*\overline{\lambda})_*$$
$$\forall\, \varphi \in \Pi_{m-1}^{\perp},\ \forall\, \overline{\lambda} \in R^{N(h)}$$

and therefore can be represented in the form

$$A_h^*\overline{\lambda} = \sum_{p\in\omega'_h} \lambda_p k_p\,. \tag{24}$$

The system (24) can be rewritten in the form $A_hA_h^*\overline{\lambda} = A_h\varphi_*^{\perp}$, and for the spline $\sigma_h^{\perp}$, which interpolates the function $\varphi_*^{\perp}$, we obtain the following:

$$\sigma_h^{\perp} = S_h\varphi_*^{\perp} = A_h^*(A_hA_h^*)^{-1}A_h\varphi_*^{\perp}\,. \tag{25}$$

In the same way, for the system (20) we have

$$\sigma_h^{\tau} = S_h^{\tau}\varphi_*^{\perp} = B_\tau A_h^*(A_hB_\tau A_h^*)^{-1}A_h\varphi_*^{\perp}\,, \tag{26}$$

where S_h is the spline operator in $\Pi_{m-1}^{\perp}$ and S_h^{τ} is the spline operator in E_τ. Let $M_h^{\tau} = A_h^*(A_hB_\tau A_h^*)^{-1}A_h$. Then the identity $C^{-1}-D^{-1} = D^{-1}(D-C)C^{-1}$ leads to

$$\begin{aligned} M_h^{\tau} - S_h &= A_h^*[(A_hB_\tau A_h^*)^{-1} - (A_hA_h^*)^{-1}]A_h \\ &= A_h^*(A_hA_h^*)^{-1}A_h(I-B_\tau)A_h^*(A_hB_\tau A_h^*)^{-1}A_h = S_h(I-B_\tau)M_h^{\tau}\,. \end{aligned} \tag{27}$$

Lemma. *If for the system of subspaces E_τ, $\tau > 0$, the asymptotic inequality*

$$\|\varphi^{\perp} - B_\tau\varphi^{\perp}\|_* \le c\tau^{\beta}\|\varphi^{\perp}\|_*, \quad \forall\, \varphi^{\perp} \in \Pi_{m-1}^{\perp},\ \beta > 0 \tag{28}$$

holds true, then the sequence of splines σ_h^{τ} is bounded by a constant indepen– dent on h and τ.

P r o o f. From (27) there follows

$$M_h^{\tau}\varphi_*^{\perp} = S_h\varphi_*^{\perp} + S_h(I-B_\tau)M_h^{\tau}\varphi_*^{\perp}\,.$$

Hence for norms we obtain

$$\|M_h^{\tau}\varphi_*^{\perp}\|_* \le \|S_h\varphi_*^{\perp}\| + \|S_h\|\cdot c\tau^{\beta}\|M_h^{\tau}\varphi_*^{\perp}\|_*$$

and the inequality $\|S_h\varphi_*^{\perp}\| \le \|\varphi_*^{\perp}\|_*$, $\|S_h\| = 1$ leads to

$$\begin{aligned} \|\sigma_h^{\tau}\|_* = \|B_\tau M_h^{\tau}\varphi_*^{\perp}\|_* &\le \|M_h^{\tau}\varphi_*^{\perp}\|_* \le \frac{\|\varphi_*^{\perp}\|_*}{1 - c\tau^{\beta}} \\ &\simeq [1+o(\tau^{\beta})]\cdot\|\varphi_*^{\perp}\|_*\,. \end{aligned}$$

To prove the main error estimate we use the lemma concerning the condensation of zeros (see [4], [6]): if the function u belongs to $W_2^m(\Omega)$ and vanishes at the points of h–net in Ω (Ω satisfies the cone condition), then we have

$$\|D^k u\|_{L_q(\Omega_\delta)} \leq C h^{m-n/2-k+n/q} \|D^m u\|_{L_2(\Omega)} \tag{29}$$

in which Ω_δ is some δ–interior of the domain Ω, constant C depends on m, n, δ, q and is independent of u and h, $2 \leq q \leq \infty$, $k-n/q \leq m-n/2$ (excluding the case $k = m-n/2$ and $q = \infty$).

We now apply (29) to the function $u = \sigma_h^\tau - \varphi_*^\perp$ vanishing (for $\tau < \tau(h)$) at the points of the h–net ω_h', to obtain

$$\begin{aligned} \|D^k(\sigma_h^\tau - \varphi_*^\perp)\|_{L_q(\Omega_\delta)} &\leq C h^{m-n/2-k+n/q} \|D^m(\sigma_h^\tau - \varphi_*^\perp)\|_{L_2(\Omega)} \\ &\leq C h^{m-n/2-k+n/q}(\|D^m \sigma_h^\tau\|_{L_2} + \|D^m \varphi_*^\perp\|_{L_2}) \, . \end{aligned}$$

Therefore from (28) we have the following error estimate:

$$\|D^k(\sigma_h^\tau - \varphi_*^\perp)\|_{L_q(\Omega_\delta)} = o(h^{m-n/2-k+n/q}) \, . \tag{30}$$

Remark 1. We have considered the interpolation process in the subspace $\Pi_{m-1}^\perp$. However, for D^m interpolation the polynomials from Π_{m-1} are restored exactly. Thus, if the projector B_τ preserves the class Π_{m-1} (a typical property of polynomial finite elements), and the meshes ω_τ of the finite–element method contain some fixed L–solvable set, which is at the same time contained in the meshes ω_h, then (30) is valid for every function $\varphi_* \in W_2^m(\Omega)$.

Remark 2. We assume that for $\tau < \tau(h)$ the interpolation conditions are non–contradictory in E_τ, so that we have some correspondence between the method of condensation of chaotic meshes ω_h and that of meshes ω_τ for finite elements. In practice, of course, we use the least squares method instead of the pure interpolation conditions (see [8]), but it seems difficult to obtain error estimates of type (30) in this situation.

We now obtain the error estimates for the finite–element approximation of the smoothing D^m splines. Let us fix the smoothing parameter $\alpha > 0$ and the set $\omega = \omega_h$ of an arbitrary point in the domain Ω. Then the problem for the smoothing spline $\sigma_\alpha \in W_2^m(\Omega)$ is written in the form

$$\alpha \|D^m \sigma_\alpha\|_{L_2}^2 + \sum_{p \in W} [\sigma_\alpha(p) - \varphi_*(p)]^2 = \min_{W_2^m} \, . \tag{31}$$

With obvious constraints on the domain $\Omega \subset R^n$ the solution of (31) exists for every $\varphi_* \in W_2^m$, $m > n/2$, and is unique if ω contains the L–solvable set of points $p_1, p_2, \ldots, p_R$.

We now consider in the space W_2^m the family of the finite–dimensional subspaces E_τ, $\tau > 0$, and formulate the problem of smoothing the spline σ_α^τ in the subspace E_τ in the form

$$\alpha \, \|D^m \sigma_\alpha^\tau\|_{L_2}^2 + \sum_{p \in \omega} [\sigma_\alpha^\tau(p) - \varphi_*(p)]^2 = \min_{E_\tau} .$$

It is well known [5] that in (32) the elements of the nullspace of the energy operator are not affected, regardless of α, so that in our case any polynomial from the space Π_{m-1} will be preserved. Let us assume that interpolation of the polynomials from Π_{m-1} with the help of finite elements from E_τ is done exactly, which allows us to consider the spline smoothing process only in the subspace $\Pi_{m-1}^\perp$. Then, with the same notation, we have

$$\sigma_\alpha = A^*(\alpha I + AA^*)^{-1} A\varphi_*^\perp = S_\alpha \varphi_*^\perp , \tag{33}$$

$$\sigma_\alpha^\tau = B_\tau A^*(\alpha I + AB_\tau A^*)^{-1} A\varphi_*^\perp = S_\alpha^\tau \varphi_*^\perp , \tag{34}$$

where A is the trace operator to the mesh ω, I is the identity operator, and B_τ is the projector to E_τ. It is clear that

$$S_\alpha^\tau - B_\tau S_\alpha = B_\tau S_\alpha (I - B_\tau) M_\alpha^\tau , \tag{35}$$

where M_α^τ is chosen from $S_\alpha^\tau = B_\tau M_\alpha^\tau$. Then

$$\|\sigma_\alpha^\tau - B_\tau \sigma_\alpha\|_V \le \|B_\tau\|_V \cdot \|S_\alpha\|_V \cdot \|(I - B_\tau M_\alpha^\tau \varphi_*^\perp)\|_V , \tag{36}$$

where $\|\cdot\|_V$ is the norm of some space V in which the embedding property of $\Pi_{m-1}^\perp$ with the norm $\|\cdot\|_*$ holds. Suppose that the family of subspaces E_τ has the property

$$\|\varphi - B_\tau \varphi\|_V \le C\tau^\gamma \|\varphi\|_*, \quad \gamma > 0 . \tag{37}$$

Then from the inequality

$$\|M_\alpha^\tau \varphi_*^\perp\|_* = \|A^*(\alpha I + AB_\tau A^*)^{-1} A\varphi_*^\perp\|_* \le \|A^*(AB_\tau A^*)^{-1} A\varphi_*^\perp\|_* \tag{38}$$

and from our lemma we have

$$\|\sigma_\alpha^\tau - B_\tau \sigma_\alpha\|_V \le \text{const}\cdot\tau^\gamma \|\varphi_*^\perp\|_* . \tag{39}$$

Now using the inequality

$$\|\sigma_\alpha - \sigma_\alpha^\tau\|_V \le \|\sigma_\alpha - B_\tau \sigma_\alpha\|_V + \|B_\tau \sigma_\alpha - \sigma_\alpha^\tau\|_V$$

we finally obtain

$$\|\sigma_\alpha - \sigma_\alpha^\tau\|_V \leq \text{const}\cdot\tau^\gamma \|\varphi_*^\perp\|_* . \quad (40)$$

Therefore, the smoothing splines in the subspaces E_τ converge to the smoothing spline σ_α at the same rate as the finite–element spaces converge to the space $W_2^m(\Omega)$.

REFERENCES

[1] Vasilenko, V.A. *Spline Functions: Theory, Algorithms, Programs* (in Russian). Novosibirsk: Nauka, 1983.

[2] Vasilenko, V.A., M.V. Zuzin, and A.V. Kovalkov. 1984. *Spline functions and digital filters* (in Russian). Computing Center of the USSR Academy of Sciences, Siberian Branch, Novosibirsk.

[3] Vasilenko, V.A. 1975. Finite-dimensional approximation in the least squares method (in Russian). In *Variatsionnye Metody v Matematicheskoj Fizike*. Computing Center of the USSR Academy of Sciences, Siberian Branch, Novosibirsk.

[4] Duchon, I. 1967. Erreur d'interpolation des fonctions de pleussieur variables par les D^m splines. Rapport no. 268, Univ. Scient. et Med., Grenoble, France.

[5] Zavyalov, Yu.S., and A. Imamov. 1978. On variational problems in the spline theory (in Russian). In *Matematicheskij Analys and Ego Primeneniya*. Novosibirsk: Nauka.

[6] Bezhaev, A.Yu. 1984. Error estimates for spline interpolation in multidimensional bounded domains (in Russian). Preprint no. 102, Computing Center of the USSR Academy of Sciences, Siberian Branch, Novosibirsk.

[7] Imamov, A. 1977. Some problems of the spline theory in Hilbert spaces (in Russian). Ph.D. diss., Computing Center of the USSR Academy of Sciences, Siberian Branch, Novosibirsk.

[8] Software Library LIDA–2: *On the Approximation of Functions and Digital Filtering* (in Russian). Computing Center of the USSR Academy of Sciences, Siberian Branch, Novosibirsk, 1983.

[9] Kovalkov, A.V. 1980. The Green function and spline approximation in multidimensional domains (in Russian). Preprint no. 70, Computing Center of the USSR Academy of Sciences, Siberian Branch, Novosibirsk.

Atmospheric Sciences

SOME PROBLEMS OF MOIST ATMOSPHERE DYNAMICS MODELLING

V.P. Dymnikov

Department of Numerical Mathematics
The USSR Academy of Sciences
Moscow, USSR

Introduction

Reviewing recent publications on dynamic meteorology, one notices increasing interest in problems involving humidity fields in the atmosphere. This is hardly surprising since humidity fields play the key role in determining the fields of heat sources in the atmosphere. Indeed, in low latitudes climatic heat sources are defined by condensation heating evolving mostly with penetrating convections in the regions linked with intertropical convergence zones and radiative cooling; moreover, being integrable by longitude, the condensation heating is essentially larger than the radiative so that in the climatic sense the low latitudes are the heat source [1]. In high latitudes in the winter, radiative cooling of the atmosphere prevails; however, its climatic significance is determined by the quantity of water vapor transferred to the pole. The situation with the middle–latitude area is more complicated (even in the climatic sense). Condensation heating is evolving here mainly (six month of winter is again a factor) in the areas connected with storm tracks over the oceans. The largest of these sources is situated along east continental coasts, and it is determined by the transfer of cold dry air from the continents. These two largest sources keep climatic temperature waves in the middle latitudes (mainly with $m = 2$) [2]. Thus, in examining the climatic regime of the atmosphere, we run into at least four problems: 1) realization of latent heat by convection; 2) realization of latent heat by large–scale condensation (in the synoptic scale of wavelength); 3) interaction between humidity fields, clouds and radiation; and 4) moisture transfer from low and middle latitudes to high ones. (We do not deal with the problem of moisture evaporation from sea surface and land.)

Problems become more complicated when we distinguish between long–term and short–term climate variability. In terms of long–term climate changes (the classification scale is a decade or more), the problem of the increasing CO_2 concentration in the atmosphere is of great importance nowadays. Some researchers even insist that the problem of adequate fitting of humidity fields in the atmosphere is the key problem [3]. It is well known that high–latitude areas are the most sensitive ones to variations of the CO_2 concentration in the atmosphere [4]. This sensitivity depends on many factors: albedo changes, small water–vapor content, decreasing ice thickness in polar regions (thus, a transfer of the heat flux from the ocean into the atmosphere), and transfers of heat and moisture flux from middle latitudes to high ones. The sensitivity of low latitudes depends first of all on the evaporation from the surface and deep convection, but it may also be due to the fact that the heat and moisture flux move from the middle–latitude to the high–latitude areas [3].

One of the important problems in short–term climate variability is that of studying the role of the ocean in the formation of these variations. The statement of the problem clearly indicates that a description of evaporation processes and formation of heat–source anomalies in the atmosphere through heat–condensation anomalies is the target of the study. We can repeat that the physics of the formation of these anomalies in low and middle latitudes are essentially different.

In middle latitudes the heat–source anomalies are defined by the season. For example, the processes involving anomalies of soil–moisture storage seem to be essential in the summer [5].

And finally, a few words about short–range and middle–range weather forecasts are in order. In middle latitudes the problem is to fit the amplitude and the phase of both long waves and synoptic disturbances. It means that in terms of dynamics the cyclogenesis in diabatic atmosphere is most crucial, and in terms of weather forecast it is the problem of forecasting precipitation fields. In fact, these two problems are closely interrelated and involve the formation of humidity fields in the atmosphere.

This paper deals only with problems of describing humidity fields with respect to weather prediction, climate formation and its changes. The paper consists of two parts. The first part treats the basic problems of formulating humidity equations as well as numerical methods of their solution. An essential result of section 1 is the equation for a special function which combines specific humidity deficit and specific water content. This equation makes it possible to solve (to a first approximation) a number of problems on the connection between the water content in nonprecipitating clouds and the cloud amount, and between the cloud amount and the mean distribution parameters of specific humidity in the atmospheric column ([1], [2]).

In section 3 we examine the numerical methods for solving the equation for humidity transfer in the atmosphere. There is a connection between these methods and numerical methods for solving hyperbolic equations. These solutions are either discontinuous functions or functions with large–space gradients. In mathematical terms, we speak of the class of the so–called monotonic schemes or schemes close, in some sense, to monotonic ones, which we shall call "quasimonotonic."

The second part of the paper is the investigation of baroclinic instability in a moist atmosphere. Methodologically the problem reduces to studying the baroclinic instability in the atmosphere with variables (in our case discontinuous) in the horizontal and vertical coordinates of the static stability parameter. We have obtained some analytical estimates (for two–dimensional Eady's problem).

The results related to the sensitivity of global atmospheric circulation to the methods of parametrization of radiation–cloudiness feedback, the role of large–scale condensation heating in formation of fundamental parameters determining global atmospheric circulation, and the parametrization of moist convection can be found in [1].

1. Humidity transfer in the atmosphere

1.1. EQUATION OF HUMIDITY TRANSFER IN THE ATMOSPHERE

In deriving the equation of humidity transfer in the atmosphere, let us assume that the water vapor and drops form a continuum in such a way that continuity obtains. To simplify, let us also assume that the medium is unturbulent.

Let $\tilde{m}$ be the condensed water content per unit of volume and time, let q_1 be the water–vapor density, and let q_2 be the water–drop density. If $f(r)$ is the distribution of a drop–radius function, then

$$q_2 = \frac{4}{3}\pi N \int_0^\infty p_0 r^3 f(r),$$

where N is the number of drops per volume unit, p_0 is the water density. If f is normalized by N, i.e., $\int_0^\infty f(r)dr = N$, then

$$q_2 = \frac{4}{3}\pi \int_0^\infty p_0 r^3 f(r)\, dr .$$

The equation for q_1 is

$$\frac{\partial q_1}{\partial t} + \operatorname{div} \vec{u}\, q_1 = -\tilde{m} . \tag{1.1.1}$$

To obtain the equation for q_2, let us first write the equation for the distribution function f:

$$\frac{\partial f}{\partial t} + \operatorname{div} \vec{u}_2 f = I_r - I_c . \tag{1.1.2}$$

Here $\vec{u}_2 = (u,v,w-w_2)$, where u, v, w are the components of the wind–velocity vector, w_2 is the sedimentation velocity of drops with radius r with respect to the air flow, I_r is the evaporation (or condensation) rate if the radius r, I_c, is the coagulation rate.

Multiply equation (1.1.2) by $4/3\pi r^3$ (we assume the f to be normalized by N) and integrate over r from 0 to ∞. We obtain

$$\frac{q_2}{t} + \operatorname{div} \vec{u}\, q_2 - \frac{\partial}{\partial z} \frac{\int_0^\infty w_2 \frac{4}{3}\pi r^3 f\, dr}{\int_0^\infty \frac{4}{3}\pi r^3 f\, dr} \cdot q_2$$

$$= \int_0^\infty (I_r - I_c)\frac{4}{3}\pi r^3\, dr\,. \tag{1.1.3}$$

Let $\overline{w}$ denote the expression

$$\overline{w} = \frac{\int_0^\infty w_2 \frac{4}{3}\pi r^3 f(r) dr}{\int_0^\infty \frac{4}{3}\pi r^3 f(r) dr},$$

where $\overline{w}$ is the mean velocity of water–gravity sedimentation in clouds. Let us consider nonprecipitating clouds in which $I_c << I_r$ and $\overline{w} << w$. Then the equation for q_2 will have the form

$$\frac{\partial q_2}{\partial t} + \operatorname{div} \vec{u}\, q_2 = \tilde{m}\,. \tag{1.1.4}$$

Using the concept of integral water content $q = q_1 + q_2$, one can easily write the equation for q, adding (1.1.1) and (1.1.4):

$$\frac{\partial q}{\partial t} + \operatorname{div} \vec{u}\, q = 0\,. \tag{1.1.5}$$

Equation (1.1.5) expresses the conservation law of integral water content in a cloud. However, in application problems we need to know the q_1 and q_2 taken separately, i.e., use the system (1.1.1, 1.1.4).

If we have a continuity equation for air density,

$$\frac{\partial \rho}{\partial t} + \operatorname{div} \rho\, \vec{u} = 0\,,$$

then introducing the concepts of specific humidity and specific water content, $\tilde{q}_1 = q_1/\rho$, $\tilde{q}_2 = q_2/\rho$, we can reduce (1.1.1) and (1.1.4) to the following form:

$$\frac{dq_1}{dt} = -\frac{\tilde{m}}{\rho}, \quad \frac{dq_2}{dt} = \frac{\tilde{m}}{\rho} = m\,. \tag{1.1.6}$$

The system (1.1.6) describes two processes: 1. transfer of vapor and water along trajectories and 2. adaptation of humidity and water content fields to each other. The characteristic time of the first process for $\overline{u} \sim 10$ m·sec^{-1}, $\overline{L} \sim 10^6$ m is $\overline{T} \sim 10^5$ sec. Let us determine the characteristic time of the second process. To do this, we consider an adaptational problem. An equation of heat transfer should be added to (1.1.6), and the expression for the condensation rate m is to be formulated. Assuming that vapor condensation occurs for drops of spherical configuration via diffusion, it is easy to obtain the following relation [6]:

$$4\pi D\bar{r}(\tilde{q}_1 - q_m) \cdot N = m ,$$

where D is the vapor–diffusion coefficient, $q_m(T,p)$ is the maximum specific humidity (a function of temperature, pressure), and $\bar{r}$ is the mean radius of drops. We will examine the adaptation process of vapor and drops over a sufficiently short interval of time; thus we can assume that $\bar{r} = r_0 =$ constant. Then the initial system of equations takes the form

$$\frac{\partial \tilde{q}_1}{\partial t} = -4\pi DNr_0(\tilde{q}_1 - q_m) = -\alpha(\tilde{q}_1 - q_m) ,$$

$$\frac{\partial \tilde{q}_2}{\partial t} = 4\pi DNr_0(\tilde{q}_1 - q_m) = \alpha(\tilde{q}_1 - q_m) , \tag{1.1.7}$$

$$\frac{\partial T}{\partial t} = \frac{L}{C_p}\alpha(\tilde{q}_1 - q_m) - \gamma_a w .$$

Here $\alpha = 4\pi DNr_0$, L = latent water–vapor–condensation heat, C_p = specific air heat at constant pressure, γ_a = dry adiabatic temperature gradient. To obtain the solution of (1.1.7) let us differentiate the first equation with respect to t and eliminate $\partial T/\partial t$, using the equation for temperature:

$$\frac{\partial^2 \tilde{q}_1}{\partial t^2} = -\alpha\frac{\partial \tilde{q}_1}{\partial t} + \alpha\frac{\partial q_m}{\partial T}\frac{\partial T}{\partial t}$$

$$= -\alpha\left(1 + \frac{L}{C_p}\frac{\partial q_m}{\partial T}\right)\frac{\partial \tilde{q}_1}{\partial t} - \alpha\frac{\partial q_m}{\partial T}\gamma_a w . \tag{1.1.8}$$

For $t = 0$ we define the initial conditions $\tilde{q}_1 = q_1(0)$, $\left.\frac{\partial \tilde{q}_1}{\partial t}\right|_{t=0} = -\alpha\Delta_H$ (Δ_H = initial supersaturation value).

The general solution assumes the form

$$q_1 = c_1 + c_2 \exp\left(-\alpha\left(1 + \frac{L}{C_p}\frac{\partial q_m}{\partial T}\right)t\right) + \gamma t ,$$

where

$$\gamma = -\frac{\partial q_m}{\partial T}\gamma_a w/\left(1 + \frac{L}{C_p}\frac{\partial q_m}{\partial T}\right)$$

(we assume $\partial q_m/\partial T$ = constant). For $D \sim 0.2\ \text{cm}^2\text{sec}^{-1}$, $r_0 \sim 10^{-4}$ cm, $N \sim 300\ \text{cm}^{-3}$, we obtain the characteristic adaptation time

$$T = 1/\alpha(1 + \frac{L}{C_p}\frac{\partial q_m}{\partial T}) \sim 1 \text{ sec.}$$

Thus we have two processes: a slow one with $T_x \sim 1$ day and a fast one with $T_x \sim 1$ sec. The latter is the process of *supersaturation adaptation to balance*. If the balanced supersaturation $(\tilde{q}_1 - q_m) << \tilde{q}_1, q_m$, then we can filtrate this fast process, assuming $\tilde{q}_1 \simeq q_m$ in clouds. In this case the system of equations is

$$\frac{d\tilde{q}_1}{dt} = -m\,, \quad \frac{d\tilde{q}_2}{dt} = m\,, \quad \tilde{q}_1 = q_m\,. \tag{1.1.9}$$

In the case when only condensation heating occurs we obtain

$$\frac{d\theta}{dt} = -\frac{\theta}{T}\frac{L}{C_p}\frac{d\bar{q}_1}{dt} \simeq \frac{L}{C_p}m\,, \tag{1.1.10}$$

where θ = potential temperature, T = absolute temperature. Thus we obtain the approximate local invariant $S = \theta + (L/C_p)\tilde{q}_1$ satisfying the equation

$$\frac{dS}{dt} = 0\,. \tag{1.1.11}$$

In dealing with fine–drop clouds, when the sedimentation of drops can be ignored, one may write the equation for the specific moisture content $\tilde{q} = \tilde{q}_1 + \tilde{q}_2$, which is also an invariant:

$$\frac{d\tilde{q}}{dt} = 0\,. \tag{1.1.12}$$

Equations (1.1.11) and (1.1.12) satisfying the conditions $\tilde{q}_1 = q_m$ in clouds can be taken as the initial system in order to find the distribution of humidity and cloudiness fields in the atmosphere. This method was suggest–ed by L.T. Matveev and used for short–term forecast of humidity and cloudiness fields in the atmosphere [8].

Using the fact that the humidity in clouds is very close to the saturation point, one can obtain very useful equations to describe the humidity and cloudiness fields [9].

To this end, let us write out the system of equations describing the transfer of specific humidity, specific water content and heat (bearing in mind that we consider here the unturbulent atmosphere, and the primes over q and T are therefore omitted):

$$\frac{dq_1}{dt} = -m\,, \quad \frac{dq_2}{dt} = m - \delta\,,$$

$$\frac{dT}{dt} = \frac{L}{C_p}m + \gamma_a\frac{RT}{gp}\frac{dp}{dt} \tag{1.1.12a}$$

(the term for the precipitation is labeled by δ.) Since q_m is the function of pressure and temperature only, then

$$\frac{dq_m}{dt} = \frac{\partial q_m}{\partial T}\frac{dT}{dt} + \frac{\partial q_m}{\partial p}\frac{dp}{dt}.$$

Set

$$\Delta = q_1 - q_m .$$

For the function Δ we have

$$\frac{d\Delta}{dt} = \frac{dq_1}{dt} - \frac{dq_m}{dt} = -m - \left(\frac{\partial q_m}{\partial T}\frac{dT}{dt}\right) - \left(\frac{\partial q_m}{\partial p}\frac{d}{dt}\right),$$

or

$$\frac{d\Delta}{dt} = -m - \frac{\partial q_m}{\partial p}\left(\frac{L}{C_p} m + \gamma_a \frac{RT}{gp}\frac{dp}{dt}\right) - \frac{\partial q_m}{\partial p}\frac{dp}{dt};$$

if $q_m = (0.622/p)e(T)$, then $\dfrac{\partial q_m}{\partial p} = -\dfrac{q_m}{p}$. Using this relation yields

$$\frac{d\Delta}{dt} = -m\left(1 + \frac{L}{C_p}\frac{\partial q_m}{\partial T}\right) - \left(\gamma_a \frac{RT}{gp}\frac{\partial q_m}{\partial T} - \frac{q_m}{p}\right)\frac{dp}{dt}. \qquad (1.1.13)$$

We can rearrange the last term using the notion of a moist adiabatic gradient

$$\gamma_{ba} = \frac{\gamma_a + \dfrac{L}{C_p}\dfrac{g q_m}{RT}}{1 + \dfrac{L}{C_p}\dfrac{\partial q_m}{\partial T}}.$$

Let us calculate the relation

$$\gamma_a - \gamma_{ba} = \frac{\gamma_a\left(1 + \dfrac{L}{C_p}\dfrac{\partial q_m}{\partial T}\right) - \gamma_a - \dfrac{L}{C_p}\dfrac{q_m}{p}\dfrac{gp}{RT}}{1 + \dfrac{L}{C_p}\dfrac{\partial q_m}{\partial T}}$$

$$= \frac{\dfrac{L}{C_p}\dfrac{gp}{RT}\left(\gamma_a \dfrac{RT}{gp}\dfrac{\partial q_m}{\partial T} - \dfrac{q_m}{p}\right)}{1 + \dfrac{L}{C_p}\dfrac{\partial q_m}{\partial T}}.$$

We obtain

$$\gamma_a\left(\frac{RT}{gp}\frac{\partial q_m}{\partial p}\right) - \frac{q_m}{p} = \left(1 + \frac{L}{C_p}\frac{\partial q_m}{\partial T}\right)\frac{C_p}{L}\frac{RT}{gp}(\gamma_a - \gamma_{ba}).$$

Thus we can rewrite (1.1.13) in the following form:

$$\frac{d\Delta}{dt} = -m\left(1 + \frac{L}{C_p}\frac{\partial q_m}{\partial T}\right) - \left(1 + \frac{L}{C_p}\frac{\partial q_m}{\partial T}\right)\frac{C_p}{L}\frac{RT}{gp}(\gamma_a - \gamma_{ba}) .$$

One can derive the expression for condensation rate m from (1.1.14). Indeed, since in the clouds $\Delta = 0$, then

$$m = -\frac{C_p}{L}(\gamma_a - \gamma_{ba})\frac{RT}{gp}\frac{dp}{dt} . \qquad (1.1.15)$$

Now multiply the second equation in (1.1.12) by $\left(1 + \frac{L}{C_p}\frac{\partial q_m}{\partial T}\right)$. We then obtain

$$\left(1 + \frac{L}{C_p}\frac{\partial q_m}{\partial T}\right)\frac{dq_2}{dt} = \left(1 + \frac{L}{C_p}\frac{\partial q_m}{\partial T}\right)m - \left(1 - \frac{L}{C_p}\frac{\partial q_m}{\partial T}\right)\delta .$$

Let us show that we can rewrite this equation with sufficient accuracy to describe the large-scale cloudiness fields as follows:

$$\frac{d}{dt}\left(1 + \frac{L}{C_p}\frac{\partial q_m}{\partial T}\right)q_2 = \left(1 + \frac{L}{C_p}\frac{\partial q_m}{\partial T}\right)m - \left(1 + \frac{L}{C_p}\frac{\partial q_m}{\partial T}\right)\delta . \qquad (1.1.16)$$

In fact,

$$\frac{d}{dt}\left(1 + \frac{L}{C_p}\frac{\partial q_m}{\partial T}\right)q_2 = \left(1 + \frac{L}{C_p}\frac{\partial q_m}{\partial T}\right)\frac{dq_2}{dt} + q_2\frac{d}{dt}\frac{L}{C_p}\frac{\partial q_m}{\partial T} .$$

Then, applying the Clausius–Clapeyron formula yields

$$\frac{d}{dt}\frac{\partial q_m}{\partial T} = \frac{d}{dt}\frac{L}{RT^2}q_m \simeq \frac{L^2}{R^2T^4}q_m\frac{dT}{dt} = \frac{L^2}{R^2T^4}q_m\,\gamma_{ba}\frac{RT}{gp}\frac{dp}{dt} .$$

This term multiplied by $(L/C_p)q_2$ should be compared with $m = C_p/L(\gamma_a - \gamma_{ba}) \times(RT/gp)(dp/dt)$, or, in other words, $(L^2/R^2C_p^2T^4)\ q_m q_2$ per unit. For the mean values of this expression we obtain

$$\frac{L^2}{R^2C_p^2T^4}q_m q_2 \sim 10^{-2} ,$$

i.e., our assumption is valid.

Now let us introduce the function ϕ

$$\phi = q_1 - q_m + \left(1 + \frac{L}{C_p}\frac{\partial q_m}{\partial T}\right)q_2 . \qquad (1.1.17)$$

Adding (1.1.16) and (1.1.14) yields the equation for this function:

$$\frac{d\phi}{dt} = -\left(1 + \frac{L}{C_p}\frac{\partial q_m}{\partial T}\right)\frac{C_p}{L}\frac{RT}{gp}(\gamma_a - \gamma_{ba})\frac{dp}{dt} - \left(1 + \frac{L}{C_p}\frac{\partial q_m}{\partial T}\right)\delta .$$

One can easily notice that this equation describes both cloudy and cloudless atmospheres. Indeed, if we assume $\Delta = 0$ in clouds, then (1.1.18) is the equation for a specific water content (multiplied by some known function); in the cloudless atmosphere $q_2 = 0$ and this equation describes a specific humidity deficit. Thus, negative values of ϕ describe specific humidity deficit, and positive values describe specific water content. The idea concerning the equations for alternating functions was propounded by Shvets [10].

Another advantage of this equation is the fact that it does not account for any difference between large values (instead of comparing q_1 with q_m, which are close to each other, one needs to compare it with q_2 as the difference $q_1 - q_m$).

Still another advantage is that the main source responsible for moisture transformation in the atmosphere is clearly defined; this permits us to solve an optimization problem. For a number of problems one can assume (1.1.18) to be linear, letting the temperature and pressure values to be independent.

And finally, the fourth advantage of this equation is that it is related to the alternating function, which essentially simplifies a numerical solution of this class of equations. In the case of turbulent atmosphere we can rewrite (1.1.15) as

$$\frac{d\phi}{dt} = \operatorname{div}(k \operatorname{grad} \phi) - \left(1 + \frac{L}{C_p}\frac{\partial q_m}{\partial T}\right)\frac{C_p}{L}\frac{RT}{gp}(\gamma_a - \gamma_{ba})\frac{dp}{dt}$$

$$- \left(1 + \frac{L}{C_p}\frac{\partial q_m}{\partial T}\right)\delta . \qquad (1.1.19)$$

The boundary conditions for (1.1.16) can be derived from boundary conditions for q_1, q_2, and T.

If we assume that $q_2 = 0$ is the boundary condition for q_2 on the low and upper atmosphere boundary, then $\phi = \Delta = q_1 - q_m$ at these levels. If the fluxes $k(\partial q_1/\partial z)$, $k(\partial T/\partial z)$ are known from the solution of the boundary layer problem, then the value $k(\partial \Delta/\partial z)$ is known as well.

1.2. PARAMETRIZATION OF MOISTURE SUBGRID PROCESSES

In calculating the atmospheric regime, one of the central problems is the parametrization of subgrid processes, in particular the problem of calculation of nonconvective cloud amounts, to determine the radiation atmospheric regime [12], [13]. A great number of general atmosphere–circulation models use an empirical relation, known as *Smagorinsky's relations* [14] or similar relations, to determine the cloud quantity [5]. These relations set a linear correspondence between the cloud quantity and the relative humidity. In general, finding this relation between a cloud quantity (within integration mesh) and mean meteorological values is a solution of an inverse problem. However, it is not clear *a priori* which values exactly define the cloud quantity. In particular, an analogue of vertical velocity in p–coordinates ($\tau = dp/dt$, see (1.1.19)) seems to be one of the main factors. We will show the domain of application of the rela–

tions analogous to Smagorinsky's relation, using the equation for the function obtained above.

Let us consider cloudiness formation in the region, in which for simplicity we assume velocity–vector projections to be constant (in this case the area size is assumed to be small enough). Going on to a moving coordinate frame, let us reduce (1.1.18) to the form:

$$\frac{\partial \phi}{\partial t} = -\left(1 + \frac{L}{C_p}\frac{\partial q_m}{\partial T}\right)\frac{C_p}{L}\frac{RT}{gp}(\gamma_a - \gamma_{ba})\frac{dp}{dt} = \alpha\tau \tag{1.2.1}$$

(we assume clouds to be nonprecipitating).

Integrating (1.2.1) by t,

$$\phi = \phi_0 + \int_0^t \alpha\tau \, d\tau . \tag{1.2.2}$$

Let $\tilde{\Omega} \times H \times t$ be the domain of definition of a function ϕ, where H is the size in the vertical coordinate. Assume that ϕ is a summable function. Then the sets $\tilde{\Omega}_1$ $(\phi > 0)$ and $\tilde{\Omega}_2$ $(\phi < 0)$ are measurable. Define the cloud amount as a ratio:

$$n = \frac{\text{mes } \tilde{\Omega}_1}{\text{mes } \tilde{\Omega}} = \frac{\Omega_1}{\Omega} \tag{1.2.3}$$

(without loss of generality one can assume mes $\tilde{\Omega} = 1$, then $n = \Omega_1$). Let us define the mean specific humidity deficit as

$$\overline{\Delta} = \frac{1}{\Omega}\int_{\Omega_2} \phi \, d\Omega = \int_{\Omega_2} \phi \, d\Omega$$

and the mean specific water content as

$$\overline{\left(1 + \frac{L}{C_p}\frac{\partial q_m}{\partial T}\right) q_2} = \int_{\Omega_1} \phi \, d\Omega .$$

Integrating (1.2.2) by Ω yields

$$\overline{\left(1 + \frac{L}{C_p}\frac{\partial q_m}{\partial T}\right) q_2} + \overline{\Delta} = \overline{\phi_0} + \int_{\Omega}\int_0^t \alpha\tau \, d\Omega , \tag{1.2.4}$$

where $\phi_0(\Omega)$ gives humidity field inhomogeneity in $\overline{\Omega}$. We have

$$\begin{aligned}\overline{\left(1 + \frac{L}{C_p}\frac{\partial q_m}{\partial T}\right) q_2} &= \int_{\Omega_1} \phi_0 \, d\Omega + \int_{\Omega_1}\int_0^t \alpha\tau \, dt \, d\Omega \\ &= \int_{\Omega_1} \phi_0 \, d\Omega + n\tau \int_0^t \overline{\alpha}^{\Omega_1} \, dt .\end{aligned}$$

Then (1.2.4) can be written in the form

$$\int_n \phi_0 \, d\Omega + n\tau\int_0^t \overline{\alpha}^{\Omega_1} \, dt + \overline{\Delta} = \overline{\phi_0}^{\Omega} + \tau\int_0^t \overline{\alpha}^{\Omega} \, dt \, . \qquad (1.2.5)$$

If $\phi_0(\Omega)$ is a given function, then $\Omega_1 = f(\phi_0, \int_0^t \alpha\tau \, dt)$, or

$$n = f(\phi_0, \int_0^t \alpha\tau \, dt). \qquad (1.2.6)$$

If ϕ is a continuous single–valued function in $\overline{\Omega}$, then $\overline{\Omega_1}$ is a monotonic function $\int_0^t \tau\alpha \, dt$ (see (1.2.2)). Consequently, (1.2.6) is solvable for $\int_0^t \tau\alpha \, dt$, i.e.,

$$\int_0^t \tau\alpha \, dt = \varphi(n,\phi_0). \qquad (1.2.7)$$

Substituting (1.2.7) in (1.2.5) yields the relation between the cloud amount and the specific humidity deficit:

$$\int_n \phi_0 \, d\Omega + n \, \overline{\varphi(n,\phi_0)}^{\Omega_1} + \overline{\Delta} = \overline{\phi_0} + \overline{\varphi(n,\phi_0)}^{\Omega} \, . \qquad (1.2.8)$$

The existence of the solution (1.2.8) for any ϕ_0 is not obvious, of course.

Let us assume that the solution (1.2.8) exists, i.e.,

$$n = \psi(\overline{\Delta},\phi_0) \, ,$$

where ϕ_0 enters parametrically, e.g. by its Fourier coefficients, i.e.,

$$n = \psi(\overline{\Delta},\alpha_1,\alpha_2,\ldots,\alpha_n,\ldots) \, . \qquad (1.2.9)$$

Let $\overline{\Delta_0}$ define $n = 0$ (provided $\overline{\Delta} > \Delta_0$, n becomes > 0). Then for sufficiently small n and with $\psi \in C^2(a,b)$, where (a,b) are the upper and lower bounds of $\overline{\Delta}$, respectively (one can see that $b = 0$, $a = -q_m$), we obtain $n = \partial\psi/\partial\overline{\Delta}(\overline{\Delta} - \overline{\Delta_0})$ or

$$n = \left.\frac{\partial\psi}{\partial\overline{\Delta}}\right|_{\overline{\Delta} = \overline{\Delta_0}} \cdot \overline{\Delta} - \left.\frac{\partial\psi}{\partial\overline{\Delta}}\right|_{\overline{\Delta} = \overline{\Delta_0}} \cdot \overline{\Delta_0} \, . \qquad (1.2.10)$$

Since Δ is a linear function of relative humidity, we obtain a linear dependence between cloud amount and relative humidity. Since these coeffi–cients are determined by the set $\{\alpha_i\}$, they are different for each layer, as we can see in Smagorinsky's charts.

In [16] we have solved the problem (1.2.8) for the case when ϕ_0 is a product of ordinary harmonic waves for every variable. Also, for the cloud content of the middle troposphere we have obtained the relation $n = 1.26r - 0.63$, which is very close to Smagorinsky's relation. A essential result is the relation between cloud amount and cloud water content

$$\left(1 + \frac{\partial q_m}{\partial T}\frac{L}{C_p}\right)q_2 \simeq n\phi_0$$

and between mean water content and cloud amount

$$\overline{\left(1 + \frac{L}{C_p}\frac{\partial q_m}{\partial T}\right)q_2} = \frac{n^2\sqrt{n}}{3\sqrt{\pi}}\overline{\phi_0}\,. \tag{1.2.12}$$

These relations allow us to calculate theoretically cloud albedo.

It is interesting to note that the relations analogous to (1.2.11)–(1.2.12) were obtained in [17] under the assumption of random distribution of humidity and temperature fields in the mesh with normal distribution. The other important problem is that of parametrization of the moist–convection—the main source of heat in low latitudes. Three approaches to the solution of this problem are currently known. The first approach was suggested by Manabe [14] and involves energy principles. The second approach is based on the principle of conditional instability of the second kind (CISK) [18], and the third approach (apparently the most promising) deals with evaluation of a convective clouds ensemble.

1.3. NUMERICAL METHODS OF THE SOLUTION OF THE HUMIDITY TRANSFER EQUATIONS

One of the main peculiarities of the equations (1.1.1)–(1.1.3) is that they describe essentially positive functions with large–space gradients and therefore require special difference schemes for their solution. Equation (1.1.18) avoids the positivity requirement; however, large–space gradients (or even derivative discontinuities) are not excepted. This means that in this case the choice of a difference scheme should not be arbitrary.

Let us illustrate a similar problem using a Cauchy problem for one–dimensional transfer equation as an example:

$$\frac{\partial \varphi}{\partial t} + u\frac{\partial \varphi}{\partial x} = 0\,, \tag{1.3.1}$$

where $u = \text{const.} > 0$.

Following the lines of [20], we say that the difference scheme changing the monotonic functions into monotonic functions with the same directional growth is a monotonic scheme.

We will consider next the class of two–layer schemes.

Theorem 1 [20]. *In order for the difference scheme*

$$\varphi_n^{j+1} = \sum_k C_{n-k}\varphi_k^j \tag{1.3.2}$$

to be monotonic, it is necessary and sufficient that all coefficients C_{n-k} in (1.3.2) are nonnegative.

Let us briefly review some properties of monotonic difference schemes. To begin with, it is positivity (nonnegativity) that guarantees the solution of the difference problem when the solution of the differential problem is essentially positive (nonnegative) and has discontinuities or large space gradients. For nonlinear hyperbolic equations,

$$\frac{\partial \varphi}{\partial t} + \frac{\partial F(\varphi)}{\partial x} = 0 \ ; \tag{1.3.3}$$

if the generalized solution is not unique, the converging monotonic schemes provide convergence to the physical solution [21].

Now let us consider the possibility of constructing a monotonic difference scheme for (1.3.1).

Let the difference scheme (1.3.2) have index p if it is accurate for the initial data, which are the polynomials of degree $\leq p$. It is proved in [20] that there are no monotonic schemes among those with index 2 (for (1.3.1)). Our theorem can easily be proved for schemes with $p > 2$. However, it does not imply that for the solution of (1.3.1) there are no monotonic difference schemes with order of accuracy higher than 1 (we mean the standard determination of the order of accuracy of converging schemes [22]). In fact, the order of scheme accuracy and its index are not interrelated in the general case. The fact that monotonic schemes of the (1.3.2) type for the solution of (1.3.1) with order of accuracy higher than 1 do not exist has been proved in [21].

It is not difficult to construct the monotonic schemes of first-order accuracy for (1.3.1) (i.e., *upstream difference schemes*). However, these schemes are hard to apply, especially for multidimensional equations since it requires a very high space and time resolution.

The nonmonotonicity of schemes with the order of accuracy higher than 1 becomes apparent, as is well known, for characteristic oscillations arising in the neighborhood of large gradients or solution discontinuities. In this connection, the notion of a scheme index concept is essential. It is proved in [23] that the solution behavior of converging schemes with odd index in the limit (as $j \to \infty$) is more advantageous in describing discontinuity solutions (see [24]–[30]).

The idea to construct nonlinear monotonic difference equations was first propounded in [31]. The essence of the method is the following: let us have a monotonic operator of first-order accuracy L_1, $\varphi^{j+1}_{(1)} = L_1 \varphi^j$, and the nonmonotonic second-order operator L_2, $\varphi^{j+1}_{(2)} = L_2 \varphi^j$. Then $\varphi^{j+1}_2 = L_1 \varphi^j + (L_2 - L_1)\varphi^j$. Let us introduce some control function $f(\zeta)$ and define the difference solution of the problem as

$$\varphi^{j+1} = L_1 \varphi^j + \Delta_2 \varphi^j \cdot f(\zeta) \ . \tag{1.3.4}$$

It is seen that for $f(\zeta) = 0$ the solution is determined from the first-order accuracy scheme, and for $f(\zeta) = 1$ from the second-order accuracy scheme.

Define ζ as $|\Delta_2\varphi/\Delta_1\varphi|$, where $\Delta_1\varphi$ is a limiting operator of first-order accuracy as yet undetermined.

We can, naturally, formulate some conditions for determining $f(\zeta)$: $f(0) = 1$ (the results for the first- and the second-order accuracy schemes coincide), $f'(\zeta) \le 0$ (the function should decrease as ζ increases, going to zero in the limit).

Let us choose some subclass of monotonic schemes for which one can write a condition for $f(\zeta)$ more precisely. Let M denote the set of all monotonic schemes for the solution of (1.3.1) (provided $r \le 1$). Let M_1 be the set of schemes the solution of which satisfies the condition

$$0 \le \frac{\varphi_n^{j+1} - \varphi_n^j}{-(\varphi_n^j - \varphi_{n-1}^j)} \le 1 . \tag{1.3.5}$$

This condition means that $\varphi_{n-1}^j \lesseqgtr \varphi_n^{j+1} \lesseqgtr \varphi_n^j$, i.e. the solution at the point $(n,j+1)$ lies inside the interval $(\varphi_{n-1}^j, \varphi_n^j)$. Let us show that $M_1 \subset M$. By the definition of a monotonic scheme we have: if $\varphi_n^j \ge \varphi_{n-1}^j$, then $\varphi_n^{j+1} \ge \varphi_{n-1}^{j+1}$. Since

$$\varphi_{n-1}^j \le \varphi_n^{j+1} \le \varphi_n^j ,$$

$$\varphi_{n-2}^j \le \varphi_{n-1}^{j+1} \le \varphi_{n-1}^j ,$$

then it is obvious that $\varphi_{n-1}^{j+1} \le \varphi_n^{j+1}$.

The converse is not valid. Indeed, the scheme

$$\varphi_n^{j+1} = (1-r-h^2)\varphi_n^j + r\varphi_{n-1}^j + h^2\varphi_{n-2}^j$$

is monotonic (provided $r < 1-\varepsilon$), but it does not fulfill (1.3.5). If we construct monotonic schemes belonging to the M_1 class, then the relation for $f(\zeta)$ becomes

$$0 \le -\frac{(L_1\varphi^j)_n - \varphi_n^j + (\Delta_2\varphi^j \cdot f(\zeta))_n}{\varphi_n^j - \varphi_{n-1}^j} \le 1 . \tag{1.3.6}$$

Choosing an explicit upstream difference scheme as $L_1\varphi^j$, we obtain,

$$0 \le -\frac{(1-r)\varphi_n^j + r\varphi_{n-1}^j - \varphi_n^j + (\Delta_2\varphi^j \cdot f(\zeta))_n}{\varphi_n^j - \varphi_{n-1}^j} \le 1 .$$

Hence we have

$$-r \le -\frac{\Delta_2\varphi^j \cdot f(\zeta)}{\varphi_n^j - \varphi_{n-1}^j} \le 1-r . \tag{1.3.7}$$

If for the operator $\Delta_1\varphi^j$ we use

$$\Delta_1\varphi_n^j = (\varphi_n^j - \varphi_{n-1}^j)\min(r,1-r)\ ,$$

then inequality (1.3.7) can be written as

$$-r \le -\frac{\Delta_2\varphi^j \min(r,1-r)\, f(\zeta)}{\Delta_1\varphi^j} \le 1-r\ . \tag{1.3.8}$$

By definition we have

$$\zeta = \left|\frac{\Delta_2\varphi^j}{\Delta_1\varphi^j}\right| ,$$

i.e.,

$$-r \le -\mathrm{sign}\left(\frac{\Delta_2\varphi^j}{\Delta_1\varphi^j}\right)\zeta \min(r,1-r)\, f(\zeta) \le 1-r\ . \tag{1.3.9}$$

If the sign of $(\Delta_2\varphi^j/\Delta_1\varphi^j)$ is negative, then the left inequality is fulfilled identically, and the right one is fulfilled under the condition

$$f(\zeta) \le \frac{1}{\zeta}\,.$$

If the sign of $(\Delta_2\varphi^j/\Delta_1\varphi^j)$ is positive, then the right inequality is fulfilled identically, and the condition $f(\zeta) \le 1/\zeta$ is required to satisfy the left inequality. In general, with the arbitrary signs of the ratio $\Delta_2\varphi^j/\Delta_1\varphi^j$ and with such choice of Δ_1, this constraint for $f(\zeta)$ cannot be reduced. We can construct the nonlinear monotonic schemes with (1.3.4), using for L_2 the operator with accuracy higher than second–order, e.g. the monotonic variant of Fromm's scheme [32]. It is worth noting that the difference schemes constructed as above are not conservative in general, whereas in the problems of general atmospheric circulation the conservation property can play a decisive role.

An example of the conservative monotonic scheme of second–order accuracy for (1.3.1) was given in [32] on the basis of Fromm's scheme.

In constructing the conservative schemes, we can formulate the necessary condition of linear value (we mean essentially nonnegative solutions) in terms of quadratic invariants [1]. Indeed, if $\varphi \ge 0$, then (1.3.1) can be written in terms of the function $\sqrt{\varphi}$ and the conservation $\int_D \varphi\, dD$ will be equivalent to the conservation $\int_D (\sqrt{\varphi})^2\, dD$. If we use a skew–symmetric representation for the space derivative approximation and the Crank–Nicolson scheme for the time approximation, the scheme in terms of the function $\psi = \sqrt{\varphi}$ will be

$$\frac{\psi^{j+1} - \psi^{j}}{\Delta t} + k\,\frac{\psi^{j+1} + \psi^{j}}{2} = 0\,, \tag{1.3.10}$$

where $(k\psi,\psi) = 0$. For the system (1.3.10),

$$(\psi^{j+1},\psi^{j+1}) = (\psi^{j},\psi^{j})\,, \tag{1.3.11}$$

where the inner product is defined as $(\psi,\zeta) = \Sigma_i\ \psi_i\zeta_i$. Relation (1.3.11) holds for any sign of ψ^{j+1}. If we next introduce the nonlinear transformation $\tilde{\psi}^{j+1}_n = ((\psi^{j+1})^2)^{1/2}$, we obtain an accurate law of conservation for the function φ^j when the condition of its nonnegativity is satisfied.

One can show that such a transformation does not change the scheme approximation order. Indeed, the transformation equivalent to the difference solution of the multiplication by a unit diagonal matrix, with the sign as that of the solution (this matrix norm is equal to 1; therefore the stability of the scheme remains unchanged), i.e.,

$$\tilde{\psi} = D(\psi)\psi\,. \tag{1.3.12}$$

Let (1.3.10) approximate the initial differential problem with respect to its second-order solution in τ and m in h, i.e.,

$$\|L^{(1)}_{h\tau}(\varphi)^{h\tau} - f^{h\tau}\|_{\phi_{h\tau}} \le C_1\tau^2 + C_2h^m\,, \tag{1.3.13}$$

where $L^{(1)}_{h\tau}$ is the difference operator, $f^{h\tau}$ is the right side of the difference scheme (in this case it is 0), $(\varphi)^{h\tau}$ is the projection of the differential problem solution onto a grid.

If we use the nonlinear transformation (1.3.24), then the operator $L_{h\tau}$ of a new scheme can assume the form of a product, $L_{h\tau} = L^{(1)}_{h\tau}\cdot D^{-1}$. Then we obtain

$$\|L_{h\tau}\,(\varphi)^{h\tau} - f^{h\tau}\|_{\phi_{h\tau}} = \|L^{(1)}_{h\tau}D^{-1}(\varphi)^{h\tau} - f^{h\tau}\|_{\phi_{h\tau}}\,.$$

Since $(\varphi)^{h\tau}$ is positive, then $D^{-1} \equiv E$ is an identical operator and the scheme approximation coincides with (1.3.13).

2. Baroclinic instability of moist atmosphere

2.1. SOME PRELIMINARY REMARKS

As has been noted, the problem of baroclinic instability is one of the key points to a better understanding of the laws which control general atmospheric circulation. First Eady [33] and Charney [34] and, later, many other researchers allowed for a great number of simplifying factors—in particular, they assumed the mean static stability parameter to be constant. However, we know that in middle latitudes the most baroclinic unstable zones are those along eastern continental coasts, where dry continental air comes into contact with moist oceanic air. These zones are characterized by a significant horizontal change of the static stability parameter. Furthermore, the baroclinic waves developing in moist atmosphere have a variable parameter of static stability. In the region of ascending vertical motions in moist-saturated atmosphere a condensation process causes a discontinuous change of the static stability parameter. Let us write the equation of heat transfer with condensation:

$$\frac{\partial T}{\partial t} + u\frac{\partial T}{\partial x} + v\frac{\partial T}{\partial y} + \tau\frac{\partial T}{\partial p} - \gamma_a\frac{RT}{gp}\tau = \frac{L}{C_p}m\,, \tag{2.1.1}$$

where $\tau = dp/dt$, $m \equiv$ water–vapor condensation rate.

Let

$$\sigma_1 = \left(\gamma_a\frac{RT}{gp} - \frac{\partial T}{\partial p}\right).$$

Since

$$\frac{\partial T}{\partial p} = \frac{\partial T}{\partial z}\left(-\frac{RT}{gp}\right),$$

we have

$$\sigma_1 = \frac{RT}{gp}\left(\gamma_a + \frac{\partial T}{\partial z}\right).$$

Since we are examining only large–scale processes, we have that $\partial T/\partial z$ in absolute value cannot exceed γ_a (dry convection occurs), i.e., σ_1 is nonnegative.

According to (1.1.15), with large–scale condensation we have

$$m = -\frac{C_p}{L}(\gamma_a - \gamma_{ba})\frac{RT\tau}{gp}$$

in the areas where $q_1 > q_m$ and $\tau < 0$.

In these areas (2.1.1) could be transformed:

$$\frac{\partial T}{\partial t} + u\frac{\partial T}{\partial x} + v\frac{\partial T}{\partial y} - \sigma_1\tau = -(\gamma_a - \gamma_{ba})\frac{RT\tau}{gp},$$

or

$$\frac{\partial T}{\partial t} + u\frac{\partial T}{\partial x} + v\frac{\partial T}{\partial y} - \sigma_2\tau = 0\,, \tag{2.1.2}$$

where

$$\sigma_2 = \frac{RT}{gp}\left(\gamma_{ba} + \frac{\partial T}{\partial z}\right). \tag{2.1.3}$$

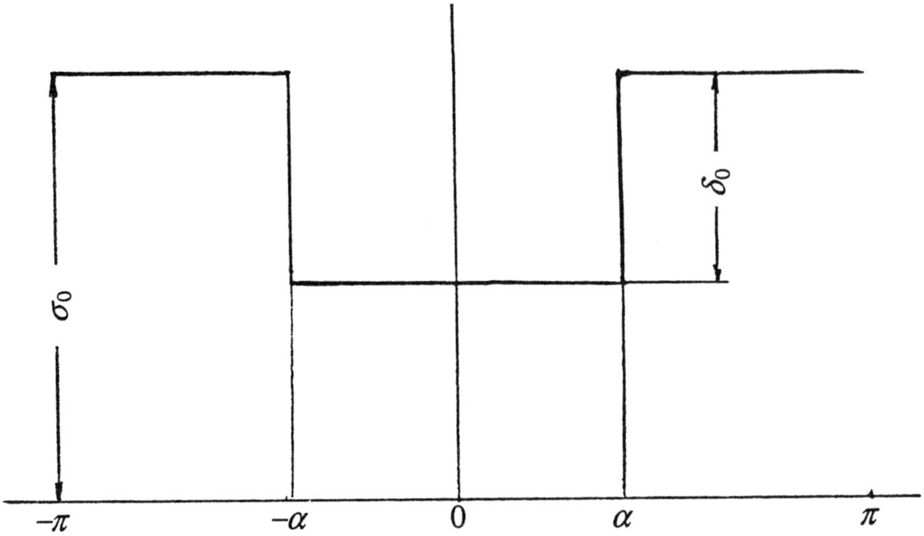

Fig. 1. The function $\overline{\sigma}(x)$

In (2.1.3) we should consider only a nonnegative σ_2 (otherwise moist convection occurs). Since $\gamma_{ba} < \gamma_a$, we have $\sigma_2 < \sigma_1$.

Thus we can reduce (2.1.1) to

$$\frac{\partial T}{\partial t} + u\frac{\partial T}{\partial x} + v\frac{\partial T}{\partial y} - \tilde{\sigma}\tau = 0\,, \tag{2.1.4}$$

where

$$\tilde{\sigma} = \begin{cases} \sigma_2 & \text{if } q_1 > q_m \text{ and } \tau < 0\,, \\ \sigma_1 & \text{otherwise}\,. \end{cases}$$

(We do not consider the processes of drop evaporation.)

One can simplify (2.1.4). Let $T = \overline{T} + T'$, where $\overline{T}$ is some standard temperature distribution which is a function of the vertical coordinate.

Then, it is easily seen that the equation for T' is

$$\frac{\partial T'}{\partial t} + u\frac{\partial T'}{\partial x} + v\frac{\partial T'}{\partial y} + \tau\frac{\partial T'}{\partial p} - \tilde{\tilde{\sigma}}t = 0\,, \tag{2.1.5}$$

where

$$\tilde{\tilde{\sigma}} = \begin{cases} \dfrac{RT}{gp}(\gamma_{ba} - \gamma) & \text{if } q_1 > q_m \text{ and } \tau < 0 \\ \dfrac{RT}{gp}(\gamma_a - \gamma) & \text{otherwise}\,. \end{cases}$$

Since in the real atmosphere we can introduce a $\overline{T}$ such that $T' << \overline{T}$, we can assume that in the first approximation $\tilde{\overline{\sigma}} = \sigma$, where the static stability parameter is defined as follows:

$$\sigma = \frac{R\overline{T}}{gp}(\gamma_i - \gamma)$$

$$\gamma_i = \begin{cases} \gamma_a \\ \gamma_{ba} \end{cases}$$

Thus, in examining the processes in the moist atmosphere we have to consider the problems with a discontinuous change of static stability parameter.

2.2. BAROCLINIC INSTABILITY IN THE ATMOSPHERE WITH VARIABILITY IN THE HORIZONTAL PARAMETER OF STATIC STABILITY

Let us examine a system of hydrothermodynamics equations on the l–plane in a p–coordinate system linearized with respect to the state $\overline{\varphi} = (\overline{u}, \overline{v}, \overline{T}, \overline{\tau}, \overline{\phi})$:

$$(\overline{u} = r(p_0 - p),\ \overline{v} = 0,\ \overline{\tau} = 0,\ \frac{\partial \overline{T}}{\partial y} = -\frac{p\ell}{R}\cdot r,\ \frac{\partial \overline{\phi}}{\partial p} = -\frac{R\overline{T}}{p})$$

$$\frac{\partial u'}{\partial t} + \overline{u}\frac{\partial u'}{\partial x} + \tau'\frac{\partial \overline{u}}{\partial p} - \ell v' = -\frac{\partial \phi'}{\partial x},$$

$$\frac{\partial v'}{\partial t} + \overline{u}\frac{\partial v'}{\partial x} + \ell v' = 0, \qquad (2.2.1)$$

$$\frac{\partial \phi'}{\partial p} = -\frac{RT'}{p}, \quad \frac{\partial u'}{\partial x} + \frac{\partial \tau'}{\partial p} = 0,$$

$$\frac{\partial T'}{\partial t} + \overline{u}\frac{\partial T'}{\partial x} + v'\frac{\partial \overline{T}}{\partial y} - \overline{\sigma}\tau' = 0$$

with $\tau' = 0$ at $p = p_0, 0$ (we assume periodicity conditions on the abscissa).

As noted in section 2.1, the problem involving baroclinic instability in the atmosphere with condensation is equivalent to the problem (2.2.1) in which static stability parameter σ changes (discontinuously) in space and time. We examine now the case where σ changes only along horizontal coordinates. Thus, let us assume that $\overline{\sigma} = \overline{\sigma}(x)$ and $\overline{\sigma}(x) = \sigma_0 - \delta(x)$, where δ_0 does not depend on x, and $\delta(x)$ is a step function (figure 1). (To simplify, we assume that a period on the abscissa is 2π; hence the wave numbers k are integers.)

To study the problem (2.2.1), we shall use Galerkin's method and choose the generalized trigonometric functions as basic functions; i.e., we shall find the solution in the form:

$$\vec{\varphi} = (u',v',T',\tau',\phi')^{\mathrm{T}} ,$$

$$\vec{\varphi} = \sum_{-\infty}^{\infty} \vec{\varphi}_k(p,t) e^{ikx} ,$$

$$\vec{\varphi}_k(p,t) = (u_k, v_k, T_k, \tau_k, \phi_k)^{\mathrm{T}} .$$

We assume that the components of the vector φ belong to the space W_2^1.

We obtain a system of equations for the nth Galerkin approximation:

$$\frac{\partial u_k^{(n)}}{\partial t} + ik\bar{u}u_k^{(n)} + \tau_k^{(n)} \frac{\partial \bar{u}}{\partial p} - \ell v_k^{(n)} = -ik\phi_k^{(n)} ,$$

$$\frac{\partial v_k^{(n)}}{\partial t} + ik\bar{u}v_k^{(n)} + \ell u_k^{(n)} = 0 ,$$

$$\frac{\partial T_k^{(n)}}{\partial t} + ik\bar{u}T_k^{(n)} - \frac{1}{2\pi} \sum_{j=-n}^{n} \int_{-\pi}^{\pi} \sigma(x)\tau_j^{(n)} e^{ijx-ikx}\, dx + v_k^{(n)} \frac{\partial \bar{T}}{\partial y} = 0 ,$$

$$iku_k^{(n)} + \frac{\partial \tau_k^{(n)}}{\partial p} = 0 , \qquad \frac{\partial \phi_k^{(n)}}{\partial p} = -\frac{RT_k^{(n)}}{p} ,$$

$$\tau_k^{(n)} = 0 \quad \text{at } p = 0, p_0 . \tag{2.2.2}$$

Let us calculate a term under the sign of the sum

$$\frac{1}{2\pi} \sum_{j=-n}^{n} \int_{-\pi}^{\pi} (\sigma_0 - \delta(x))\tau_j^{(n)} e^{i(j-k)x}\, dx$$

$$= (\sigma_0 - \frac{a\delta_0}{\pi})\tau_k^{(n)} - \sum_{-n}^{n} \tau_j^{(n)} \frac{\sin (j-k)a}{(j-k)a}\, \delta_0 .$$

We can reduce system (2.2.2) for the quasigeotrophical motions (we neglect the term $(\partial/\partial t + ik\bar{u})\bar{u}_k^{(n)}$ from the first equation) to the second-order system in p for $\tau_k^{(n)}$:

$$\frac{D}{ik}\frac{\partial^2 \tau_k^{(n)}}{\partial p^2} - 2\frac{\partial \bar{u}}{\partial p}\frac{\partial \tau_k^{(n)}}{\partial p} - \frac{Rk^2}{\ell^2}\frac{D}{ik}\Big((\delta_0 - \frac{a\delta_0}{\pi})\tau_k^{(n)}$$

$$- \sum_{-n}^{n} \tau_j \frac{\sin (j-k)a}{(j-k)a}\, \delta_0\Big) = 0 , \tag{2.2.3}$$

$$D \equiv \frac{\partial}{\partial t} + ik\bar{u} , \quad \tau_k^{(n)} = 0 \ \text{ at } p = 0, p_0 .$$

Note that we can exclude from (2.2.3) the case where $k = 0$ since $\tau_k^{(n)} = 0$. In fact, using the fourth equation of (2.2.1) we have $\partial\tau_0^{(n)}/\partial p = 0$ and by virtue of zero boundary conditions we obtain that $\tau_0^{(n)} \equiv 0$.

Let us transform system (2.2.2) to vector form. Introduce the vector

$$\vec{\tau}_1^{(n)} = \begin{vmatrix} \tau_{-n}^{(n)} \\ \vdots \\ \tau_{-1}^{(n)} \\ \tau_1^{(n)} \\ \vdots \\ \tau_n^{(n)} \end{vmatrix}$$

the diagonal matrices $D_1 = \text{diag}\left(\frac{1}{ik}\right)$, $D_2 = \text{diag}\,(k^2)$, and the symmetric matrix

$$S = \left[\frac{\sin\, ma}{m\pi}\delta_0 \quad \sigma_0 - \frac{a\delta_0}{\pi} \quad \frac{\sin\, ma}{m\pi}\delta_0\right].$$

The dimension of all matrices is equal to n, the $(\sin\, ma/m\pi)\delta_0$ in matrix S are on the mth diagonal, and the $\sigma_0 - a\delta_0/\pi$ are on the principal diagonal. This notation allows us to reduce (2.2.3) to the form

$$\frac{\partial}{\partial t} D_1 \frac{\partial^2 \vec{\tau}_1^{(n)}}{\partial p^2} - \frac{R}{\ell^2} D_1 D_2 S \vec{\tau}_1^{(n)} = -\bar{u}\frac{\partial^2 \vec{\tau}_1^{(n)}}{\partial p^2}$$

$$+ \bar{u}\frac{R}{\ell^2} D_2 S \vec{\tau}_1^{(n)} + 2\frac{\partial \bar{u}}{\partial p}\frac{\partial \vec{\tau}_1^{(n)}}{\partial p}. \tag{2.2.4}$$

Let

$$\frac{\partial^2 \vec{\tau}_1^{(n)}}{\partial p^2} - \frac{R}{\ell^2} S_1 \vec{\tau}_1^{(n)} = \vec{V}_1,$$

where $S_1 = D_2 S$. Then subsystem (2.2.4) can be transformed to two subsystems

$$\frac{\partial^2 \vec{\tau}_1^{(n)}}{\partial p^2} - \frac{R}{\ell^2} S_1 \vec{\tau}_1^{(n)} = \vec{V}_1,$$

$$\frac{\partial}{\partial t} D_1 \vec{V}_1 = -u\vec{V}_1 + 2\frac{\partial \bar{u}}{\partial p}\frac{\partial \vec{\tau}_1^{(n)}}{\partial p}. \tag{2.2.5}$$

Before turning to direct investigation of the behavior of the solution of (2.2.5), let us prove some preliminary statements. Note that we examine only the case $\sigma_0 > \delta_0$, to exclude the possibility of convection.

Lemma 1. *Every eigenvalue of the matrix S_1 is positive, and a system of eigenvectors is complete.*

First let us show that the symmetric matrix S has positive eigenvalues for any (n). Since S is the sum of a scalar matrix and the symmetric matrix S_2 with zeros at the principal diagonal, with $(\sin(ma)/m\pi)$ on the mth diagonal, we have

$$\lambda_{\min}(S) \geq \sigma_0 - \frac{a\delta_0}{\pi} - \rho(S_2) ,$$

where $\rho(S_2)$ is the spectral radius of the matrix S_2.

Since $\rho(S_2)$ is the norm of the matrix S_2 due to its symmetry, $\rho(S_2)$ will be a monotonic increasing function of dimension (n). It follows that $\rho(S_2)$ will be limited by $\lim \rho(S_2)$ as $n \to \infty$.

In the infinite–dimensional case, we find eigenvectors in the form $\psi_m = e^{im\alpha}$, where ψ_m is the mth component of the eigenvector. For the eigenvalues we have

$$\begin{aligned} \lambda_{S_2} &= -\delta_0 \sum_{m=1}^{\infty} \frac{\sin ma}{m\pi} (e^{im\alpha} + e^{-im\alpha}) \\ &= -\frac{2\delta_0}{\pi} \sum_{m=1}^{\infty} \frac{\sin ma}{m} \cos m\alpha \\ &= -\frac{\delta_0}{\pi} \sum \left(\frac{\sin m(a+\alpha)}{m} + \frac{\sin m(a-\alpha)}{m} \right) . \end{aligned} \tag{2.2.6}$$

Due to the convergence of both series (2.2.6) hold. We can easily see that for any a and α, λ_{S_2} lies inside the interval

$$\left(-\frac{a\delta_0}{\pi}, \frac{(\pi-a)\delta_0}{\pi}\right) .$$

For $a \leq \pi/2$ (this assumption does not contradict the general reasoning; otherwise, one needs to change the notation in fig. 1) we have the inequality

$$\lambda_{\min}(S) \geq \sigma_0 - \delta_0 . \tag{2.2.7}$$

Since $\sigma_0 > \delta_0$, it follows from (2.2.7) that all the eigenvalues are positive. We have thus shown that S is positive definite since S is a symmetric matrix. The matrix $S_1 = D_2 S$, where D_2 is symmetric and positive definite as well. We can determine the square root of every positive definite matrix. Making a similar transformation of S with $D_2^{1/2}$ yields

$$\lambda_{S_1} = \lambda(D_2^{-1/2} D_2 S D_2^{1/2}) = \lambda(D_2^{1/2} S D_2^{1/2}) .$$

Since the matrix $D_2^{1/2} S D_2^{1/2}$ is symmetric and positive definite, its eigen-values are positive, too.

The eigenvectors S_1 are given by

$$D_2 S \psi_i = \lambda_{S_1} \psi_i . \tag{2.2.8}$$

Multiplying (2.2.8) on the left by $D_2^{-1/2}$, we rewrite it as follows:

$$D_2^{1/2} S D_2^{1/2} D_2^{-1/2} \psi_i = \lambda_{S_1} D_2^{-1/2} c_i . \tag{2.2.9}$$

It is seen from the matrix (2.2.9) that $D_2^{-1/2}\psi_i$ are eigenvectors of the symmetric matrix $D_2^{1/2} S D_2^{1/2}$. Therefore the vector system $D_2^{-1/2}\psi_i$ is orthogonal and complete. To obtain ψ_i, we must multiply $D_2^{-1/2}\psi_i$ by a nonsingular matrix $D_2^{1/2}$. This implies that the system ψ_i is complete.

The lemma is proved.

Let $\{\vec{\psi}_i\}$ and $\{\vec{\psi}_i^*\}$ be the system of eigenvectors for S_1 and S_1^* and let $\{\lambda_i\}$ be their eigenvalues (S_1^* is the transpose of matrix transposed to S_1 since the S_1 is real–valued).

Expanding $\vec{\tau}_1^{(n)}$ and $\vec{V}_1$ as a Fourier series by $\{\vec{\psi}_i\}$, we obtain

$$\vec{\tau}_1^{(n)} = \sum_i \tau_{1i} \vec{\psi}_i , \quad \vec{V}_1 = \sum_i V_{1i} \vec{\psi}_i . \tag{2.2.10}$$

Multiplying (2.2.5) by $\vec{\psi}_i^*$, we have the system of equations

$$\begin{aligned} \frac{\partial^2 \tau_{1i}}{\partial p^2} - \frac{R^2}{\ell^2} \lambda_i \tau_{1i} &= V_{1i} , \\ \frac{\partial}{\partial t}(D_1 \vec{V}_1, \vec{\psi}_i^*) &= -\bar{u} V_{1i} + 2 \frac{\partial \bar{u}}{\partial p} \frac{\partial \tau_{1i}}{\partial p} . \end{aligned} \tag{2.2.11}$$

We have $(D_1 \vec{V}_1, \vec{\psi}_i^*) = \underline{i}(\tilde{D}_1 \vec{V}_1, \vec{\psi}_i^*) = \underline{i}(\vec{V}_1, \tilde{D}_1 \vec{\psi}_i^*)$. Here $\underline{i}$ is the imaginary unit.

Since $\tilde{D}_1$ is a real nonsingular matrix, scalar product $(\vec{V}_1, D_1 \vec{\psi}_i^*) = V_{1i}$ can be thought of as coefficients of expansion into a Fourier series via a system of functions $\{\tilde{D}_1^{-1} \vec{\psi}_i\}$.

Let us transform system (2.2.11) into the form

$$\begin{aligned} \frac{\partial^2 \tau_{1i}}{\partial p^2} - \frac{R^2}{\ell^2} \lambda_i \tau_{1i} &= V_{1i} , \\ \underline{i} \frac{\partial}{\partial t} \tilde{V}_{1i} &= -\bar{u} V_{1i} + 2 \frac{\partial \bar{u}}{\partial p} \frac{\partial \tau_{1i}}{\partial p} . \end{aligned} \tag{2.2.12}$$

We shall find the solutions V_{1i}, $\tilde{V}_{1i}$, τ_{1i} such that relations

$$\frac{\partial}{\partial t} V_{1i} = -\underline{i}c_i V_{1i} \tag{2.2.13}$$

are satisfied.

From (2.2.12) we have

$$(\bar{u} - c)\, V_{1i} = 2\frac{\partial \bar{u}}{\partial p}\frac{\partial \tau_{1i}}{\partial p}. \tag{2.2.14}$$

Substituting (2.2.14) into (2.2.12) we obtain the equation

$$\begin{gathered}(\bar{u} - c_i)\frac{\partial^2 \tau_{1i}}{\partial p^2} - 2\frac{\partial \bar{u}}{\partial p}\frac{\partial \tau_{1i}}{\partial p} - (\bar{u} - c_i)\frac{R\lambda_i}{\ell^2}\tau_{1i} = 0\,, \\ \tau_{1i} = 0 \ \text{ at } \ p = 0, p_0\,.\end{gathered} \tag{2.2.15}$$

This equation has already been examined in [33]. If we assume that

$$\frac{\partial \bar{u}}{\partial p} = -r\,, \qquad \frac{\sqrt{R\lambda_i p_0}}{\ell} = \alpha_i\,,$$

then the eigenvalue problem (2.2.15) has a nontrivial solution with

$$c_{i_{1,2}} = \frac{rp_0}{2}\left(1 \pm \sqrt{1 - 4/\alpha_i^2(\alpha_i c^{\text{th}}\alpha_i - 1)}\right).$$

The values c_i become complex (and complex conjugate pairs always exist) when $\alpha_i < 2.4$. Since we choose $r > 0$, then if the c_i are real they are positive.

Now let us turn to equation (2.2.13). We have a representation for $\tilde{V}_{1i}$: $\tilde{V}_{1i} = (\vec{V}_{1i}, \tilde{D}_1\vec{\psi}_i^*) = \Sigma_j\, V_{1j}(\psi_j, \tilde{D}_1\psi_i^*)$. Let A be a matrix whose elements are $a_{ij} = (\psi_j, D_1\psi_i^*)$. It is obvious that the elements of A^{-1} are $(\tilde{D}_1^{-1}\psi_j, \psi_i^*)$. Then we can rewrite (2.2.13) in vector form:

$$A\frac{\partial \vec{w}}{\partial t} = ic\vec{w}$$

or

$$\frac{\partial \vec{w}}{\partial t} = iA^{-1}c\vec{w}\,, \tag{2.2.16}$$

where $\vec{w}$ is a vector with components V_{1i}, and $c = \text{diag}(c_i)$.

Lemma 2. *The matrix A is symmetric.*

To prove the lemma we have to show that $(\tilde{D}_1\vec{\psi}_j,\vec{\psi}_i^*) = (\tilde{D}_1\vec{\psi}_i,\vec{\psi}_j^*)$. $\vec{\psi}_i$ and $\vec{\psi}_j$ are determined from the relations

$$D_2 S\vec{\psi}_i = \lambda_i\vec{\psi}_i\,, \quad SD_2\vec{\psi}_i^* = \lambda_i\vec{\psi}_i^* \tag{2.2.17}$$

(λ_i is a real positive value). We can represent the matrix D_2 in the form of a product $\tilde{D}_1^{-1}\tilde{D}_1^{-1}$.

We shall have $\tilde{D}_1^{-1}\tilde{D}_1^{-1}S\vec{\psi}_i = \lambda_i\vec{\psi}_i$ or

$$\tilde{D}_1^{-1}S\tilde{D}_1^{-1}\tilde{D}_1\vec{\psi}_i^* = \lambda_i\tilde{D}_1\vec{\psi}_i\,. \tag{2.2.18}$$

From the second equation of (2.2.17) we obtain

$$\tilde{D}_1^{-1}S\tilde{D}_1^{-1}\tilde{D}_1^{-1}\vec{\psi}_i^* = \lambda_i\tilde{D}_1^{-1}\vec{\psi}_i^*\,. \tag{2.2.19}$$

It follows from (2.2.19) that

$$\tilde{D}_1\vec{\psi}_i = \gamma_i\tilde{D}_1^{-1}\vec{\psi}_i^*\,. \tag{2.2.20}$$

The case when $\tilde{D}_1\vec{\psi}_i$ and $\tilde{D}_1^{-1}\vec{\psi}_i^*$ are two different vectors corresponding to a single eigenvalue is impossible, for these two vectors should be orthogonal due to the symmetry of matrix $\tilde{D}_1^{-1}S\tilde{D}_1^{-1}$, i.e., $(\tilde{D}_1\vec{\psi}_i,\tilde{D}_1^{-1}\vec{\psi}_i^*) = 0$. Consequently $(\vec{\psi}_i,\vec{\psi}_i^*) = 0$, and that contradicts the condition of biorthogonality for the system $\{\vec{\psi}_i\}$ and $\{\vec{\psi}_i^*\}$. Let us normalize the vectors $\vec{\psi}_i$ and $\vec{\psi}_i^*$ in such a way that $\gamma_i = 1$. The equalities $(\tilde{D}_1\vec{\psi}_i,\tilde{D}_1\vec{\psi}_j) = \delta_{ij}$, $(\tilde{D}_1^{-1}\vec{\psi}_i^*,\tilde{D}_1^{-1}\vec{\psi}_j^*) = \delta_{ij}$ also follow from (2.2.18) and (2.2.19). Now the lemma proof implies from an obvious equality chain

$$(\tilde{D}_1\vec{\psi}_j,\vec{\psi}_i^*) = (\tilde{D}_1^{-1}\vec{\psi}_j^*,\tilde{D}_1\tilde{D}_1^{-1}\vec{\psi}_i^*) = (\tilde{D}_1^{-1}\vec{\psi}_j^*,\tilde{D}_1\tilde{D}_1\vec{\psi}_i) = (\vec{\psi}_j^*\tilde{D}_1\vec{\psi}_i)\,.$$

Theorem. *The solution of system* (2.2.2) *becomes unstable when the problem* (2.2.15) *has at least one complex conjugate pair of eigenvalues.*

To begin with, we shall prove that if all c_i are real, i.e., C is a positively determined matrix, then the solution (2.2.2) will be stable. Indeed, as A^{-1} is a symmetrical matrix, then the eigenvalues of $A^{-1}C$ coincide with those of symmetric matrix $C^{1/2}A^{-1}C^{1/2}$, i.e., they are real.

If an eigenvector system is complete (see Lemma 1), then as a consequence the solution of the system (2.2.16) is stable. Due to the fact that the components of vector $\vec{w}$ are connected with $\tau_i^{(n)}$ by the equation

$$\frac{\partial^2\tau_i^{(n)}}{\partial p^2} - \frac{R}{\ell^2}\lambda_i\tau_i^{(n)} = V_{1i}\,,$$

where the norm of the inverse to the operator

$$L \equiv \frac{\partial^2}{\partial p^2} - \frac{R}{\ell^2}\lambda_i$$

is limited (zero boundary conditions), then consequently $\vec{\tau}_1^{(n)}$ is stable.

If at least one diagonal element $c_i = d_i + \underline{if_i}$ (we can always choose the necessary sign of f_i) situated on the ith row of matrix C appears in C, the ith column of matrix $A^{-1}C$ will contain values of the type $\tilde{a}_{ji}(d_i + \underline{if_i})$, and all the rest of the columns will be real.

From this it follows that the spur of matrix $A^{-1}C$ is equal to

$$\text{Sp}\, A^{-1}C = k + a_{ii}(d_i + \underline{if_i}) ,$$

where k is real.

As far as $\text{Sp}\, A^{-1}C = \Sigma_i\, \lambda_i(A^{-1}C)$, it means that the matrix $A^{-1}C$ has at least one complex eigenvalue with imaginary part having sign $a_{ii}f_i$. Due to the arbitrariness of sign f_i, we shall always have the eigenvalue providing exponentially increasing solution V_{1i}. By repeating the reasoning concerning the connection between V_{1i} and $\tau_1^{(n)}$, we complete the proof of the theorem.

Hence, we can formulate a condition of instability of the solution of problem (2.2.2)

$$\frac{\sqrt{R\lambda_{\min}^{(n)}}}{\ell} \cdot p_0 < 2.4 . \tag{2.2.21}$$

For minimum eigenvalue $\lambda_{\min}^{(n)}$ of the matrix D_2S we can write a relation

$$\lambda_{\min}^{(n)}(D_2)\lambda_{\min}^{(n)}(S) \le \lambda_{\min}^{(n)}(D_2S) \le \lambda_{\min}^{(n)}(D_2)\lambda_{\max}^{(n)}\, S .$$

Remembering the estimates for the eigenvalues of S, we obtain

$$\sigma_0 - \delta_0 \le \lambda_{\min}^{(n)} \le \sigma_0 . \tag{2.2.22}$$

However, this estimate is practically non–informative as it does not contain a dependence on parameter α.

Before turning to this dependence calculation, it is necessary to show the convergence $\lambda_{\min}^{(n)} \to \lambda$ for $n \to \infty$. This convergence was tested directly by numerical calculation. The minimum eigenvalue of matrix D_2S was calculated by Lusternik's method [22]. The calculations showed that $\lambda_{\min}$ changed by 0.2 percent when changing the matrix dimension from 20 to 40 (further on we assume n to be equal to 40). Let us substitute the matrix in the form of a product of a scalar matrix $(\sigma_0 - a\sigma_0/\pi)E$ by the matrix S_2 with ones on the main diagonal and the rest of the elements given by

$$\frac{\sin\, ma}{ma}\left(\frac{a\delta_0/\pi\sigma_0}{1-a\delta_0/\pi\sigma_0}\right)$$

for the mth diagonal. We see that the eigenvalues of matrix D_2S are determined by two parameters α/π and δ_0/σ_0. The calculations of λ_{min} were conducted for a wide range of parametric changes (see tables 1 and 2).

Here

$$\gamma = \frac{[\lambda_{min} - (\sigma_0 - \frac{a\delta_0}{\pi})]}{\sigma_0 - \frac{a\delta_0}{\pi}}.$$

One can easily note that the calculated values λ_{min} are very close to $(\sigma_0 - a\delta_0/\pi)$ which is equal to the average value of parameter σ by an interval of 2π.

TABLE 1: $\frac{a}{\pi} = \frac{1}{2}$

σ_0/δ_0	8	4	3	2.5	2	1.5	1.4	1.3	1.2
λ_{min}	8.24	8.06	7.82	7.57	7.2	5.88	5.38	4.69	3.7
γ	3.0%	7.3%	9.0%	10.0%	10.0%	2.8	–2.3%	–11.0%	–26.0%

TABLE 2: $\frac{a}{\pi} = \frac{1}{3}$

σ_0/δ_0	3	2	1.5	1.2	1.1
λ_{min}	8.11	7.62	6.92	5.99	5.56
γ	6.4%	6.4%	3.8%	–2.7%	–7.0%

In fact,

$$\bar{\sigma} = \frac{1}{2\pi}\int_{-\pi}^{\pi} \sigma(x)\,dx = \sigma_0 - \frac{\delta_0 a}{\pi}.$$

Note that as the value of α/π decreases, so does γ. This means that a process of stability loss in the system (2.2.2) proceeds in such a way if we use $\bar{\sigma}$ instead of $\sigma(x)$, i.e., a process of stability loss is controlled by an integral parameter of static stability.

Now let us estimate a growth rate of unstable mode. With this aim we have to calculate the imaginary part of the complex eigenvalues of operator $A^{-1}C$. Divide the matrix into two parts, $C = C_g + \underline{i}C_m$, where C_g is a diagonal matrix containing real parts c_i, and C_m is a matrix containing imaginary parts. In our case C_g is a positively determined matrix with a single nonzero element on the diagonal.

Introduce a new dependent variable in the equation

$$\partial w/\partial t = \underline{i}A^{-1}Cw$$

using

$$\tilde{w} = e^{-\underline{i}A^{-1}C_g t}w\underline{i}A^{-1}(C-C_g)e^{-\underline{i}A^{-1}C_g t}\tilde{w} = M\tilde{w} . \qquad (2.2.23)$$

The eigenvalues of the matrix M in (2.2.23) coincide with the eigenvalues of the matrix $\underline{i}A^{-1}(C-C_g) = -A^{-1}C_m$. By the definition of the matrix C_m, $A^{-1}C_m$ will be a matrix with one nonzero column and one eigenvalue equal to $\tilde{a}_{ii}\mathrm{Im}(c_i)$.

Recalling the definition A^{-1}, we obtain

$$\lambda = \tilde{a}_{ii}\mathrm{Im}(c_i) = (\tilde{D}_1^{-1}\psi_i,\psi_i^*)\mathrm{Im}(c_i) .$$

REFERENCES

[1] Marchuk, G.I., et. al. *Matematicheskoe Modelirovanie Obshchej Tsirkulyatsii Atmosfery* (Mathematical Modelling of General Atmosphere Circulation). Leningrad: Gidrometeoizdat, 1984.

[2] Kurbatkin, G.P. 1982. The role of middle–latitudes ocean in short–term climate variations (in Russian). Paper presented at the Conference on Large–Scale Oceanographic Experiments in WCRP, Tokyo.

[3] Dymnikov, V.P., Galin, V.Ya., and Perov, V.L. 1980. The investigation of climate sensitivity to doubling the CO_2 concentration by zonal averaged model of general circulation (in Russian). Pt. II. In *Matematicheskoe Modelirovanie Atmosfernykh Dvizhenij* (Mathematical Modelling of Atmospheric Motions), 15–21. Novosibirsk: Nauka.

[4] Manabe, S., and Wetherald, R. 1975. The effects of doubling the CO2 concentration on the climate in a general circulation model. *J. Atmosph. Sci.* 32, no. 1:3–15.

[5] Kurbatkin, G.P., Manabe, S., and Han, D.G. 1979. On moisture content of the continents and intensiveness of summer monsoon circulation (in Russian). *Meteorologiya i Gidrologiya* 11:5–11.

[6] Sedunov, Yu.S. *Physics of Liquid–drop Phase Formation in the Atmosphere* (in Russian). Leningrad: Gidrometeoizdat, 1972.

[7] Dymnikov, V.P. 1969. On some specific features of numerical solution of humidity–transfer equations in the atmosphere (in Russian). *Izvestiya Akademii Nauk SSSR, ser. FAiO*, vol. 5, no. 6:649–52.

[8] Matveev, L.T. *Obshchaya Meteorologiya. Atmosfernaya Fizika* (General Meteorology. Atmospheric Physics). Leningrad: Gidrometeoizdat, 1965.

[9] Dymnikov, V.P. 1971. The statement of the problem of humidity fields in the atmosphere forecast (in Russian). *Izvestiya Akademii Nauk, ser. FAiO*, 7, no. 12:1311–14.

[10] Gandin, L.S., Dubov, A.S. *Numerical Methods for Short–term Weather Forecast*. Leningrad: Gidrometeoizdat, 1968.
[11] Dymnikov, V.P., and Ishimova, A.V. 1979. Diabatic model for the short–term weather forecast. *Meteorologiya i Gidrologiya* 6:5–14.
[12] Kondrat'ev, K.Ya. *Aktinometriya* (Actinometry). Leningrad: Gidtometeoizdat, 1965.
[13] Fejgelson, E.M. *Radiation Heat Exchange and Clouds*. Leningrad: Gidrometeoizdat, 1970.
[14] Manabe, S., Smagorinsky, J., and Strickler, R.F. 1965. Simulated climatology of a general circulation model with a hydrologic cycle. *Mon. Wea. Rev.* 93, no. 12:769–98.
[15] January and July simulation experiments with 2.5° latitude–longitude version of the NCAR general circulation model NCAR/TN–123–STR, 1977.
[16] Dymnikov, V.P. 1974. On parametrization of inconvective cloud amount in the problems of weather forecast and general atmosphere circulation. *Trudy Zapadno–Sibirskogo RNIGMI* 11:62–68.
[17] Sommeria, G., and Deardorf, J.W. 1977. Subgrid–scale condensation in models of nonprecipitating clouds. *J. Atmosp. Sci.* 34, no. 2:344–55.
[18] Kuo, H.L. 1974. Further studies of the parametrization of the influence of cumulus convection of large–scale flows. *J. Atmosph. Sci.* 31, no. 7:1232–40.
[19] Arakawa, A., and Schubert, H. 1974. Interaction ensemble with the large–scale environment cloud of cumulus. *J. Atmosph. Sci.* 31, no.3.
[20] Godunov, S.K. A method of numerical solution of hydrodynamics equations (in Russian). *Mathematical Collected Articles*, vol. 47, no. 3:271–306.
[21] Harten, A., Hyman, J.M., and Lax, P.D. 1976. On finite–difference approximations and enthropy conditions for shocks. *Comm. Pure & Applied Math.*, vol. 29, no. 3:297–322.
[22] Marchuk, G.I. *Methods of Numerical Mathematics*. New York Berlin Heidelberg Tokyo: Springer–Verlag, 1978.
[23] Zhukov, A.I. 1959. A limit theorem for difference operators (in Russian). *Uspekhi Matem. Nauk*, vol. 14, no. 3:129–36.
[24] Yanenko, N.N., and Shokin, Yu.I. 1968. On the correctness of the first differential approximation of difference schemes (in Russian). *Doklady Akademii Nauk SSSR* 182, no. 4.
[25] Lax, P.D., and Wendroff, B. 1960. Systems of conservation laws. *Comm. Pure & Applied Math.* 13:217–37.
[26] Fromm, J.E. 1968. A method for reducing dispersion in convective difference schemes. IBM Research Lab. Report.
[27] McCormac, R.W. The effect of viscosity in hypervelocity impact cratering. AIIAA Paper, 69–353.
[28] Rusanov, V.V. 1968. Difference schemes of third–order accuracy for direct count of discontinuous solutions (in Russian). *Doklady Akademii Nauk SSSR* 180, no. 6:1303–5.
[29] Anderson, D., and Fattahi, B. 1974. A comparison of numerical solutions of the advective equations. *J. Atmosph. Sci.* 31, no. 6:1500–6.

[30] Kries, H.O., and Oliger, J. 1972. Comparison of accurate methods for the integration of hyperbolic equations. *Tellus* 24, no. 3.
[31] Goldin, V.Ya., Kalitkin, N.N., and Shishova, T.B. 1965. Nonlinear difference schemes for hyperbolic equations. *J. Comp. Ath. and Math. Phys.* 5, no. 5.
[32] Van Leer, B. 1974. Towards the ultimate conservative difference scheme. II. Monotonicity and conservation combined in a second–order scheme. *J. Comp. Phys.* 14:361–70.
[33] Charney, J.C. 1947. The dynamics of long waves in a baroclinic western current. *J. Met.* 4, no. 5:135–62.

SATELLITE OBSERVATIONS OF THE EARTH'S RADIATION BUDGET COMPONENTS AND THE PROBLEM OF THE ENERGETICALLY ACTIVE ZONES OF THE WORLD OCEAN (EAZO)

K.Ya. Kondrat'ev and V.V. Kozoderov
Moscow, USSR

Introduction

In studying short–term climate variability, ERB observations from space are of great significance. The high stability of the global climate implies that the global mean heat loss caused by long wave emission of the earth–atmosphere system is in approximate balance with the absorbed solar radiation. Both of these earth's radiation–budget components determine the sources and sinks of energy, which govern the general circulations of the atmosphere and world ocean.

Observations from satellites have opened the possibility of continuous modelling of the earth's radiation budget. The polar–orbiting satellites provide complete coverage of the globe with observational data for short enough time intervals, and geostationary satellites permit an almost continuous monitoring of very large territories.

The observations from space are becoming more important due to the need for detection of specific zones in the world ocean which are the main source of long–term weather anomalies and short–term climatical changes—the so–called energetically active zones (EAZO). The mathematical formalism of conjugate equations of thermohydrodynamics [1], [2] permits one to describe the climatical changes in terms of the observed anomalies of the processes in the EAZOs. It has now become possible to apply the larger volume of observational data (primarily, ship data) to a detailed monitoring of the processes occurring in the EAZOs [3], and the data obtained by satellites to a more accurate evaluation of the processes governing the long–term weather anomalies and short–term climatical changes [4]. The application of these two kinds of observational data to a study of climate changes is part of the research program "Sections," the objective of which is to examine the role that the ocean plays in short–term climatical changes [5]. This program is based on the notion of EAZO. It uses the observational data on the most important climatic regions of the world, as well as computer modelling.

The analysis of mean square deviations (MSD) of satellite data on the monthly mean radiation budgets and their components, using the observational data for a period of 45 months (1974–78) [6], showed the zones of substantial year–to–year variability, closely connected with EAZO [7]. Evaluating measurement accuracy and representing the satellite data in the form of mean monthly maps of total outgoing radiation fluxes shows the statistical value of the results obtained. In [8], it has been established that the zonality of MSDs of the radiation budget and its longwave components in energetically active zones has changed. Statistically significant is also a reduction of the data on the radiation–budget components to the earth's surface level, and a solution of boundary–value problems of radiation transfer in the atmosphere [9]. Characteristic horizontal scales of the effect of EAZO (the northern Atlantic) have been estimated in [10]. The influence of the cloud–cover inhomogeneity on the formation of radiation–budget anomalies in EAZO has been analyzed in [11]. All these results is an empirical verification of the EAZO characteristics in analyzing the ERB and its components [12]. This paper is a further study of the ERB observations from space.

Annual change of MSDs

Using the northern Atlantic as an example, we shall consider in more detail the origin of characteristic patterns of MSD, which serve as a measure of year–to–year variability of the radiation budget and its components. Their mean values are defined by zonal changes (the inconsistency of zonal changes mainly depends on the distribution of continents and oceans). However, the year–to–year variations of MSDs of the radiation budget and its longwave component have a clearly expressed nonzonal character: clusters of isolines are observed in the region of the Sargasso Sea (the amplitude of the radiation budget is about 20 W/m^2), in the region of Newfoundland and near the equator at 40° W (the amplitudes reach 15 W/m^2), as well as in the Norwegian Sea (13 W/m^2), with mean annual values for the territory considered (10° S–70° N; 0°–80° W) about 10–12 W/m^2 (except for the territory of Africa where the amplitudes also reach 20 W/m^2).

Compared with the annual mean values of the radiation budget and its components for the central parts of the above EAZOs, those for the oceanic basins along 30° W and the regions near the eastern coastlines of Greenland and North and South America show that the annual change of the radiation budget and its longwave component vary marginally in these three energetically active zones, unlike the tropics, where these variations are more substantial. The annual mean values are considerably varied in the case of the shortwave ERB component, which may have been due to the cloudiness variations in the EAZOs under consideration.

Quite different are the annual changes of the year–to–year MSDs of the radiation budget and its components (figs. 1–3). Here the month–to–month change of the radiation budget and its longwave component for all of the three EAZOs, with the exception of the tropical zone, is inhomogeneous (fig. 1). A characteristic bimodal distribution of the annual change of MSD with two maxima in April and October is also manifested in the case of oceans near the Newfoundland EAZO and east of the Gulf Stream (fig. 2), and is not seen in the Norwegian Sea and in the region of the equator. The annual distribution of the radiation budget and its longwave component for the land adjacent to an EAZO (fig. 3) greatly differs from that presented in figures 1 and 2.

A specific feature of the foregoing bimodal distributions (fig. 1) is that in the case shown in figure 1(a) the contributions of individual components to the year–to–year variability are almost equal in April and October, whereas in the case shown in figure 1(b) these contributions equal that of the abnormal year, 1976. This has led to the excessive longwave component's MSDs versus the radiation budget in the case shown in figure 1(b). From figure 1(c) one can see that the amplitude of the year–to–year variability for all the 45–month observational data of the radiation budget is 20 W/m^2 (for the longwave component it is 15 W/m^2) and basically given by the two maxima in April and October and by minima in July and December. These changes of the ERB longwave component can lead to temperature variations of the surface–atmosphere system by 3–4° C with respect to adjacent territories, with a month–to–month variability of about 10 W/m^2.

The temperature variations of the system at a given scale of averaging can hardly be explained by specific tracks of cyclones or by anomalies of heating sources outside the territory in question, which affect it through advection. Also hardly probable is the influence of the polar–front shifting, as well as other dynamic effects. The ERB variability diagrammed in figures 1(a), 1(b), and 1(c) is perhaps due to the impact of the ocean in the zone of the Gulf Stream, the cold Labrador current near Newfoundland and the Northern Atlantic current in the Norwegian Sea. The absence of a marked correlation between the variabilities of the short– and longwave ERB components supports the hypothesis of the oceanic origin of this variability. As is seen in figures 1 and 3, the origin of the year–to–year variability for the continental territories adjacent to EAZO is clearly different from the origin for oceans: in figure 3 the bimodal distribution typical of figure 1 disappears. Under the assumption that the data variability in figures 1(d) and 2(d) is also of oceanic origin, the respective maxima in the winter Northern hemisphere can be due to the warm water coming from the Southern hemisphere across the equator.

These assumptions must be further verified both experimentally and theoretically from independent observations and modelling. The ERB values considered are undoubtedly more sensitive to variations in the ocean–atmosphere system occurring during transition periods (spring, fall) than to the dynamic effects of the heating source anomalies, which are more charac–

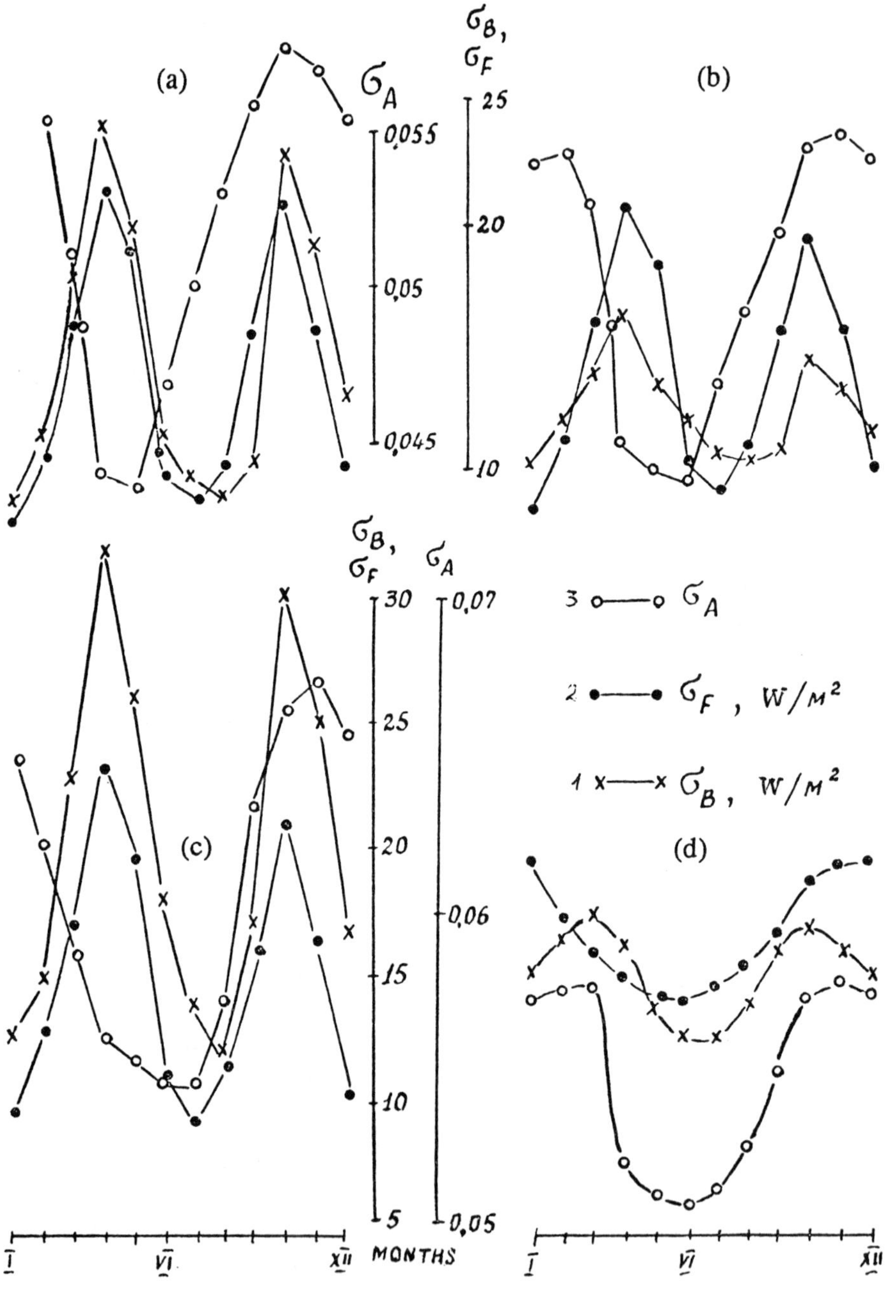

Fig. 1. Monthly distributions of MSDs of the radiation budget (1), its shortwave (3) and longwave (2) components for the Newfoundland EAZO (a), Norwegian EAZO (b), Gulf Stream area (c) and tropical Atlantic EAZO (d).

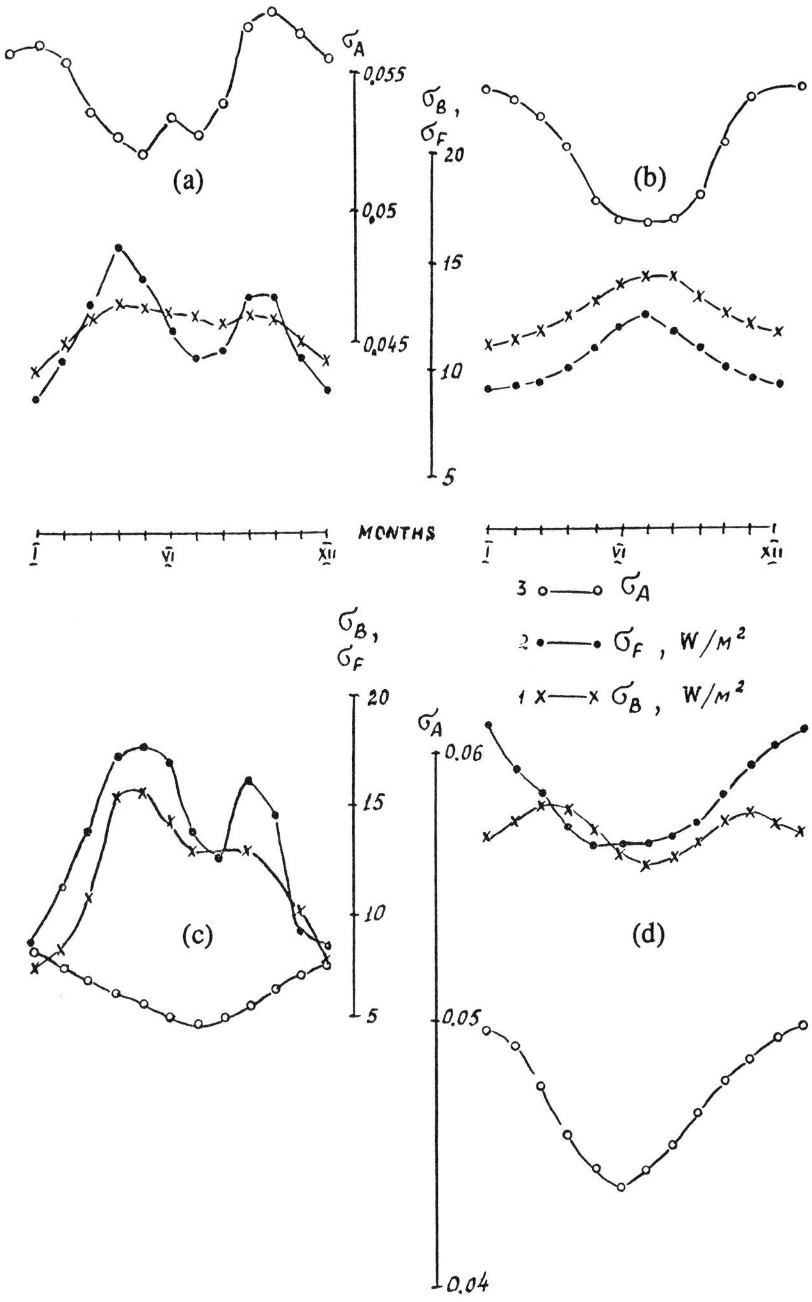

Fig. 2. The same distributions (see fig. 1) along the 30°W longitudinal section; the latitudes correspond to the EAZOs enumerated in fig. 1.

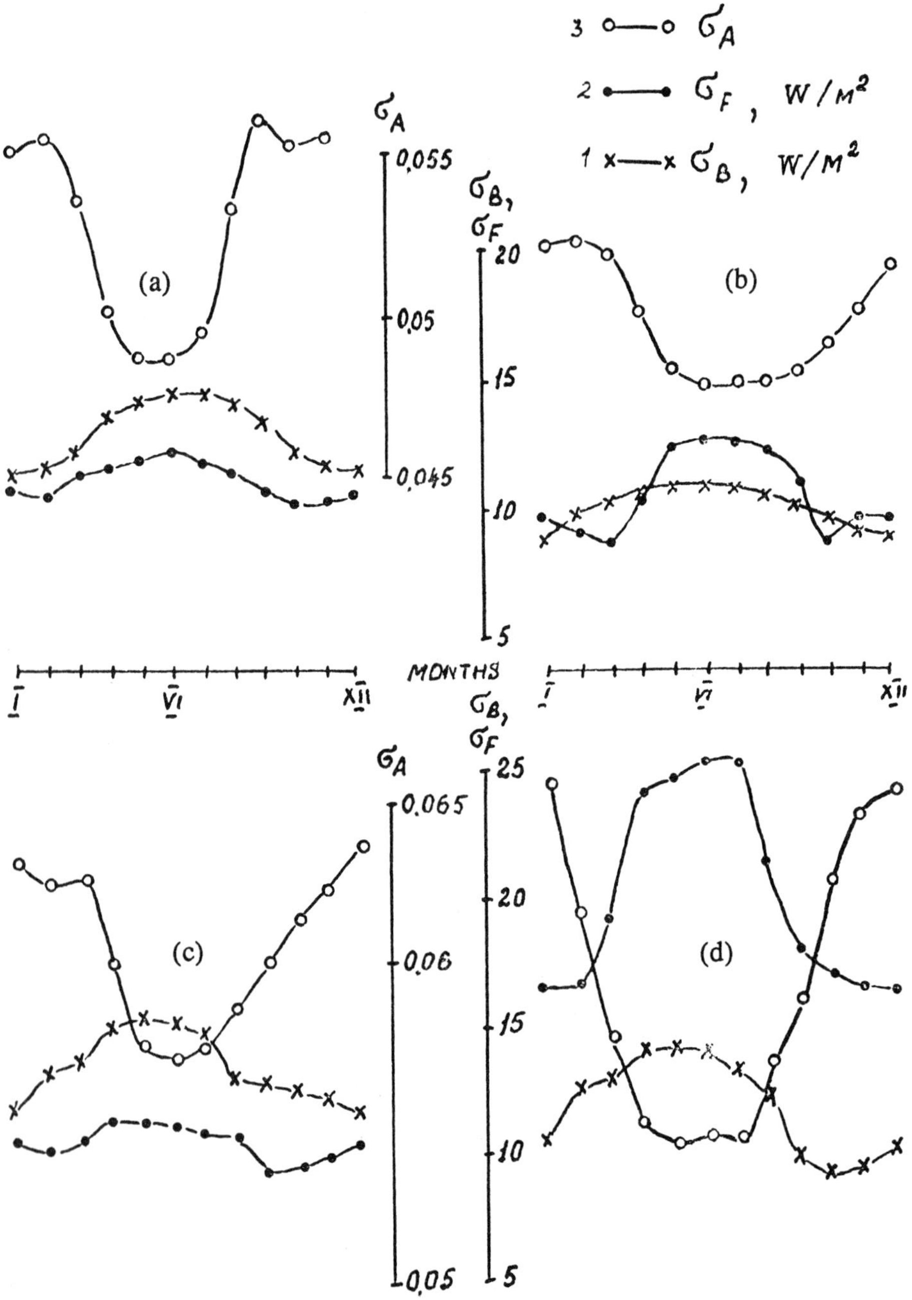

Fig. 3. The same distributions as in fig. 1 for coastal land areas, corresponding to those enumerated in fig. 1.

teristic of the winter and summer conditions. This suggests that the influence of seasonal variations of the oceanic thermocline in the northern Atlantic during the transition periods are of crucial importance. These variations, although not typical for some other scales of averaging, are present in the case of monthly averaging of the ERB observations.

These results are preliminary since the satellite data were insufficient and restricted to the given scales of a monthly averaging. The data for the longwave ERB component was obtained by means of averaging, for every 2.5°×2.5° lat.–long. grid, with respect to measurements at 09:00 and 21:00 local time, and for the shortwave component with respect to measurements at 09:00 only. More errors could occur in analyzing the data while passing from the radiance case to the irradiance one and in determining the hemispherical total short- and longwave radiation fluxes from the observational data in narrow spectral intervals (NOAA satellites).

Teleconnections between the ERB anomalies in the tropical and middle latitudes

The problem of applying the time series of satellite measurements to climate studies is closely related to the problem of estimating a climate noise level and subsequently analyzing the statistical significance of the anomalies of the ERB and its components in different regions of the globe. This problem is reduced to the identification of the geographical regions where the observed year–to–year variability is much higher than the climate noise level. The detection of teleconnections between the ERB anomalies helps solve the problem of identification of various "signals" of short–term climatical changes.

In this connection, we will review the analysis of the year–to–year variability of the radiation budget and of the noise component in the data of NOAA and TIROS–N. The sampled variability of measurement data makes us go from the theoretical statistics techniques (with an infinite number of realizations with respective asymptotic transitions) to a realistic estimation from limited samples. The climate noise results from limited samples. Like the natural variability of the measured fields, it may be estimated from the autocorrelation function.

Practically, lower daily variabilities and longer times of correlation are observed at a large spatial averaging [13]. As a result, a combination of data for certain territories at grid points permits one to enlarge the volume of sampling and to obtain the distributions of anomalies, which will be smoothed as if an analysis were made with long observation series. This methodological approach together with analysis of the instrumental errors, sensitivity trends of sensors and cloudiness variations, broadens the possibility of using the satellite information for detecting a climate signal against noise.

The mathematical expectation of the square difference between current data and monthly means is [13]:

$$\mathrm{Var}\,(\overline{X}_T) = \frac{S_{\mathcal{D}}^2}{n}\left[1 + 2\sum_{\tau=1}^{n}\left(1 - \frac{\tau}{n}\right) R_x(\tau)\right], \tag{1}$$

where X_k, $k = 1,2,...n$, is the set of n observations for a given month (it can be the radiation–budget components as well as other parameters); $\overline{X}_T = 1/n\sum_{k=1}^{n} X_k$ is the monthly mean; τ is determined by the number of independent samplings. The measure of variability, a sample dispersion, is

$$S_{\mathcal{D}}^3 = \frac{1}{n-1}\sum_{k=1}^{n} (X_k - \overline{X}_T)^2, \tag{2}$$

and the autocorrelation function is

$$R_X(\tau) = \frac{1}{n-\tau}\sum_{k=1}^{n-\tau} (X_k - \overline{X}_\tau)(X_{k+\tau} - \overline{X}_T)/S_{\mathcal{D}}^2. \tag{3}$$

Here the $S_{\mathcal{D}}$ is a measure of observational data variability, provided they are independent day–to–day, and $\mathrm{Var}(\overline{X}_T)$ is a measure of observational data variability in the case of autocorrelation with the function $R_x(\tau)$: the greater the values of this function, the greater the amount of noise data, i.e., $\mathrm{Var}(\overline{X}_T)$ is also a measure of climate noise. If the observations are uncorrelated, then the expected variability of the monthly means only depends on the number of observations used to obtain monthly means, i.e., the expected variability of monthly means is determined by day–to–day variations. The climate noise level can be estimated from the dispersions and the autocorrelation functions.

It has been shown [13] that despite the fact that mean daily variability in summer and in winter for the central tropical Pacific is approximately equal, a substantial difference of the autocorrelation functions for these seasons has led to substantially different values of the signal/noise ratio, which is 2.7 for summer and 4.0 for winter. Along with noise data characterized by the $\mathrm{Var}(\overline{X}_T)$ parameter, dispersions for current monthly means were calculated:

$$S_{0,\ell}^2 = \frac{1}{n-1}\sum_{k=1}^{n} (X_k^{(\ell)} - \overline{X}^{(\ell)})^2, \tag{4}$$

where

$$X^{(\ell)} = \frac{1}{y}\sum_{i=1}^{y} X_i^{(\ell)}, \quad \ell = 1,2,...,12;$$

y is the number of monthly means used in observations.

In analyzing spectral density curves for different seasons, it was determined that the variability of mean July values of this characteristic was greater than that of the mean January values [10]. This can be attributed to the more pronounced climatic manifestations of radiation–budget anomalies in the summer. However, the summertime noise data do not allow us to conclude with certainty that climate "signals" are crucial in the analysis of summertime anomalies. Further studies in this direction are needed.

Note that for the Gaussian process, 95% of measurement data variability fall within $\pm\mathrm{Var}(\overline{X}_T)^{1/2}$, i.e., in this case the confidence interval is estimated by means of the well–known criteria of significance level, taking account of a varying dispersion. The expected variability (in contrast to the "observed" one to be found) is determined by the character of variations from one realization to another. If observations are uncorrelated, then $\mathrm{Var}(\overline{X}_T)$ will only depend on the number of measurements, n, used to find mean values of $\overline{X}_T$. An efficient number of independent measurements is given by τ and governs the summation law in the expression for $\mathrm{Var}(\overline{X}_T)$. A 95% confidence interval characterizes the limits within which the true values of anomalies (with an 0.95 probability) from the calculated sample dispersion lie, accounting for the noise in data.

The analysis of data in [13] is based on the nature of their interrelation, including individual measurements within each month. The analysis in [4], [7], [8], [10] is based on monthly mean values which could not account for the monthly variability. We had at our disposal only 45 time realizations for each of the points at which annual changes can be filtered. However, a methodological approach suggested in [13] can be used, which increases the number of points by enlarging the region of analysis. On the other hand, the time correlation (the expected covariance) of monthly means can be estimated from 45 realizations with the annual distribution filtered. The corresponding expression for the

$$R_{\overline{X}_T\overline{Y}_T}(0) = \frac{\mathrm{Cov}(\overline{X}_T, \overline{Y}_T)}{[\mathrm{Var}(\overline{X}_T)]^{1/2}\,[\mathrm{Var}(\overline{Y}_T)]^{1/2}} \tag{5}$$

$$= \frac{R_{XY}(0) + \sum\limits_{\tau=1}^{n-1}(1-\frac{\tau}{n})R_{XY}(\tau) + \sum\limits_{\tau=1}^{n-1}(1-\frac{\tau}{n})R_{XY}(-\tau)}{[1+2\sum\limits_{\tau=1}^{n-1}(1-\frac{\tau}{n})R_X(\tau)]^{1/2}[1+2\sum\limits_{\tau=1}^{n-1}(1-\frac{\tau}{n})R_Y(\tau)]^{1/2}},$$

where $R_X(\tau)$ and $R_Y(\tau)$ are the autocorrelations of observations made at different times, $\mathrm{Cov}(\overline{X}_T,\overline{Y}_T)$ is the covariance of observations at different times, $R_{XY}(\tau)$ and $R_{YX}(\tau)$ are the cross–correlations of observations at different shifts, τ:

$$R_{XY}(\tau) = \frac{1}{n-\tau}\sum_{k=1}^{n-\tau}(X_k - \overline{X}_T)(Y_{k+\tau} - \overline{Y}_T)/S_{XY}, \tag{6}$$

$$R_{YX}(\tau) = \frac{1}{n-\tau}\sum_{k=1}^{n-\tau}(X_{k+\tau} - \overline{X}_T)(Y_k - \overline{Y}_T)/S_{XY}, \tag{7}$$

$$S_{XY} = [\frac{1}{n-1}\sum_{k=1}^{n}(X_k - \overline{X}_T)^2\,\frac{1}{n-1}\sum_{k=1}^{n}(Y_k - \overline{Y}_T)^2]^{1/2}. \tag{8}$$

Here $T = n\Delta t$ is the sequence of observations ($n = 45$), Δt is the interval between observations (1 month), $R_{XY}(0) = R_{YX}(0)$ are the coefficients of mutual correlation of observations made at different times.

Now we review the analysis of teleconnections between monthly means anomalies for the radiation budget and its components at different points. Simultaneous observations at adjacent grid points are mutually correlated due to a finite size of weather disturbances manifested in radiation measurements from satellites. Monthly means have a natural trend to increased correlation at certain directions of disturbance motion.

The "signal" of the short–term climate variability, visible in the tropics as clouds and the ERB longwave component field, has been proven in [13], [14], among others. These and other studies lay the foundation of the TOGA research program. The teleconnections between key regions, obtained from the longwave component fluctuations in the equatorial central Pacific using correlations with a zero–shift from (6) and (7), are shown in figure 4 [14].

The importance of the mutual correlation coefficients, corresponding to a 95% significance level, was determined from the condition

$$R_{XY}(0) > 2\mathscr{SD}(C_{XY})/\sigma_F , \tag{9}$$

where the standard deviation of the covariance of two different time observations, which can be represented in the form of a Markov process of the first order [14], is equal to

$$\mathscr{SD}(C_{XY}) = \sigma_F \left[\frac{2}{n\{1 - \exp[-(\lambda_x+\lambda_y)]\}}\right]^{1/2} , \tag{10}$$

C_{XY} is the sampled estimate of the cross–covariance of two discrete processes X and Y:

$$C_{XY}(\tau) = \frac{1}{n-|\tau|} \sum_{k=1}^{(n-|\tau|)} (X_k - \overline{X}_T)(Y_{k+\tau} - \overline{Y}_T) , \tag{11}$$

λ_X and λ_Y are the indices of the exponent of the Markov random processes.

Expression (10) follows from a theoretical representation of the covariance of the estimates of $C_{XY}(\tau_1)$ and $C_{XY}(\tau_2)$ in the form

$$\begin{aligned} \mathrm{Cov}[C_{XY}(\tau_1),C_{XY}(\tau_2)] = \frac{1}{n_{XY}} \sum_{k=+\infty}^{\infty} [&\gamma_{XX}(k)\gamma_{YY}(k+\tau_1+\tau_2) \\ &+ \gamma_{XY}(k+\tau_1)\gamma_{YX}(k-\tau_2)] , \end{aligned} \tag{12}$$

where γ_{XX}, γ_{YY}, γ_{XY}, γ_{YX} are non–normalized autocorrelation and cross–covariance functions related to the numerators of (6) and (7); n_{XY} is an effective number of the pairs of processes X and Y at shifts τ_1 and τ_2, respectively. If we assume that the processes are uncorrelated ($\gamma_{XY} = \gamma_{YX} = 0$), then we have (9) from (12) and from the assumption that these processes are first–order autoregressive (Markov). The parameters λ_X and λ_Y are incorporated in the expressions:

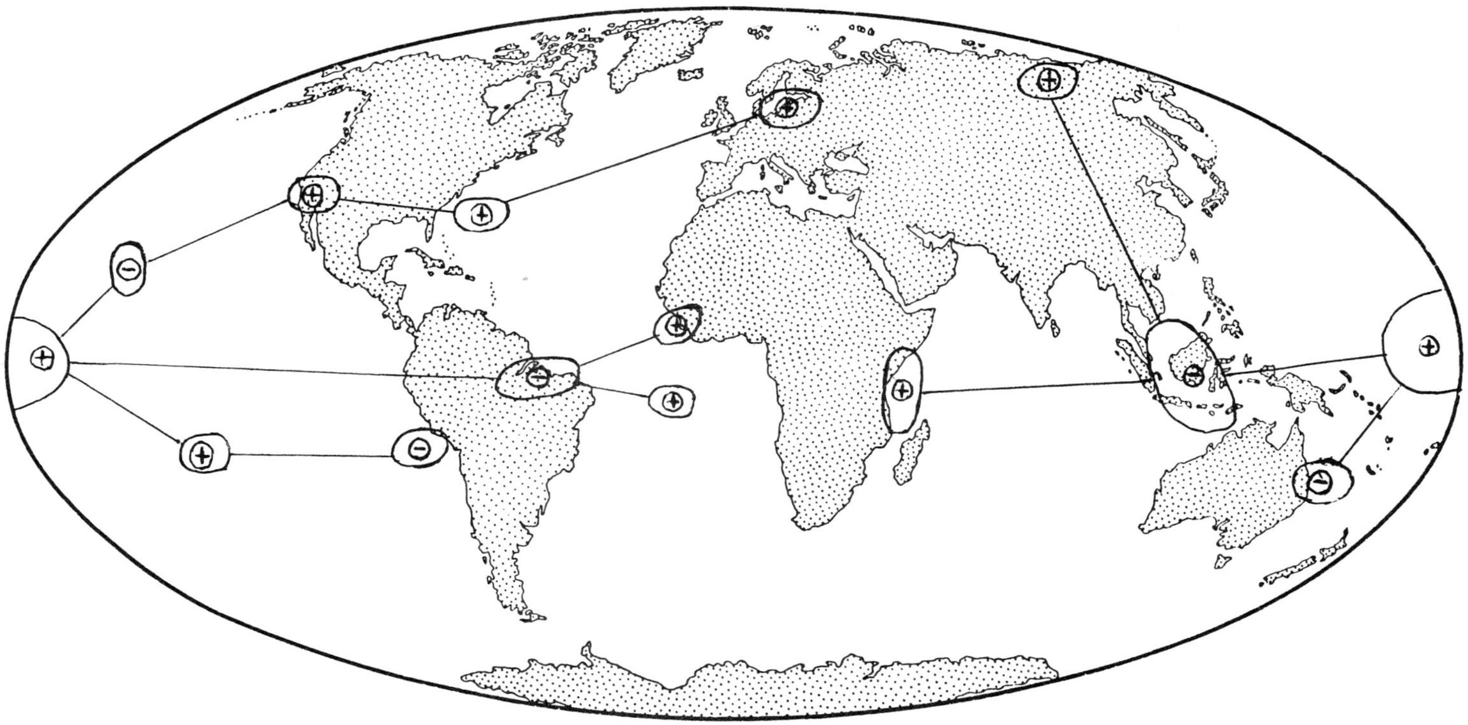

Fig. 4. A scheme of the key regions of the globe (energetically active zones) from the viewpoint of teleconnections between anomalies of the radiation budget longwave component and initial fluctuations in the tropical central Pacific.

$$\gamma_{XX}(\tau) = \sigma_F^2(X)e^{-\lambda_X|\tau|} , \qquad (13)$$

$$\gamma_{YY}(\tau) = \sigma_F^2(Y)e^{-\lambda_Y|\tau|} , \qquad (14)$$

where $\sigma_F^2(X)$ and $\sigma_F^2(Y)$ are dispersions of the ERB longwave component for different time observations.

In figure 4, the quantitative measure of data teleconnectivity was determined using the expression

$$Q(X,\tau=0) = \frac{1}{N(X,\tau=0)} \sum_Y H(|R_{\overline{X}_T,\overline{Y}_T}(0)| - |\hat{R}_{\overline{X}_T,\overline{Y}_T}(0)|) \times |R_{\overline{X}_T,\overline{Y}_T}(0)| , \qquad (15)$$

where

$$\hat{R}_{\overline{X}_T,\overline{Y}_T}(0) = 2\mathcal{SD}(C_{XY}) , \qquad (16)$$

$H(\alpha)$ is the Heaviside step function [14]; $N(X,\tau=0)$ is the total number of observations for which $|R_{\overline{X}_T,\overline{Y}_T}(0)| \geq |\hat{R}_{\overline{X}_T,\overline{Y}_T}(0)|$.

It is seen from figure 4 that the most significant teleconnections are those between the equatorial Pacific and the following geographical regions (the sign +/– corresponds to sinphase/counterphase variations):

	(+)	(–)
Tropics:	Equatorial Central Pacific, East Africa	Polynesia, Australia, Peru coastline, north–eastern Brazil
Extratropical latitudes:	North west Atlantic, west Europe, Siberia	Hawaii, arid zone of the southern Pacific

Most important to us are teleconnections between the regions of the tropical Pacific and the energetically active zone of the Gulf Stream, in terms of maximal amplitudes of the radiation budget and its longwave component. Figure 5 illustrates the delay correlation of the radiation budget, with zero shift, using formula (10).

It is seen from figure 5 that the effect of the Gulf Stream EAZO (in the case of the radiation budget) is at the limit of climate significance level, determined from (9) and corresponding to a 95% confidence level. In accordance with (9), the indicated limit is determined by significance coefficients of mutual correlation, reaching maximum values close to 0.6, moving (in the case of the radiation budget) along the Gulf Stream current at a

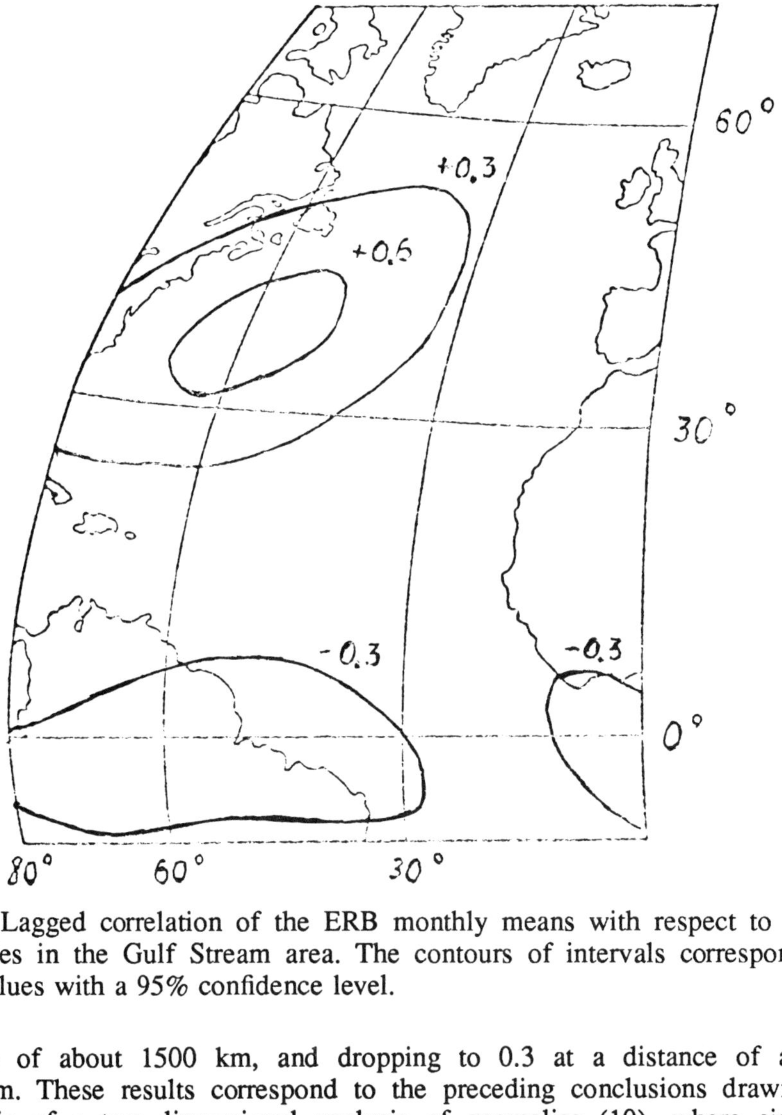

Fig. 5. Lagged correlation of the ERB monthly means with respect to ERB anomalies in the Gulf Stream area. The contours of intervals correspond to 0.3—values with a 95% confidence level.

distance of about 1500 km, and dropping to 0.3 at a distance of about 2500 km. These results correspond to the preceding conclusions drawn on the basis of a two–dimensional analysis of anomalies (10), where similar regularities are observed for the correlation function calculated over the entire territory (10°S–70°N; 0°–80°W), without special selection of a Gulf Stream area, using the mathematical formalism of two–dimensional filtration.

Despite some uncertainty of the computational procedure used (this uncertainty is due to the absence of "instant" measurements and estimation involving smoothed mean monthly fields) and of the estimates obtained for 45 mean monthly fields characterized by smooth monthly observations, one may make the assumption that a further increase of the time series will increase the significance and make it possible to study the correlations between the EAZO considered and other mid–latitude regions. This proves the assumption concerning the existence of cross–correlation about ± 5 months for radiation–budget anomalies with initial reference level in the Gulf Stream EAZO (fig. 6).

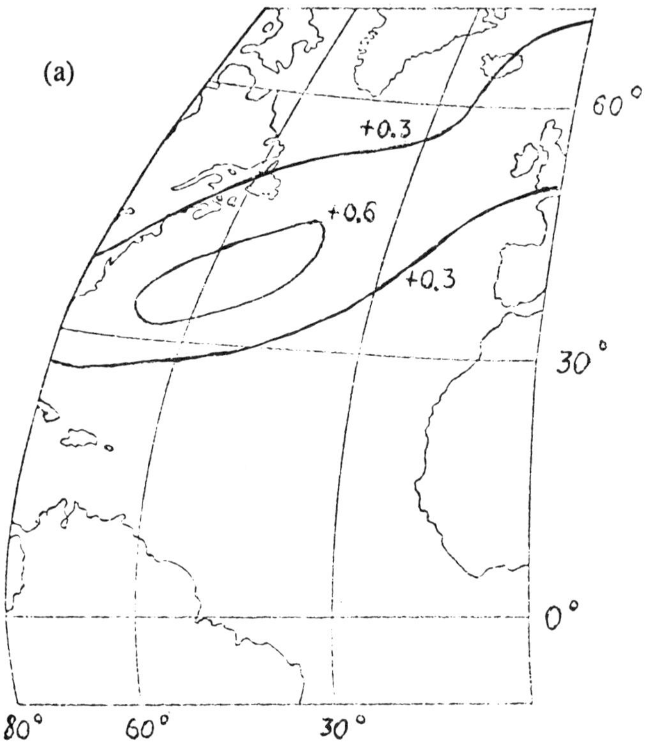

Figure 6 shows, in particular, the presence of delay correlation in mid–latitudes of the northern Atlantic with respect to the Gulf Stream EAZO, where the effect of disturbances, as follows from figure 4, is secondary (the original source of ERB anomalies is the tropical Pacific manifested in the Southern Oscillation/El Nino events [13], [14], etc.) Figure 6 shows a larger region of the effect of Gulf Stream EAZO telecon– nections with a delay correlation versus a zero shift (fig. 5). Further studies in this direction will allow a more detailed analysis of correla– tions between anomalies of the radiation budget and its components in the northern Atlantic and the respective anomalies of meteorological parameters in continental Europe.

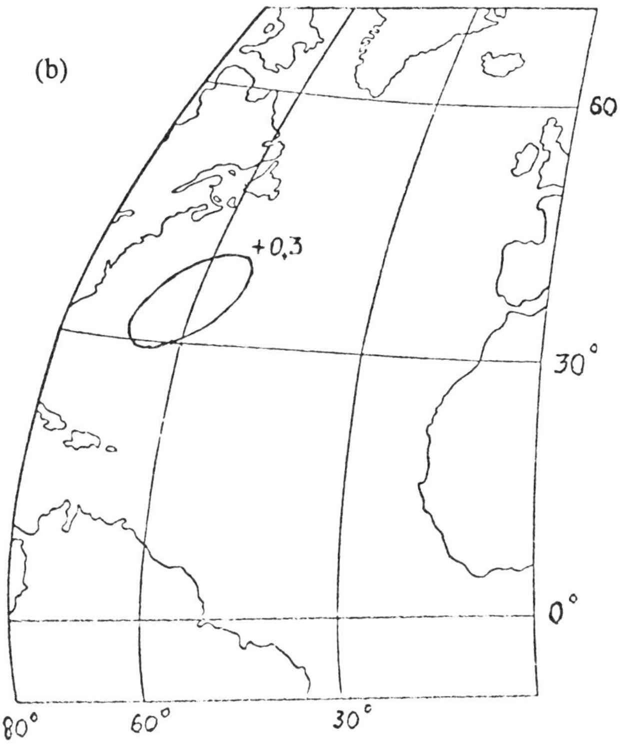

Fig. 6. Lagged cross–correlation of ERB anomalies with respect to the Gulf Stream area of +5 months (a) and –5 months (b).

ERB and cloudiness

In the interpretation of satellite data, of particular importance is the development of climate models which incorporate the estimates of the "signals" of short–term climate changes and the estimates of the noise in the observational data. The analysis of the year–to–year variability of the radiation budget and its components can form a methodological basis for such studies. The key problem is then to better understand the nature of correlations between radiation and cloudiness.

Let us consider, as an example, the problem of sensitivity of climate models incorporating the ERB data, to variations in cloudiness.

Usually, in radiation climatology we study the sensitivity of the radiation budget, B, to variations in the cloud amount, n_c, determined in the following way:

$$\delta = \frac{\partial B}{\partial n_c} = \frac{\partial G}{\partial n_c} - \frac{\partial F}{\partial n_c},$$

where G is the absorbed shortwave radiation, F the outgoing longwave emission, and n_c the cloud amount.

The partial derivative $\partial G/\partial n_c$ characterizes the albedo (shortwave) effect of clouds and $\partial F/\partial n_c$ the effect of clouds on the outgoing emission (the greenhouse effect). It has been shown in most of the studies that variations in the shortwave component dominate those in the longwave component ($\delta < 0$). However, in some studies the mutual compensation of these effects ($\delta \approx 0$) has been suggested [16].

The planetary albedo can be represented as

$$A = A_c n_c + A_s(1-n_c) ,$$

where A_c, A_s are the albedos of clouds and cloud–free territories, respectively. With the assumed independence of A_c and A_s of cloud amount, n_c, we obtain

$$\frac{\partial G}{\partial n_c} = -S_0 \frac{\partial A}{\partial n_c} = -S_0(A_c - A_s) , \tag{18}$$

where S_0 is the solar constant.

Since

$$\frac{\partial F}{\partial n_c} = \frac{\partial F}{\partial A}\frac{\partial A}{\partial n_c} = (A_c - A_s)\frac{\partial F}{\partial A}, \tag{19}$$

the problem of analysis of the radiation–budget sensitivity to cloudiness variations is reduced to finding the difference A_c–A_s and estimating the derivative $\partial F/\partial A$.

Despite the theoretical possibility of estimating the difference A_c–A_s from satellite observations, reliable estimates have not yet been obtained. The main reason is twofold: the difficulty of cloudiness classification and the derivation of surface albedo from satellite data. For this purpose the concept of minimum albedo [15], [16] is usually used, with A_s determined from a minimum value of the measured brightness within horizontal scales of about 250–500 km, and the values of A and n_c are taken from climatological data, and A_c is estimated with the use of binar classification.

The results obtained in [4], [9] make it possible to solve this problem in general, without these assumptions. In this case, four classes of cloud formations are selected [4] by respective brightness levels obtained from a geostationary satellite. There is also the possibility of obtaining A_s for given classes of cloud formation and atmospheric aerosol with the use of a calculation scheme for the surface radiation budget [9]. An additional analysis of regressive correlations between the year–to–year variability of the ERB longwave component and the albedo opens the possibility of estimating the derivative $\partial F/\partial A$.

Figure 7 illustrates regressive estimates of derivatives $\partial F/\partial A$ for 45 mean monthly ERB values in the four EAZOs of the northern Atlantic, used in the program "Sections."

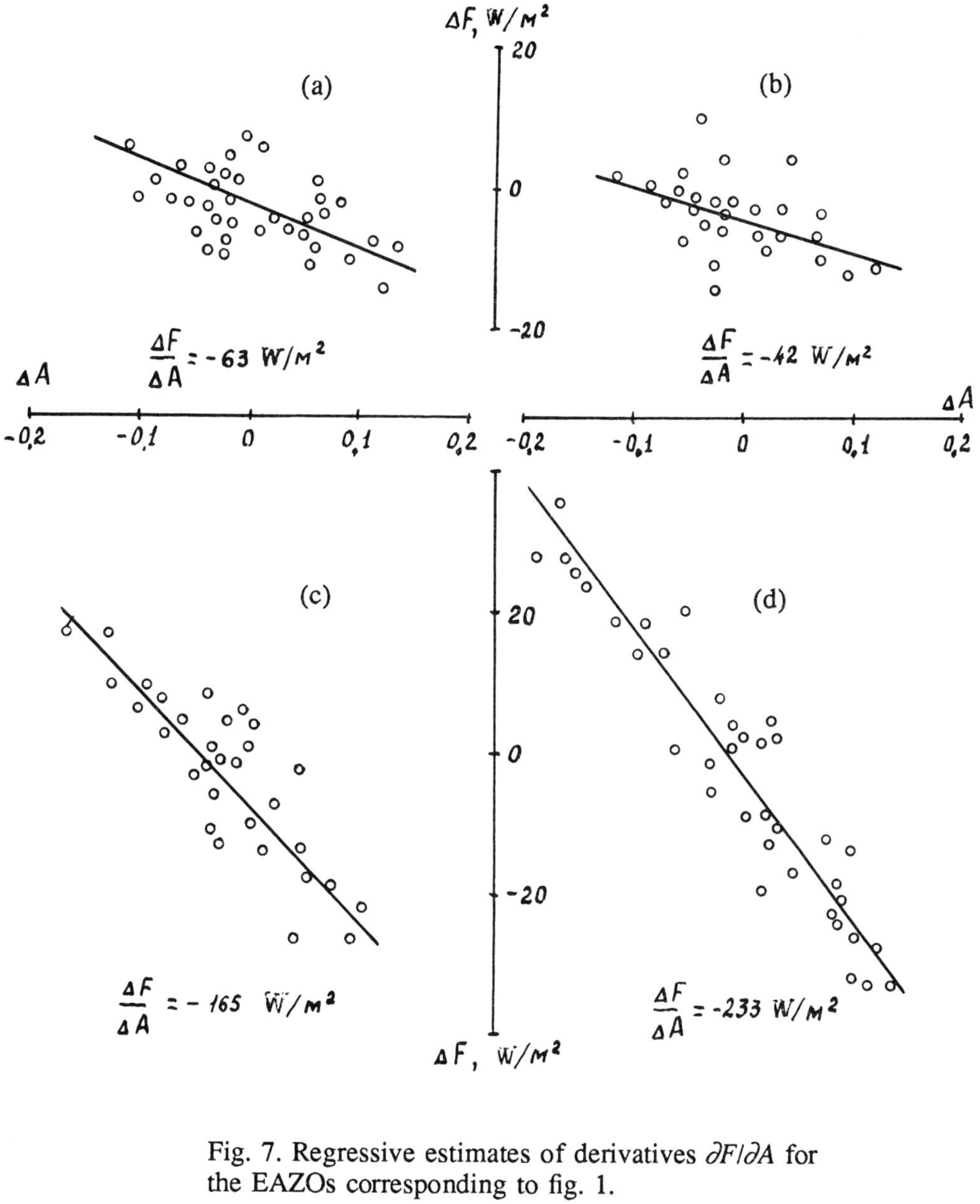

Fig. 7. Regressive estimates of derivatives $\partial F/\partial A$ for the EAZOs corresponding to fig. 1.

Figure 7 allows us to see essentially different effects of cloudiness in the EAZOs under consideration: the slope of the regression line varies from –42 W/m^2 for the Norwegian EAZO to –233 W/m^2 for the tropical range. These variations are, apparently, explained by quite different effects of cirrus clouds in the first case and powerful convective clouds in the second case. The derivatives were estimated to determine the following climatological characteristic:

$$\varepsilon = \frac{\partial F / \partial n_c}{\partial G / \partial n_c} = \frac{\partial F}{\partial G},$$

incorporating combined variations in the long– and shortwave components of the radiation budget with varying cloudiness. In calculations of the ε parameter from (20), (18) and (19) are used.

Figure 8 shows the isolines of this characteristic. It is seen that $\varepsilon > 1$ only in a narrow area of the oceans of South America and the Gulf Stream

$$\varepsilon = \frac{\partial F / \partial n_c}{\partial G / \partial n_c} = \frac{\partial F}{\partial G}$$

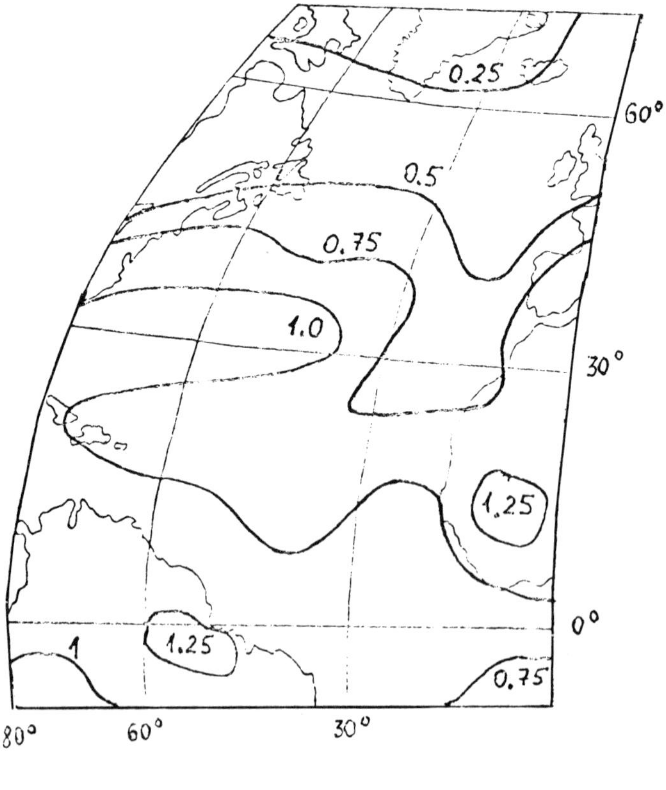

Fig. 8. Isolines of the sensitivity of the ERB components to variations in cloud amount.

with a maximum value of $\varepsilon \approx 1.25$. For the rest of the region considered $\varepsilon < 1$ and reaches a minimum of 0.3 in Greenland. On the average, for the whole area considered (10°S– 70°N; 0°–80°W) $\varepsilon \approx 0.74$, which confirms the conclusion about the prevailing effect of the ERB shortwave component over the longwave one. At the same time, an analysis of the isolines in figure 8 does not permit one to conclude that the sensitivity of climate to variations in cloudiness substantially depends on specific features of EAZO. Further studies are needed to better comprehend the relation between the year–to–year variability of the ERB components and respective variability in cloudiness in the EAZOs of land and ocean.

Conclusion

Using the variability of ERB and its components as an example, specific manifestations of EAZO, constituting a methodological basis for a study of short–term climatical changes, are discussed. This concept combines theoretical studies of climate variability and forecast analysis of observations in key regions of the world ocean. The EAZO concept makes the application of observational data to studies of the short–term climatical changes more efficient.

Here are the major results:

1. In analyzing the ERB year–to–year variability, we established that the EAZOs appear as characteristic clusters of the isolines of dispersions of the ERB and its componets with respect to their monthly means.

2. For the annual distribution of the radiation budget and its components for central parts of the four EAZOs of the northern Atlantic, used in the research program "Sections," and for distant regions toward open ocean and land, the year–to–year variability of the ERB and its longwave component in the EAZOs is maximal in April and October; it is zero in the adjacent land areas, and is only marginal in the adjacent oceanic areas. This allows one to conjecture that the characteristic fields of ERB anomalies in these EAZO are of oceanic origin.

3. There are global key regions in terms of maximum teleconnections with the central tropical Pacific. These regions are closely connected with EAZOs. One of these key regions is the Gulf Stream area, the effect of which, in contrast to other regions of the northern Atlantic, is more significant in terms of teleconnections between anomalies in tropical and middle latitudes, being at the limit of climatic significance (in continuous 45–month satellite observations of the ERB and its components). A further analysis of the auto– and cross–correlation, both "instant" and mean monthly ERB values together with a larger time series, may help demonstrate in more detail the concept of teleconnections between the ERB anomalies in different regions of the globe.

4. Further studies are needed on the mechanisms of the radiation–cloudiness feedback in EAZOs, to be applied to climate models. The application of satellite data to climate studies requires, in particular, solution of the following problems: better understanding of the mechanisms of the relation (feedback) between cloudiness and ERB components; improving reliability and enlarging the satellite database, including data from polar–orbiting and geostationary satellites; increasing the length of satellite–data time series; the development of climate models which incorporate data from satellites.

REFERENCES

[1] Marchuk, G.I. 1974. Long–range weather forecast techniques based on the solution of basic and conjugate problems (in Russian). *Meteorologiya i Gidrologiya* 3:17–34.

[2] ——————. 1979. Climate–change modelling and the problem of long–range weather forecast (in Russian). *Meteorologiya i Gidrologiya* 7:25–36.

[3] Lappo, S.S., S.K. Gulev, A.P. Metalnikov, A.E. Rozhdestvenskij, V.A. Sokolov, G.P. Volkov, T.N. Kopejkina, Yu.A. Reva, V.A. Tikhonov, and M.V. Semenov. 1984. Energetically active zones of the world ocean (in Russian). *Doklady Akademii Nauk SSSR*, ser. matem. fiz. 275, no. 4:1018–21.

[4] Marchuk, G.I., K.Ya. Kondrat'ev, and V.V. Kozoderov. 1984. Energetically active zones of the ocean as manifestations of the interannual variability of the ERB components (in Russian). *Studies of the Earth from Space* 1:3–15.

[5] Marchuk, G.I., ed. 1983. The program of studies on the atmosphere–ocean interaction to study short–term climate changes ("Sections"). *Adv. in Sci. and Technol., ser. Atmosphere, ocean, space,* vol. 1, VINITI, Moscow.

[6] Winston, J.S., et al. 1979. Earth atmosphere radiation budget analyses derived from NOAA satellite data, June 1974–February 1978. U.S. Department of Commerce, NOAA/NESS.

[7] Marchuk, G.I., K.Ya. Kondrat'ev, and V.V. Kozoderov. 1983. Variability of the north Atlantic radiation budget on the basis of observations from space (in Russian). *Doklady Akademii Nauk SSSR,* ser. matem. fiz. 272, no. 5:1099–1102.

[8] Marchuk, G.I., K.Ya. Kondrat'ev, O.A. Avaste, V.V. Kozoderov, and O.Yu. Kiarner. 1985. The interannual variability of the Earth's radiation–budget components on the basis of satellite observations (in Russian). *Doklady Akademii Nauk SSSR,* ser. matem. fiz. 280, no. 1:65–70.

[9] Kozoderov, V.V. 1983. On the retrieval of the Earth's radiation–budget components from satellite observations (in Russian). *Studies of the Earth from Space* 2:65–75.

[10] Kondratyev, K.Ya., and V.V. Kozoderov. 1984. Statistical characteristics of anomalies of the 2–D fields of the north Atlantic radiation budget (in Russian). *Doklady Akademii Nauk SSSR*, ser. matem. fiz. 275, no. 2:338–42.
[11] Marchuk, G.I., K.Ya. Kondrat'ev, and V.V. Kozoderov. 1984. Cloudiness as a factor of interannual variability of the Earth's radiation budget from satellite data and the problem of energetically active zones of the ocean (in Russian). *Proc. of the 9th International Conference on Cloud Physics*, Tallin, vol. 3, 689–92.
[12] Kondratyev, K.Ya., and V.V. Kozoderov. 1983. Anomalies of the Earth's radiation budget and the heat content of the upper oceanic layer as manifestations of the energetically active zones (in Russian). *Adv. in Sci. and Technol., ser. Atmosphere, ocean, space,* program "Sections," vol. 4, VINITI, Moscow.
[13] Short, D.A., and R.F. Cahalan. 1983. Interannual variability and climate noise in satellite–observed outgoing longwave radiation. *Mon. Weather Rev.* 111, no. 3:572–77.
[14] Ka–Ming Lau, and P.H. Chan. "Short–term Climate Variability and Atmospheric Teleconnection from Satellite–observed Longwave Radiation." Pt I: Simultaneous relationships. *J. Atmos. Sci.* 40, no. 12 (1983): 2735–50. Pt. II: Lagged correlations. *J. Atmos. Sci.* 40, no. 12 (1984): 2751–67.
[15] Kondrat'ev, K.Ya. *Satellite Climatology* (in Russian). Leningrad: Gidrometeoizdat, 1983.
[16] ————. 1983. The Earth's radiation budget, aerosols, and cloudiness (in Russian). *Adv. in Sci. and Technol., Meteorology and Climatology* 10.

PROPOSAL FOR A NUMERICAL MODEL OF THE BIOSPHERE FOR USE WITH NUMERICAL MODELS OF THE ATMOSPHERE

Yale Mintz and Piers J. Sellers
Department of Meteorology
University of Maryland

Gurij Ivanovich has been fearless and bold in developing numerical methods for the solution of difficult problems in extremely complex physical and biological systems. In his honor we present this proposal for a numerical model of the earth's vegetation cover, the biosphere, which, when used with a numerical model of the atmosphere (and a suitable ocean model), will provide a closed set of governing equations for the simulation and prediction of weather and climate.

1. Importance of the biosphere for weather and climate

The temperature, rainfall and circulation of the atmosphere are in large measure determined by the transfers of energy, water mass and momentum across the lower boundary of the atmosphere. The earth's vegetation cover, the *biosphere*, influences these transfers in the following ways:

(i) The leaves of the vegetation trap the incident solar radiation by multiple reflections and absorptions, so that it is the structure of the vegetation, as well as the optical properties of the individual leaves, that influences the radiational heating of the vegetated land surface. Typically, bare ground absorbs 60 to 70% of the daily insolation, grass cover absorbs 75 to 85%, and tree canopies absorb 80 to 90%.

(ii) The roots of the vegetation extract moisture from the soil, the stems transport the moisture to the leaves, and the stomata in the leaves transpire the moisture into the air. In addition, the leaves intercept and retain some of the rainfall, which returns to the air by direct evaporation from the wet surface of the leaves. On average, about 70% of all the precipitation that falls on the continents is returned to the atmosphere by the combined transpiration and interception loss; and only about 30% of the continental precipitation is transferred to the oceans by river drainage.

(iii) Vegetation, and especially the elevated canopies of the trees, acts as a layer of porous material which extracts momentum from the air that streams through it. The vegetation, in this way, influences the surface–wind stress and the curl of the stress. It is mainly the curl of the surface stress that determines the horizontal mass convergence in the atmospheric boundary layer and, thereby, the convergence of the horizontal water–vapor transport in the boundary layer. In this way vegetation influences the horizontal distribution of convective clouds and convective precipitation, which draw most of their water vapor from the boundary layer. The surface–roughness length, z_0, on which the surface–wind stress depends, is typically about one tenth of the vegetation height; so that z_0 is less than 1 cm for bare ground, of the order of 1 to 10 cm for a grass cover, and of the order of 100 to 300 cm for a forest.

It is clear, therefore, that the earth's vegetation cover has an influence on the boundary forcing of the atmosphere and that numerical models of the biosphere should be combined with numerical models of the atmosphere (and with numerical models of the oceans) for the simulation and prediction of weather and climate.

Until now there have been only separate numerical evaluations of the ways in which the vegetation–dependent processes influence the atmospheric circulation and rainfall: (i) the absorption of insolation (the albedo effect); (ii) the extraction of soil moisture (the evapotranspiration effect); and (iii) the wind stress (the surface roughness effect).

Various numerical models of the atmosphere have been used to examine (i) the albedo effect (starting with the study by Charney et al., 1977) and (ii) the soil–moisture effect (starting with Walker and Rowntree, 1977). Some of these studies have been analyzed and compared in two review papers (Mintz, 1984; and Rowntree, 1985). More recently, Sud et al., (1986) examined (iii) the surface–roughness effect. All of the studies showed that the simulated atmospheric circulation and rainfall were sensitive to the prescribed land–surface albedo, available soil moisture and surface roughness.

Fig. 1 shows how different vegetation structures produce different transfers of energy and water mass across the lower boundary of the atmosphere. It compares the water and energy budgets of a grass covered and a tree–covered land surface, as measured in two adjacent catchment basins which have nearly the same atmospheric conditions (data from Calder and Newson, 1979, and Shuttleworth and Calder, 1979). The total evapotranspiration from the tree–covered area was more than twice as large as that from the grass–covered area. With the grass cover, 58% of the net radiational heating of the surface was used for evapotranspiration and 42% for sensible heat transfer to the atmosphere. The Bowen ratio was positive: 0.72. With the trees, however, the energy used for evapotranspiration exceeded the radiational heating from the atmosphere. The Bowen ratio was negative: −0.13. This was due to the large interception loss from the trees. In the tree–covered catchment, where it was possible to measure the two components of the evapotranspiration separately, the interception loss was 1.7 times larger than the transpiration.

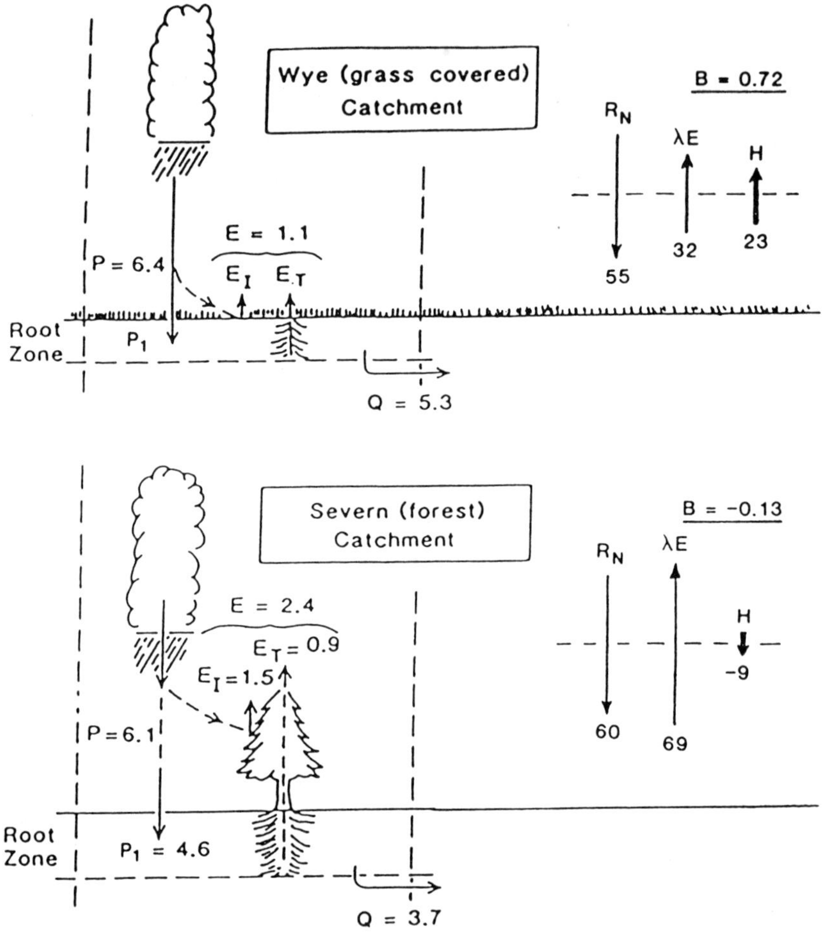

WATER BUDGET (mm/day)
P = precipitation
P_1 = surface infiltration
Q = runoff
E_T = transpiration
E_I = interception loss
E = $(E_T + E_I)$ = evapotranspiration

ENERGY BUDGET (watt/m^2)
R_N = net radiational heating
λE = latent heat transfer
H = sensible heat transfer
B = $(H/\lambda E)$ = Bowen ratio

Fig. 1. Measured mean annual water and energy balance of adjacent grass–covered and forest–covered catchments in central Wales, U.K. (Data from Calder and Newson, 1979; Shuttleworth and Calder, 1979.)

Although atmospheric conditions were about the same for the two adjacent areas, the net radiational heating was about 10% larger with the trees than with the grass cover. This is not only because the trees absorb more solar radiation, but also because the larger evapotranspiration rate lowers the temperature of the leaves and they emit less longwave radiation. This rather extreme example, from a region where the surface is wet for a large part of the time, is not representative of all climate regimes, but it shows the importance of treating the biosphere in a realistic way when simulating and predicting weather and climate.

In terms of its influence on the behavior of the atmosphere, the basic discrimination is between tall vegetation and short vegetation. This is because tall vegetation, as compared with short vegetation, typically

(i) traps and absorbs more solar radiation;
(ii) has both a larger rainfall–interception storage capacity and larger rate of interception loss;
(iii) has deeper roots and, consequently, a larger available soil–moisture storage capacity; and
(iv) has a larger surface–roughness length, which produces a larger surface–wind stress.

2. Vegetation structure of the Simple Biosphere

The *tall* vegetation components in the proposed *Si*mple *B*iosphere model (SiB) are *trees* (perennial, tall woody plants with stems or trunks that branch out into a canopy at some distance from the ground); and the *short* vegetation components are *shrubs* (perennial woody plants, shorter than trees, with stems that branch out into a canopy at or close to the ground) and *ground cover* (grass and other annual, herbacious plants that carpet the ground). As shown in fig. 2, these are arranged in six combinations: trees only, trees and ground cover, ground cover only, shrubs with ground cover, shrubs with bare soil, and bare soil. This is almost the same as in the Küchler (1979, 1983) classification of the world's natural vegetation, except that his has one small region in northeast India where there are trees with shrubs.

From a 1° by 1° digitized version of the Küchler map provided by Dr. C.J. Willmott, we have derived the distribution of the ten natural biomes shown in fig. 3.

Corresponding to the number code in fig. 3, the ten biomes are

Tall Vegetation

1. broadleaf trees (evergreen and deciduous)
2. broadleaf and needleleaf trees
3. needleleaf trees (evergreen and deciduous)
4. broadleaf trees with ground cover

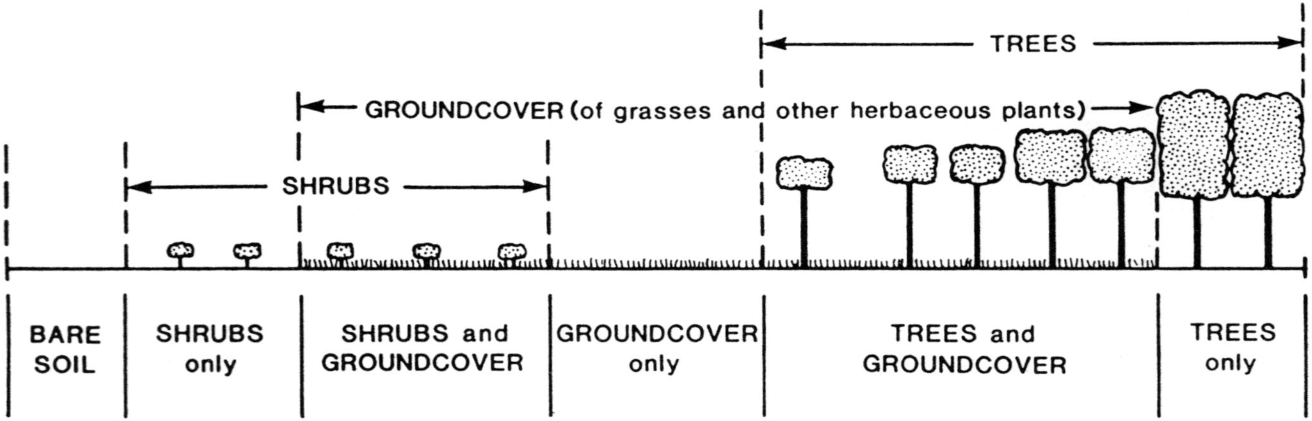

Fig. 2. Vegetation structure of the Simple Biosphere (SiB).

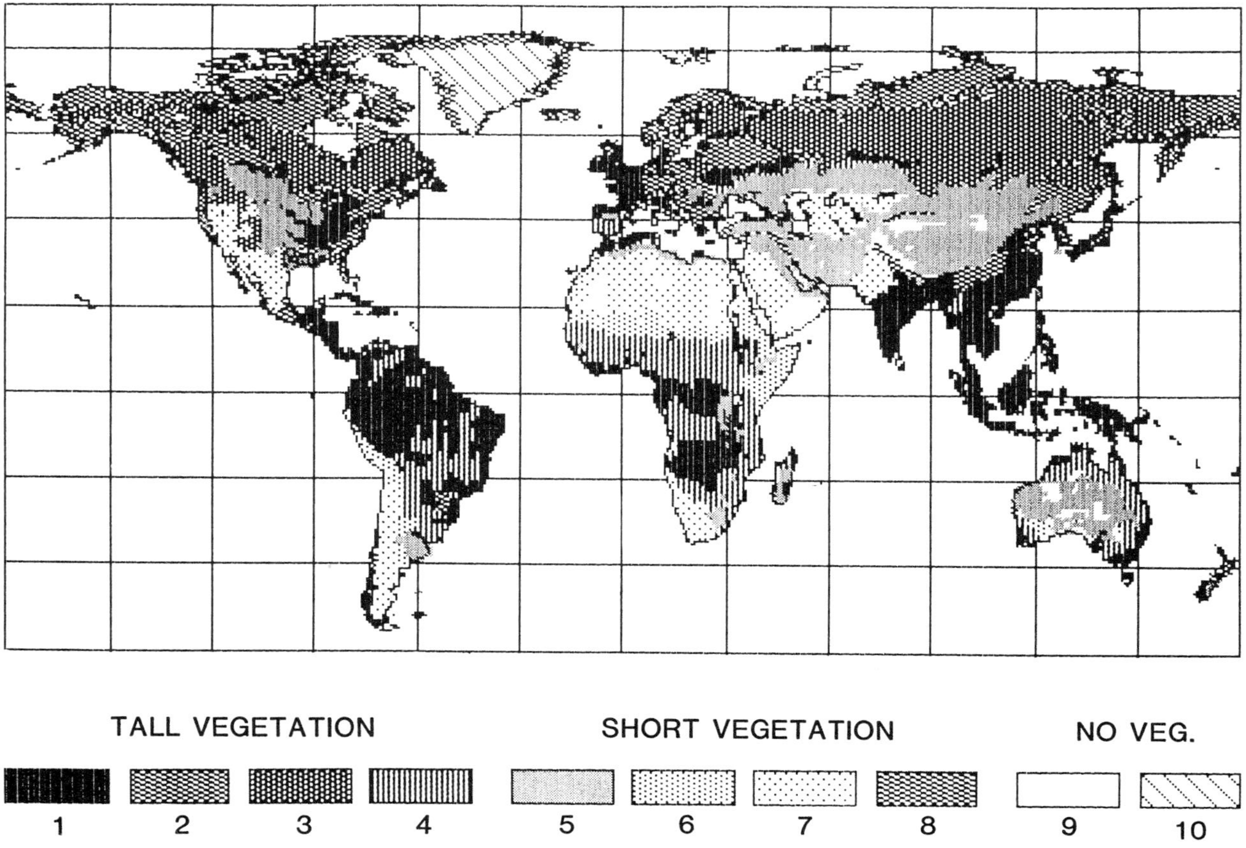

Fig. 3. World Map of the Simple Biosphere.

Short Vegetation

5. ground cover
6. broadleaf shrubs with ground cover
7. broadleaf shrubs with bare soil
8. dwarf trees and shrubs with ground cover (tundra vegetation)

No Vegetation

9. bare soil
10. perpetual ice

The biomes, which represent only the predominant vegetation in the 1° by 1° areas, are quantitatively defined by morphological, physical and physiological parameters (see Sellers et al., 1986). The vegetation morphology is given by the fractional areas of the surface independently covered by the canopy vegetation and ground cover; by the height of the canopy top and canopy bottom and the height of the ground cover; and by the root depths and root–length densities of the canopy vegetation and ground cover. All of these may vary from grid area to grid area of the numerical model; so that there can be a large variation within the same biome. At present, global numerical models of the atmosphere have grid areas of the order of $(100\ km)^2$ to $(500\ km)^2$.

In some regions of the world the natural biomes shown in Figure 3 have been substantially modified by man. In western Europe and the eastern United States, for example, something like 75% of the trees have been removed. When SiB is used for simulating and predicting contemporary weather and climate, therefore, the biomes shown in Figure 3 must be modified wherever contemporary land use has made a substantial modification of the natural vegetation.

The principal physiological parameter in SiB, the stomatal resistance to transpiration, is controlled mainly by the photosynthetically active radiation, the soil moisture and the leaf temperature (Sellers et al., 1986), which makes SiB physiologically interactive with the atmosphere on all time scales.

With respect to the morphological parameters, the leaf–area densities of most broadleaf trees and shrubs and almost all of the morphological parameters of the ground cover vary phenologically (i.e., they vary periodically and aperiodically on a seasonal and subseasonal time scale). For some purposes, such as diagnostic studies of the global hydrologic cycle and weather predictions on a short–time scale (7–10 days), the phenologically changing state of the vegetation morphology may be prescribed from observations: either observations of climatological normals or a time series of observations made with the help of satellite observations. But for other purposes, such as climate simulations (and, perhaps, climate predictions) on the time scale from weeks up to the order of 10^0 years, governing biophysical equations must be added that will make the phenologically changing parameters of the morphology interactive with the soil moisture, leaf temperature and photosynthetically active radiation. For example, instead of prescribing when the broadleaf trees and shrubs are "deciduous" (i.e., when their leaves "fall down"), that will be determined by the calculated soil moisture and leaf temperature and the amount of daylight.

For long–term climate simulations, of the order of 10^1 years and more, it will be necessary to add governing equations that will determine the distribution of the biomes themselves, which may not remain the same as that shown in fig. 3. For climate simulations on this long–time scale, there must also be an interactive model of the world ocean.

3. Governing equations for the ground cover

The forthcoming paper by Sellers et al. (1986) presents the full set of governing equations for the *S*imple *B*iosphere (SiB): equations for the absorption, transmission, reflection and emission of radiation by the vegetation canopy, ground cover and soil; equations for the precipitation interception, storage and interception loss by the leaves of the canopy and ground cover; equations for the infiltration, movement and storage of water in the soil; equations for the stomatal control over the transpiration of the soil moisture by the leaves of the canopy vegetation and ground cover; equations for the sensible heat transfer between the boundary–layer air and the canopy, ground cover and soil; and equations for the extraction of momentum from the boundary–layer air by the canopy, ground cover and soil.

Here, for the purpose of illustration, we present the governing equations when the ground cover is a continuous carpet on the soil and there is no canopy of trees or shrubs. With this very simple vegetation structure, the first subset of equations are

$$\lambda E_g = [e^*(T_g) - e_r] \frac{\rho c_p}{\gamma} \left[\frac{1 - W_g}{r_g + r_a} + \frac{W_g}{r_a} \right] \quad (1)$$

$$H_g = \frac{[T_g - T_r]}{r_a} \rho c_p \quad (2)$$

$$H_g + \lambda E_g = R_{n_g} - c_g \frac{\partial T_g}{\partial t} \quad (3)$$

$$R_{n_g} = S_a(1-\alpha) + R_{La} - \sigma T_g^4 \quad (4)$$

$$r_a = r_a[L_{d(z)}, u_r, (T_g - T_r)] \quad (5)$$

$$r_g = r_g[r_s, 0(\xi,\theta), S_a, \psi_{\ell g}, e_r, T_g, L_g] \quad (6)$$

E_g = evapotranspiration from the ground cover, kg m^{-2} s^{-1}

$e^*(T_g)$ = saturation vapor pressure at temperature T_g, mb

e_r = given vapor pressure at the reference height in the atmosphere, mb

W_g = fraction of the ground–cover leaves covered with water

r_g = bulk stomatal resistance of the ground cover, s m^{-1}

r_a = aerodynamic resistance between the ground cover and the reference height in the atmosphere, s m^{-1}

T_g = ground cover temperature, K

T_r = given air temperature at the reference height, K

H_g = sensible heat flux from the ground cover to the atmosphere, W m^{-2}

R_{n_g} = net radiation absorbed by the ground cover, W m^{-2}

c_g = heat capacity of the ground cover and soil, J m^{-2} K^{-1}

R_{La} = given longwave downward radiation from the atmosphere, W m^{-2}

S_a = given downward solar radiation, W m^{-2}

α = surface albedo

$L_{d(z)}$ = leaf area density as a function of height, m^2 m^{-3}

u_r = given wind speed at the reference height in the atmosphere, m s^{-1}

r_s = leaf stomatal resistance, s m^{-1}

$0(\xi,\theta)$ = leaf angle distribution function

ξ,θ = leaf azimuth angle and inclination angle

$\psi_{\ell g}$ = leaf–water potential, m

L_g = leaf–area index of the ground cover, m^2 m^{-2}

λ = latent heat of vaporization, J kg^{-1}

γ = psychrometric constant, mb K^{-1}

σ = Stefan–Boltzmann constant, W m^{-2} K^{-4}

Given e_r, T_r, u_r, S_a, and R_{La} as output from the numerical model of the atmosphere; W_g from the solution for the interception storage (as described below); and $\psi_{\ell g}$ from the solution for the moisture in the soil (as described below); the six equations provide the solution for the six unknowns: E_g, T_g, H_g, R_{n_g}, r_a and r_g.

As shown schematically in Figure 4, the transpiration, E_T, is the water that evaporates from the walls of the mesophyll cells that surround the substomatal cavities within the leaves of the plants and then diffuses to the atmosphere through the stomatal openings. The stomatal openings on the leaf surface, and hence the rate of transpiration, are under the active control of the plant. The function of the stomata is to regulate the influx of carbon dioxide (from atmosphere to the photosynthesizing structures within the leaf mesophyll) in such a way as to minimize the contemporaneous water loss

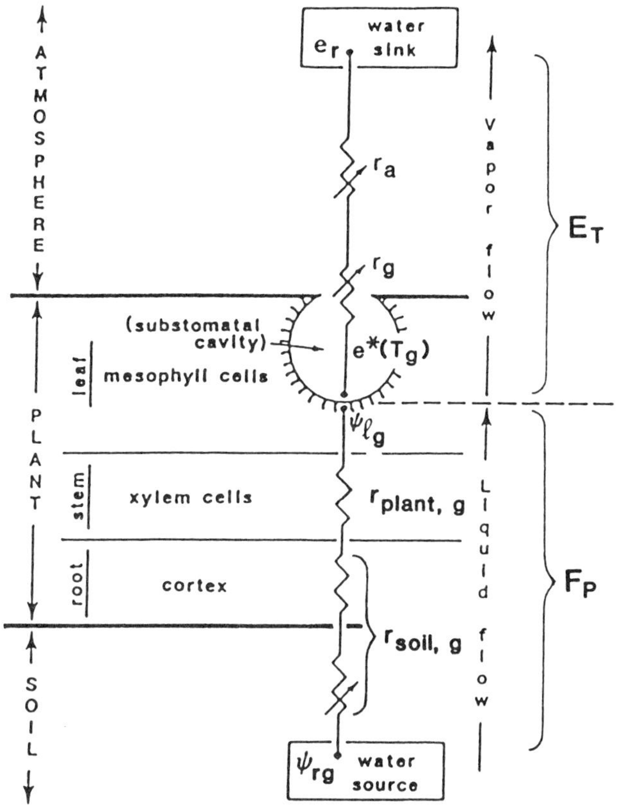

Fig. 4. Electrical analog representation of potentials and resistances, and of the flow of liquid water and water vapor through the soil, ground cover, atmosphere system. (For definitions of the symbols, see text.)

over the same route. Accordingly, the stomata close under nonphotosynthesizing conditions (low levels of shortwave radiation, extremes of temperature, etc.) in order to conserve moisture. Transpiration may therefore be regarded as the inevitable loss of moisture associated with maintaining an open gas-transfer pathway between the atmosphere and saturated leaf interior. The rate at which the water is transferred from its origin in the substomatal cavities to the free atmosphere is given by the "dry part" of equation (1), the part where $(1-W_g)$ is the numerator. The interception loss, E_I, which is independent of r_g, is given by the "wet part" of equation (1), (the part with W_g as the numerator). The vapor pressure within the leaf interior is taken as the saturation vapor pressure, e^*, given by the Clausius–Clapyron equation for the temperature of the leaf, T_g, which is assumed to be constant throughout the leaf (whose thickness is typically about 1 mm). The unknowns in (1) are E_g, T_g, r_a, r_g.

T_g is obtained from equation (2), the diffusion equation for the sensible heat transfer from the surface of the leaves, at temperature T_g, to the air at the reference level, at temperature T_r. It is assumed that r_a is the same for the diffusion of sensible heat and water vapor. Equation (2) adds the unknown, H_g.

The combined flux of sensible heat, H_g, and latent heat, λE_g, is obtained from the energy–conservation equation (3), where R_{n_g} is the net downward total radiation flux, and the second term on the right–hand side is the rate of heat storage in the ground cover and soil. The net radiation absorbed by the ground cover is calculated from (4), where S_a and R_{La} are the downward components of the solar and longwave radiation from the atmosphere, α is the calculated albedo of the ground cover, and σT_g^4 is the emitted longwave radiation.

The incident solar radiation, S_a, is divided into two spectral components: the visible, or photosynthetically active radiation (0.4–0.7μ) and the near infrared radiation (0.7–3.0μ). Each of these components is divided into a direct beam and a diffuse contribution. The fate of the incident radiation (the interception, scattering and absorption by the plant elements) is calculated separately for each spectral and angular component using a two stream approximation method (see Dickinson, 1983; Sellers, 1985). The sum of all the reflectances, weighted by the total incident solar radiation, yields the global shortwave surface albedo, α.

The aerodynamic resistance, r_a, depends on the vertical distribution of the leaf–area density, which determines the value of the zero–plane displacement height, d, and the roughness length, z_0; on the wind speed at the atmospheric reference level, u_r, and on the thermal stability of the air, (T_g-T_r), (for example, see Goudriaan, 1977). Typically, with wind speeds in the atmospheric boundary layer of a few meters per second and midday unstable lapse rates, r_a is of the order of 50 s m^{-1} for ground–cover vegetation (0.1 to 1 m high).

The bulk stomatal resistance, r_g, is given as the integrated value of the stomatal resistance of the individual leaves, r_s, summed over all the leaf orientations, $0(\xi,\theta)$, and irradiances within the ground cover. Typically, when the leaf–area index is about four, r_g is also of the order 50 s m^{-1} for ground–cover plants which are not under moisture stress.

The stomata close when there is no shortwave radiation, S_a; when the relative humidity of the air, $RH_a = RH[e_a,T_a]$, falls below a critical value; or when under extremes in leaf temperature, T_g. The stomata also begin to close when the water potential, $\psi_{\ell g}$, in the guard cells that surround the stomatal opening falls below a limiting value. (What controls the magnitude of $\psi_{\ell g}$ is discussed below.) When the stomata are closed, transpiration takes place only through the cuticle of the leaf, whose resistance to the water–vapor transfer is typically about two orders of magnitude larger than r_g (about 10^4 s m^{-1}, when L_g equals four).

Conservation of water mass requires that the water vapor which moves away from the cell walls of the substomatal cavities be replaced by a flow of liquid water toward the walls from the other side. If we neglect the small time rate of change of the water stored in the cells of the plants, we have $E_T = F_p$, where E_T is the rate of transpiration and F_p is the rate of liquid water flow through the plant.

$$E_T = F_p = \frac{(\psi_{rg} - \psi_{\ell g})}{(r_{\mathrm{soil}_g} + r_{\mathrm{plant}_g})} \cdot \rho_w \tag{7}$$

$$\psi_{rg} = \psi_s \left(\frac{\theta_{rg}}{\theta_s}\right)^{-B} \tag{8}$$

$$r_{\mathrm{soil}} = r_{\mathrm{soil}}[\theta, RT_D(z)] \tag{9}$$

E_T = transpiration from the ground cover, kg m^{-2} s^{-1}

F_P = flow of liquid water through soil–root–stem system of the ground cover, kg m^{-2} s^{-1}

ψ_{rg} = soil–moisture potential in the root zone, m

ρ_w = density of water, kg m^{-3}

r_{soil_g} = combined soil and root resistance, s

r_{plant_g} = plant xylem resistance, s

ψ_s = soil–moisture potential at saturation, m

θ_s = soil–moisture content at saturation, m^3 m^{-3}

B = soil–moisture potential parameter

θ_{rg} = soil–moisture content in root zone, $m^3\ m^{-3}$

$RT_D(z)$ = root–length density, $m\ m^{-3}$

From $F_P = E_T$, with E_T obtained from the solution of equations (1–6); and θ_{rg} obtained from the solution for the soil–water budget (as described below), these three equations provide the solution for the unknowns $\psi_{\ell g}$, ψ_{rg} and r_{soil_g}.

The transpiration rate may be reduced in response to a fall in $\psi_{\ell g}$, to which the stomatal guard cells are directly sensitive. Equations (1) and (6) show that the magnitude of $\psi_{\ell g}$ varies directly with the transpiration rate; (7) and (8) show that it varies inversely with the soil moisture in the root zone, θ_{rg}. Thus, the bulk stomatal resistance, r_g, increases with *either* an increase in the transpiration rate *or* a decrease in the soil–moisture content. The dynamics of the system ensures that the transpiration rate is limited to a maximum value, typically about 1.5mm per hour for a continuous ground cover, even when there is no soil–moisture stress.

The time rate of change of the water stored on the surface of the leaves of the continuous ground cover can be taken as

$$\frac{\partial M_g}{\partial t} = P - \frac{E_I}{\rho_w} \tag{10}$$

$$\lambda E_I = \frac{[e^*[T_g] - e_r}{r_a} \frac{\rho c_p}{\gamma} \cdot W_g \tag{11}$$

$$W_g = M_g/S_g\,, \qquad 0 \le W_g \le 1$$

M_g = water held on the ground–cover leaves, m

S_g = maximum value of M_g, m

P = precipitation rate, $m\ s^{-1}$

E_I = interception–loss rate, $kg\ m^{-2}\ s^{-1}$

The soil moisture is stored in three zones: a small near–surface store (from which not only root uptake but also direct evaporation can take place if the ground cover is not continuous); an intermediate soil–moisture store, which is drawn on mainly by the root uptake; and a deep store, from which only capillary rise can bring water toward the surface.

When the ground cover is continuous, the governing equations for the three soil–moisture stores are

$$\frac{\partial W_1}{\partial t} = \frac{1}{\theta_s D_1}\left(P_1 - Q_{1,2} - \frac{E_{T,1}}{\rho_w}\right) \tag{12}$$

$$\frac{\partial W_2}{\partial t} = \frac{1}{\theta_s D_2}\left(Q_{1,2} - Q_{2,3} - \frac{E_{T,2}}{\rho_w}\right) \tag{13}$$

$$\frac{\partial W_3}{\partial t} = \frac{1}{\theta_s D_3}(Q_{2,3} - Q_3) \tag{14}$$

W_i = wetness of soil in the ith layer

= θ_i/θ_s

θ_i = soil–moisture content of the ith layer, $m^3\ m^{-3}$

P_1 = infiltration of precipitation into upper soil moisture store, m s^{-1}

$Q_{i,i+1}$ = moisture flow between the i and the i+1 soil layers, m s^{-1}

D_i = depth of ith soil layer, m

Q_3 = drainage of water through the bottom of soil layer 3, m s^{-1}

P_1, the infiltration of precipitation into the upper soil–moisture store, is taken as the smaller of (K_s, P_0), and zero when $W_1 = 1$. K_s is the saturated hydraulic conductivity of the soil; $P_0 = (P - E_I - \partial M_g/\partial t)$, $P_0 > 0$, is the rate at which the water precipitated from the atmosphere drains through the ground cover and reaches the soil surface; D_i is the thickness of the ith layer. Typically, $D_1 \approx 5$ cm, $D_2 \approx 50$ cm (the typical root depth of ground cover), and $D_3 \approx 500$ cm. $Q_{i,i+1}$ is the transfer of water from the ith to the $i+1^{\text{th}}$ soil layer by hydraulic diffusion; and Q_3 is the gravitational drainage of water through the bottom of soil layer 3.

The water excess at the surface, $(P_0 - P_1)$, joins the gravitational drainage, Q_3, to produce the "runoff"

$$Q_r = (P_0 - P_1) + Q_3 \,. \tag{15}$$

For the transfer of soil moisture by hydraulic diffusion and gravitational drainage, we let

$$Q_{i,i+1} = \overline{K}\left[2\,\frac{\psi_i - \psi_{i+1}}{D_i + D_{i+1}} + 1\right], \quad i = 1,2 \tag{16}$$

$$\overline{K} = \frac{D_i K_i + D_{i+1} K_{i+1}}{D_i + D_{i+1}}$$

and

$$Q_3 = K_s W_3^{(2B+3)} \tag{17}$$

K_i = hydraulic conductivity of ith soil layer, m s^{-1}

K_i = $K_s W_i^{(2B+3)}$

K_s = saturation hydraulic conductivity of the soil, m s^{-1}

ψ_i = soil–moisture potential of ith soil layer, m

$\overline{K}$ = mean hydraulic conductivity for two adjacent soil layers, m s^{-1}

From the empirical relationship given by Clapp and Hornberger (1978), $\psi_i = \psi_s / W_i^B$ is the soil–moisture potential of the ith layer, where ψ_s is the soil–moisture potential at saturation and B is an empirical constant.

The rate of heat storage in the ground cover and the soil, G, which is required for the solution of (4), is estimated with a slab model, as

$$G = c_g \frac{\partial T_g}{\partial t} \tag{18}$$

where c_g is the heat capacity of the ground cover together with that part of the soil which participates in the diurnal temperature variation. Typically, c_g is of the order of 10^5 J m^{-2} K^{-1}.

In going from the soil–moisture store to the substomatal cavities of the plant leaves, the transpiration flux must traverse two resistances: the combined soil and root resistance, r_{soil_g}, and the xylem resistance, r_{plant_g}.

The soil and root resistance have been combined into a single term by Federer (1979), whereby

$$r_{\text{soil}} = (R/D_d + \alpha_f/K_r) 1/z_d \tag{19}$$

$$\alpha_f = \frac{1}{8\pi D_d} \left(V_r - 3 - 2 \ln\left[\frac{V_r}{1-V_r}\right]\right) \tag{20}$$

R = root resistance per unit length, s m^{-1}

D_d = root density, m m^{-3}

V_r = volume of root per unit volume of soil, m^3 m^{-3}

K_r = mean soil hydraulic conductivity in the root zone, m s^{-1}

z_d = root depth, m

The xylem resistance, r_{plant}, has been variously reported as constant or slightly dependent on environmental conditions in a number of studies. Its absolute value is of some importance when the soil is saturated and the transpiration rate high, but its relative importance declines as the soil dries out and r_{soil} increases.

The bulk stomatal resistance, r_g, is the integral of all the individual leaf stomatal resistances over all leaf orientations throughout the depth of the ground cover. The stomatal resistance of a single leaf is closely related to its photosynthetic function and thus its *inverse* (equivalent to a conductance) has a form close to a rectangular hyperbola. Thus

$$r_s = \left[\frac{a}{b+F\downarrow} + c\right] \cdot [f(\psi_{\ell g}) \cdot f(T_g) \cdot f(RH)]^{-1} \tag{21}$$

a,b,c = species dependent constants

$f(\psi_{\ell g}), f(T_g), f(RH)$ = adjustment factors for the effects of leaf–water potential, $\psi_{\ell g}$, leaf temperature, T_g, and relative humidity, RH.

$F\downarrow$ = incident photosynthetically active radiation (0.4–0.7μ), W m^{-2}

Equation (21) is derived from a similar expression proposed by Jarvis (1976). The form of the adjustment factors, which vary from 1 (optimal conditions) to 0 (conditions inimical to photosynthesis or liable to lead to excessive transpiration loss) have been expressed in a number of different ways by different researchers (see, for example, Jarvis (1976) or Federer (1979)). Generally speaking, low values of $\psi_{\ell g}$, extreme values of leaf temperature, T_g, and low values of the relative humidity lead to stomatal closure by lowering the respective adjustment factor towards zero.

Equation (21) describes the dependence of stomatal resistance upon environmental conditions for one leaf only. In order to obtain the bulk stomatal resistance, we must integrate this function for all the different photosynthetically active radiation (PAR) flux densities incident on all the leaves in the ground cover. This can be done quite easily for a number of leaf angle distributions provided that the PAR flux is assumed to decay down through the vegetation layer in a near exponential fashion. Thus,

$$\frac{1}{r_g} = \int_0^{L_g} \frac{1}{r_s}\, dL \tag{22}$$

L_g = leaf–area index of ground cover, m^2 m^{-2}

$$\frac{1}{r_g} = f(A) \cdot \int_0^{L_g} \int_0^{\pi/2} \int_0^{2\pi} \frac{0(\xi,\theta)}{r_s(F\downarrow,\xi,\theta)} \sin\theta \, d\xi \, d\theta \, dL \tag{23}$$

$0(\xi,\theta)$ = leaf angle distribution function

ξ,θ = leaf azimuth, inclination angles

$f(A)$ = $f(\psi_{\ell g}) \cdot f(T_g) \cdot f(RH)$

Solutions to the integral part of (23) are given in Sellers (1985). The factor $f(A)$ may be placed outside the integral because the leaf–water potential, leaf temperature and air relative humidity exhibit only small variations within the ground cover compared to the swift exponential extinction of PAR.

Finally, the ground–cover component of the surface wind stress (which is the only component in this simple case) is taken as

$$\boldsymbol{\tau}_g = \rho C_{D,g} u_r \cdot \mathbf{u}_r \tag{24}$$

$\boldsymbol{\tau}_g$ = vector wind stress on the ground cover, kg m^{-1} s^{-2}

ρ = air density, kg m^{-3}

$C_{D,g}$ = drag coefficient of the ground cover

$\mathbf{u}_r$ = given vector wind at the atmospheric reference level, m s^{-1}

u_r = magnitude of $\mathbf{u}_r$, m s^{-1}

To obtain the solution for the five prognostic variables (T_g, M_g, W_1, W_2, and W_3), we first calculate ΔT_g from

$$c_g \frac{\Delta T_g}{\Delta t} = R_{n_g} + \frac{\partial R_{n_g}}{\partial T_g} \Delta T_g - H_g - \frac{\partial H_g}{\partial T_g} \Delta T_g - \lambda E_g - \frac{\partial \lambda E_g}{\partial T_g} \Delta T_g \tag{25}$$

and add this ΔT_g to the initial value of T_g at time t_0 to obtain T_g at $(t_0 + \Delta t)$.

T_g at $(t_0 + \Delta t)$, together with the calculated value of P_1 at time t_0, are then used in the finite–difference equivalents of equations (10) through (15) to obtain the changes in M_g, W_1, W_2 and W_3 over the time step Δt.

In summary, from

(i) the initial state of the five prognostic variables T_g, M_g, W_1, W_2 and W_3;

(ii) the boundary conditions T_r, e_r, u_r, $F_{\Lambda,\mu(0)}$ (the spectral and angular components of S_a and R_{La}), and P;

(iii) the given morphological, physiological and physical properties of the ground cover and soil, we calculate

(i) the net fluxes of energy, water mass and momentum across the lower boundary of the atmosphere, in the form of: radiation (R_{n_g}), sensible heat (H_g), interception loss ($E_{I,g}$), transpiration ($E_{T,g}$), and vector wind stress (τ_g) ; and

(ii) the time rate of change and future state of the five prognostic ground cover and soil variables: T_g, M_g, W_1, W_2, W_3, in preparation for the next time step.

4. The complete structure of SiB

Figure 5, from Sellers et al. (1986), shows the complete structure of the *Si*mple *B*iosphere (SiB). The addition of the canopy layer (of trees or shrubs) adds two additional prognostic variables, T_c and M_c, corresponding to T_g and M_g; and the solution requires additional governing equations. There is a second flux of water vapor, E_c, consisting of interception loss and transpiration from the canopy; and, when bare soil is exposed between the ground–cover plants, a third flux of water vapor, E_s, which is a direct evapor–ation from the pores of the uppermost layer of the soil. It is assumed that the exposed soil and the evenly spaced ground–cover plants have the same temper–ature T_{gs}, and this controls the sensible heat flux, H_{gs}. The other sensible heat flux, H_c, is from the canopy. Also calculated are R_{n_c}, the net radiation absorbed by the canopy, and τ_c, the horizontal momentum that the canopy extracts from the air.

Acknowledgements

The authors thank Drs. Robert Dickinson, Thomas Schmugge, Yogesh Sud and Cort Willmott for their interest and suggestions, and Jeffrey Dorman and Gregory Walker for technical assistance.

The research was supported by grants to the University of Maryland from the U.S. National Science Foundation and the U.S. National Aeronautics and Space Administration.

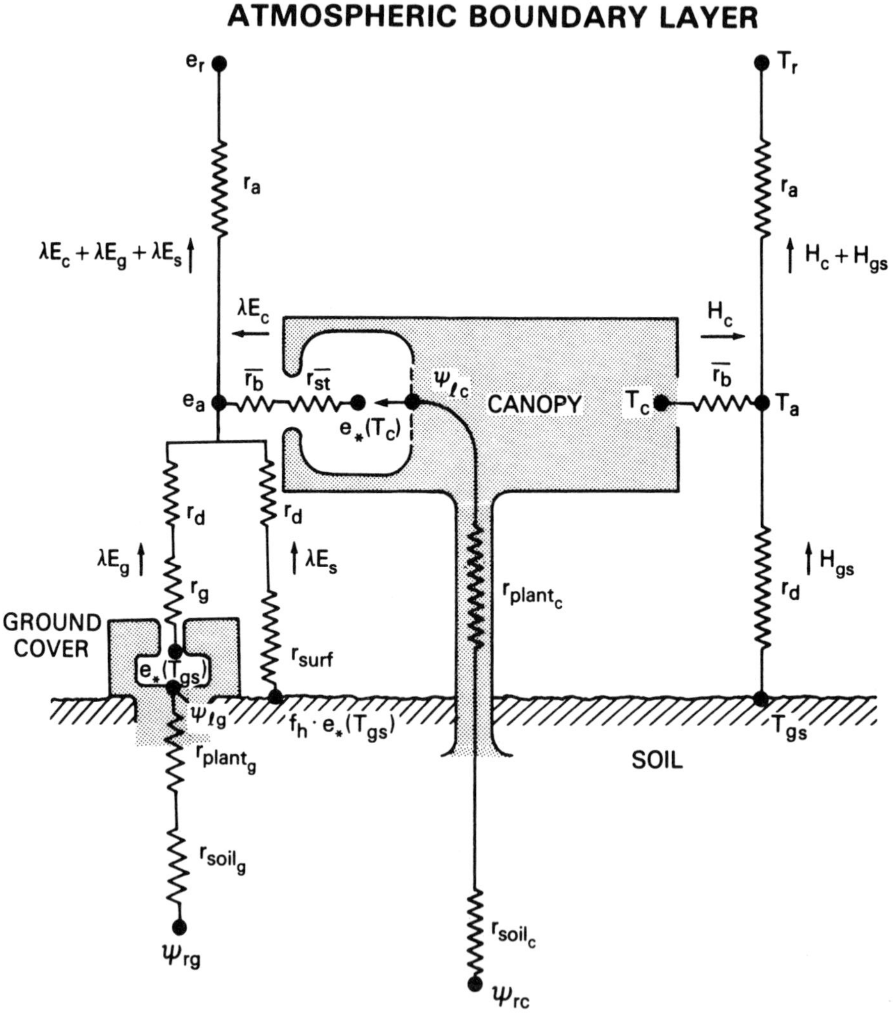

Fig. 5. The Simple Biosphere (SiB) when it has a canopy of trees or shrubs, ground cover and bare soil. (From Sellers, et al., 1985.)

REFERENCES

Calder, I.R., Newson, M.D. 1979. Land use and upland water resources in Britain–a strategic look. *Water Resources Bull.*, American Water Resources Assoc. 15:1628–39.

Charney, J.G., Quirk, W.J., Chow, S.H., and Kornefield, J. 1977. A comparative study of the effects of albedo change on drought in semi–arid regions. *J. Atmosph. Sci.* 34:1366–85.

Clapp, R.B., and Hornberger, G.M. 1978. Empirical equations for some soil hydraulic properties. *Water Resources Research* 14, no. 4:601–604.

Dickinson, R.E. 1983. Land surface processes and climate– surface albedoes and energy balance. *Advances in Geophysics* 25:305–53.

Federer, C.A. 1979. A soil–plant–atmosphere model for transpiration and availability of soil water. *Water Resources Res.* 15, no. 3:555–62.

Goudriaan, J. 1977. *Crop Micrometeorology: A Simulation Study.* Wageningen, Holland: Wageningen Center for Agricultural Publishing and Documentation.

Jarvis, P.G. 1976. The interpretation of the variations in leaf water potential and stomatal conductance found in canopies in the field. *Phil. Trans. Roy. Soc. London*, Ser. B, 273:593–610.

Küchler, A.W. 1983. World Map of Natural Vegetation. Scale 1:75,000,000. In *Goode's World Atlas*, 16–17. 16th ed. New York: Rand McNally. (Also available as a wall map. Scale 1:30,000,000.)

Küchler, A.W. 1949. A physiognomic classification of vegetation. *Ann. Assoc. Amer. Geogr.* 39:201–10.

Mintz, Y. 1984. The sensitivity of numerically simulated climates to land–surface boundary conditions. In *The Global Climate*, 75–105, ed. J. Houghton. Cambridge London New York: Cambridge University Press.

Rowntree, P.R. 1985. Review of general circulation models as a basis for predicting the effects of vegetation change on climate. *The Proceedings of the United Nations University Workshop on Forests, Climate, and Hydrology*, Oxford.

Sellers, P.J. 1985. Canopy reflectance, photosynthesis and transpiration. Intern. *J. Remote Sensing* 6, no.8. In press.

Sellers, P.J., Mintz, Y., and Sud, Y.C. 1985. A simple biosphere model (SiB) for use with numerical models of the atmosphere. Submitted to the *J. Atmosph. Sci.*

Shuttleworth, W.J., and Calder, I.R. 1979. Has the Priestly–Taylor equation any relevance to forest evaporation? *J. Appl. Meteorology* 18:639–46.

Sud, Y., Shukla, C.J., and Mintz, Y. 1985. Influence of land surface roughness on atmospheric circulation and rainfall: a sensitivity study with a general circulation model. Submitted to the *J. Atmosp. Sci.*

Walker, J.M., and Rowntree, P.R. 1977. The effect of soil moisture on circulation and rainfall in a tropical model. *Q. J. Roy. Met. Soc.* 103:29–46.

LARGE–SCALE OCEAN CIRCULATION MODELLING

A.S. Sarkisyan

Department of Numerical Mathematics
The USSR Academy of Sciences
Moscow, USSR

The current theoretical methods for ocean investigation can be divided into two categories. The first one we shall call the classical theory of ocean circulation. The essence of this approach is the following: we state a problem on determining all the internal ocean characteristics, proceeding from a certain closed system of ocean thermohydrodynamics equations and the sea surface boundary conditions. To illustrate this direction in some detail, we proceed from the following simplified system of the ocean thermohydrodynamics equations.

Equations of motion:

$$\frac{\partial u}{\partial t} + u\frac{\partial u}{\partial x} + v\frac{\partial u}{\partial y} + w\frac{\partial u}{\partial z} - \ell v$$

$$= -\frac{1}{\rho_0}\frac{\partial P_1}{\partial x} + \frac{\partial}{\partial z}\nu\frac{\partial u}{\partial z} + \frac{\partial}{\partial x}A_\ell\frac{\partial u}{\partial x} + \frac{\partial}{\partial y}A_\ell\frac{\partial u}{\partial y}\,; \qquad (1)$$

$$\frac{\partial v}{\partial t} + u\frac{\partial v}{\partial x} + v\frac{\partial v}{\partial y} + w\frac{\partial v}{\partial z} + \ell u$$

$$= -\frac{1}{\rho_0}\frac{\partial P_1}{\partial x} + \frac{\partial}{\partial z}\nu\frac{\partial u}{\partial z} + \frac{\partial}{\partial x}A_\ell\frac{\partial v}{\partial x} + \frac{\partial}{\partial y}A_\ell\frac{\partial v}{\partial y}\,. \qquad (2)$$

Equations of statics:

$$\frac{\partial P_1}{\partial z} = \rho_1 g\,. \qquad (3)$$

The continuity equation of incompressible liquid:

$$\frac{\partial u}{\partial x} + \frac{\partial v}{\partial y} + \frac{\partial w}{\partial z} = 0 . \tag{4}$$

Equation of heat and salt transfer:

$$\frac{\partial T}{\partial t} + u\frac{\partial T}{\partial x} + v\frac{\partial T}{\partial y} + w\frac{\partial T}{\partial z}$$

$$= \frac{\partial}{\partial z}\mathcal{K}_T\frac{\partial T}{\partial z} + \frac{\partial}{\partial x}A_T\frac{\partial T}{\partial x} + \frac{\partial}{\partial y}A_T\frac{\partial T}{\partial y} ; \tag{5}$$

$$\frac{\partial S}{\partial t} + u\frac{\partial S}{\partial x} + v\frac{\partial S}{\partial y} + w\frac{\partial S}{\partial z}$$

$$= \frac{\partial}{\partial z}\mathcal{K}_T\frac{\partial S}{\partial z} + \frac{\partial}{\partial x}A_S\frac{\partial S}{\partial x} + \frac{\partial}{\partial y}A_S\frac{\partial S}{\partial y} . \tag{6}$$

Equation of state:

$$\rho = a_{1_k}T + a_{2_k}S + a_{3_k}T^2 + a_{4_k}TS + a_{5_k}S^2 + a_{6_k}T^3 + \cdots . \tag{7}$$

The system of equations (1)–(7) contains seven unknown functions: flow velocity components u, v, w along the axes O_x, O_y, O_z; pressure p_0; density $\rho_1 = \rho + \rho_0$; temperature T, and salinity S. When solving any problem on nonstationary circulation, it is sufficient to have the initial values of only four functions u, v, T, S, from which the other three initial fields are determined.

The boundary conditions in the vertical direction are the following.

At sea surface, at $z = -\zeta_1(x,y,t)$:

$$p_1 = p_a , \tag{8}$$

$$\rho_0\, \nu\frac{\partial u}{\partial z} = -\tau_x, \quad \rho_0\, \nu\frac{\partial v}{\partial z} = -\tau_y , \tag{9}$$

$$w = -\left(\frac{\partial \zeta_1}{\partial t} + u\frac{\partial \zeta_1}{\partial x} + v\frac{\partial \zeta_1}{\partial y}\right) , \tag{10}$$

$$\frac{\partial T}{\partial z} = Q , \tag{11}$$

or

$$T = T(x,y,t) , \tag{12}$$

$$\frac{\partial S}{\partial z} = Q_1 , \tag{13}$$

or

$$S = S(x,y,t) . \tag{14}$$

At the bottom, at $z = H(x,y)$, we assume the non–slip conditions

$$u = v = w = 0 \tag{15}$$

or free–slip conditions

$$\frac{\partial u}{\partial n} = \frac{\partial v}{\partial n} = 0\,, \tag{16}$$

$$w = u_H \frac{\partial H}{\partial x} + v_H \frac{\partial H}{\partial y}\,. \tag{17}$$

The conditions for temperature and salinity

$$\frac{\partial T}{\partial n} = \frac{\partial S}{\partial n} = 0 \tag{18}$$

or

$$T = T_H; \qquad S = S_H\,, \tag{19}$$

where n is a normal to the sea bottom surface. For the sake of generality, two versions of some of the boundary conditions are given, each version for a specific problem.

Now, let us consider the boundary conditions in the horizontal direction. The lateral boundaries of the basin are assumed to be vertical. u and v, as the functions of coordinates and time, are specified on the liquid part of the lateral boundaries. On the solid boundaries we assume the non–slip or free–slip conditions. However, we will solve sequential problems taking into account the lateral exchange; in this case it is sufficient to specify the velocity component normal to the boundary. In investigating the large–scale and middle–scale currents, the vertically average velocity value is often specified. This "softened" boundary condition causes the distortion of the coastal current fields, but apparently its effect is marginal in off–shore regions. In the horizontal plane the boundary is usually approximated by a broken line, every link of which is parallel to one of the coordinates. Thus, for u and v in this case, the boundary conditions are the following:

$$\frac{1}{H}\int_0^H u\,dz = U_1\,,$$
$$\frac{1}{H}\int_0^H v\,dz = V_1\,. \tag{20}$$

At the solid part of the boundary and at the island contours $U_1 = V_1 = 0$. For temperature and salinity at the lateral boundaries we assume:

$$\frac{\partial T}{\partial N} = Q'\,; \qquad \frac{\partial S}{\partial N} = Q_1' \tag{21}$$

or

$$T = T_b\,; \qquad S = S_b, \tag{22}$$

where N is a normal to the lateral boundary. At the solid lateral boundary $Q' = Q_1' = 0$.

The above equations and boundary conditions can provide the basis for solving any problem on concerning sea–current dynamics. However, this is rarely feasible since we deal with complicated systems of nonlinear equations, which are difficult to solve even on a high–speed computer. Therefore, one should, naturally, try to simplify these equations without essential loss of accuracy.

Let us first transform the static equation (3). To this end, let us integrate it in the vertical direction from ζ_1 to z, taking into account the boundary condition (8):

$$P_1 = P_a + g\int_{-\zeta_1}^{z} \rho_1\, dz = P_a + g\int_{-\zeta_1}^{0} \rho_1\, dz + g\int_0^z \rho_1\, dz$$

$$\approx P_a + g\int_{-\zeta_1}^{0} \rho_0\, dz + g\int_0^z (\rho_0 + \rho)\, dz$$

$$= P_a + \rho_0 g\zeta_1 + \rho_0 g z + g\int_0^z \rho\, dz .$$

Excluding the hydrostatic pressure of a homogeneous liquid column, we obtain the following relation for pressure anomaly:

$$p = p_a + \rho_0 g\zeta_1 + g\int_0^z \rho\, dz . \tag{23}$$

It is more convenient to use a conventional sea–surface topography elevation:

$$\zeta = \zeta_1 + \frac{P_a}{\rho_0 g} . \tag{24}$$

Thus, equation (3) and the boundary condition (8) are transformed to the simple formula for pressure anomaly:

$$p = \rho_0 g\zeta + g\int_0^z \rho\, dz . \tag{25}$$

It is also easy to show that for practically all problems of large–scale sea and ocean circulation (and even for large lakes) the boundary condition (10) can be replaced by the condition $w = 0$ at $z = 0$. Furthermore, using equation (4) and boundary conditions for w yields

$$\frac{\partial S_x}{\partial x} + \frac{\partial S_y}{\partial y} = 0 , \tag{26}$$

where $S_x = \int_0^H u\, dz$, $S_y = \int_0^H v\, dz$.

Using (26), we introduce the total mass flux stream function:

$$S_x = -\frac{\partial \psi}{\partial y}, \quad S_y = \frac{\partial \psi}{\partial x} . \tag{27}$$

Thus, instead of a pressure field we can introduce one of the two functions: ζ or ψ.

These transformations and simplifications are cited, for instance, in [29], but we will write the equations in complete form.

The equation for sea–surface topography:

$$- A_\ell \, \Delta\zeta + \frac{\partial}{\partial t}\Delta\zeta + \frac{g}{\ell}\mathcal{J}(\zeta,\Delta\zeta) + \frac{\ell}{2\alpha H}\Delta\zeta + \frac{\ell}{H}\mathcal{J}(H,\zeta) + \beta\frac{\partial\zeta}{\partial x}$$

$$= \frac{\ell}{\rho_0 g H}\,\mathrm{rot}\,\tau + \frac{1}{\rho_0 g H}\,[\beta\tau_x + \frac{\partial}{\partial t}\mathrm{div}\,\tau] + f_1 \,, \tag{28}$$

where

$$f_1 = \frac{1}{H}\left(\frac{g}{\rho_0\ell}\right)^2 \mathcal{J}\left(\int_0^H (H-z)\,\rho\,dz\,,\int_0^H (H-z)\Delta\rho\,dz\right)$$

$$- \frac{g}{\rho_0\ell H}\int_0^H (H-z)\,\mathcal{J}(\zeta,\Delta\rho)\,dz - \frac{1}{\rho_0 H}\int_0^H (H-z)\,\frac{\partial}{\partial t}\Delta\rho\,dz$$

$$- \frac{g}{\rho_0^2\ell H}\int_0^H \mathcal{J}\left(\int_0^z \rho\,dz,\int_0^z \Delta\rho\,dz\right)dz - \frac{\rho}{2\alpha\rho_0 H}\int_0^H \Delta\rho\,dz$$

$$- \frac{\rho}{\rho_0 H}\int_0^H \mathcal{J}(H,\rho)\,dz - \frac{\beta}{\rho_0 H}\int_0^H (H-z)\,\frac{\partial\rho}{\partial x}\,dz\,. \tag{29}$$

The equation for the total mass flux stream function:

$$- A_\ell\Delta\Delta\psi + \frac{\partial}{\partial t}\Delta\psi + \frac{1}{H}\mathcal{J}(\psi,\Delta\psi) + \frac{\rho}{2\alpha H}\Delta\psi + \frac{\ell}{H}\mathcal{J}(H,\psi) + \beta\frac{\partial\psi}{\partial x}$$

$$= \frac{1}{\rho_0}\,\mathrm{rot}\,\tau + \frac{1}{\rho_0 H}\left(\frac{\partial H}{\partial y}\mathcal{T}_x - \frac{\partial H}{\partial x}\mathcal{T}_y\right) + f_2 \,, \tag{30}$$

where

$$f_2 = \frac{1}{H}\left(\frac{g}{\rho_0\ell}\right)^2 \mathcal{J}\left(\int_0^H (H-z)\rho\,dz,\int_0^H (H-z)\Delta\rho\,dz\right)$$

$$- \left(\frac{g}{\rho_0\ell}\right)^2 \int_0^H \mathcal{J}\left(\int_0^z \rho\,dz,\int_0^z \Delta\rho\,dz\right)dz$$

$$- \frac{g}{2\alpha\rho_0 H}\int_0^H z\Delta\rho\,dz - \frac{g}{\rho_0 H}\int_0^H z\,\mathcal{J}(H,\rho)\,dz\,. \tag{31}$$

The classical theory of ocean circulation and other ocean characteristics has been treated in Bryan [2], Cox [3], Han and Gates [6], Haney [7], O'Brien et al. [24], Semter and Holland [36], Veronis [38], etc. A significant contribution in the research in this area belongs to Academician G.I. Marchuk and his associates [11]–[22].

There are two groups of publications in this field. The first group includes works of Marchuk himself [11]–[15] and many articles he wrote jointly with his associates [16]–[19], [22], [23], and works of other authors—all characterized by high mathematical accuracy: proofs of uniqueness and existence of solutions, stability of integrals, high–order approximations, as an example.

The second group of publications includes, among others, works of Academician Marchuk's associates—his students (some of them written jointly with Gurij Ivanovich) [20], [21], [28], [29], [35]; they deal with the modelling of geophysical characteristics of ocean systems.

This classification is, however, arbitrary and inessential—all of the works are complementary and of equal interest.

The research done by G.I. Marchuk and his associates, on the physical and mathematical problems of modelling hydrological characteristics of the world ocean provided the answer to the question as to which of the factors are essential and which are not in a system of equations and boundary conditions; we now better understand the role of the sea water nonhomogeneity and geometry of the world ocean and the necessity of most accurate calculation of the vertical velocity component, and are able to determine the climatic characteristics of the world ocean.

Let us briefly discuss some of the disadvantages of the classical approach of investigation of the world ocean. The latest research shows that to take into account the jet–like currents, upwelling zones, synoptic scale eddies, and large variability of currents, one needs to solve finite–difference equations in space and time with higher resolution than the available computers are capable of. The parametrization problem of subgrid processes has not been solved yet, either. Furthermore, the calculations have been made roughly with rough parametrization of turbulence, with overestimated computational or turbulent viscosity. For these and other reasons all of the computational results under the classical approach are too smoothed in time and space. Researchers in many countries are now working to improve the existing and develop new models and computational methods.

The objective of the diagnosis of the ocean dynamics consists in optimal application of the observed data in modelling the ocean thermo–hydrodynamics. The theoretical foundation of this approach was laid early this century and concerned the dynamics method of determining the current [4], [27]. Studying the diagnostic observations of the current (see the bibliography in [29]) was the first step in this direction, as illustrated in figure 1. Stommel's beta–spiral method may be viewed as a diagnostic method, too [37].

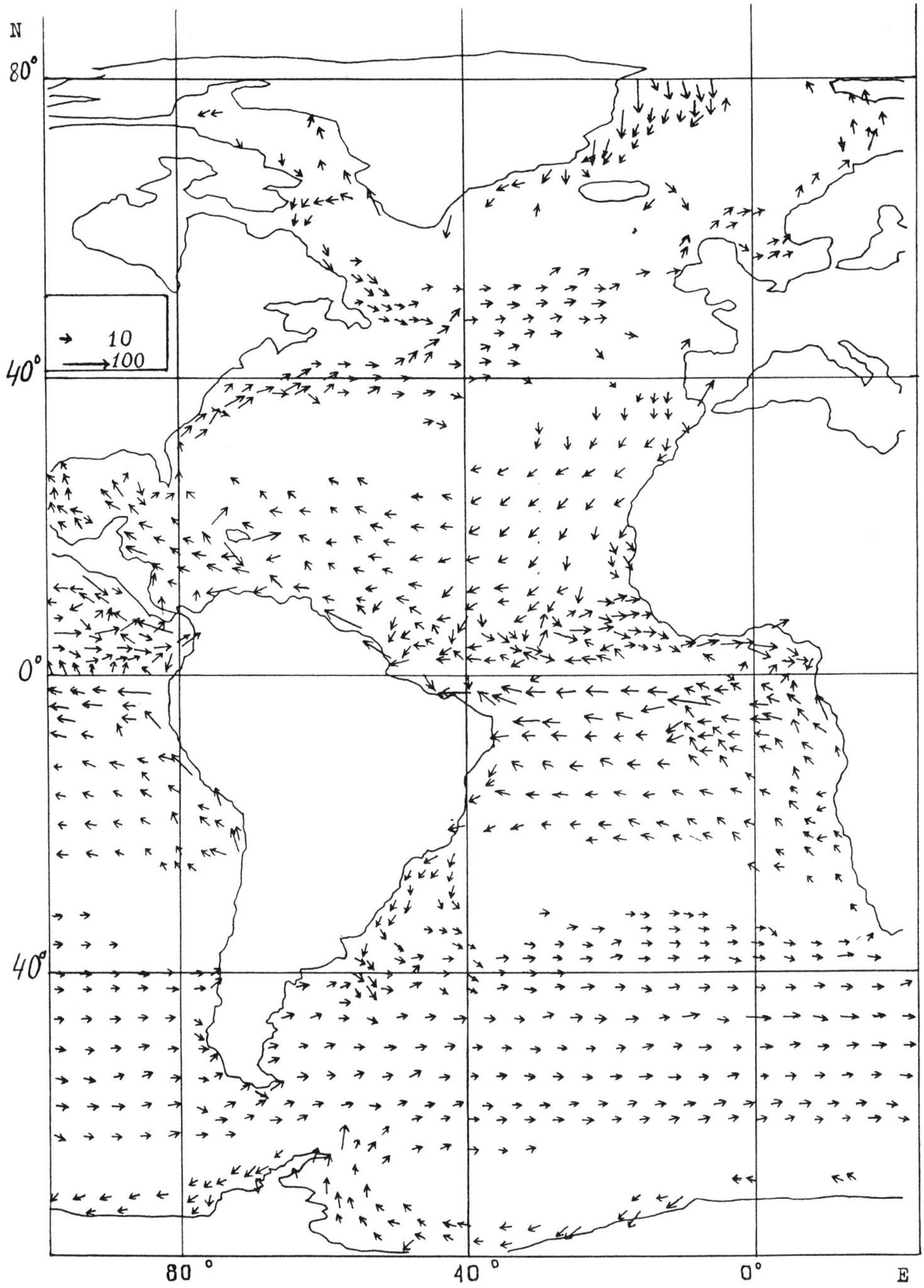

Fig. 1. Surface currents of the Atlantic Ocean in the summer

The so–called semi–diagnostic, or adaptational, calculations is the second step. They are used in applying the observational data to the model equations, boundary conditions, space–time scale of the process considered and to the basin geometry. The theory of the adaptational calculations of oceanic currents and its first practical application are presented in [30], [31]. Figures 2–4 illustrate the process of temperature field adaptation.

Next we will discuss in more detail another, essential step in developing the method of the ocean dynamics diagnosis, that is the dynamic–stochastic method of four–dimensional analysis of the ocean thermohydrodynamic characteristics.

This approach is based on the Kalman–Bucy theory of optimal filtering [8], and was first applied to systems with distributed parameters by Balakrishnan and Lions [1]. Later, the optimal filter equations for measurements of different types were obtained [10], [25], [26]. In the case when measurements are made discretely both in time and space—which is of great significance for oceanology—optimal estimation procedure involves two stages: prediction and analysis.

The prediction stage is between the observations of the internal ocean characteristics (state vector)

$$\mathbf{U}(\mathbf{x},t) = \|u(\mathbf{x},t),\ v(\mathbf{x},t),\ \rho(\mathbf{x},t),\ \zeta(x,y,t)\|^{\mathrm{T}},\quad \mathbf{x} = (x,y,z) \tag{32}$$

and of the correlation function of the state vector estimation error. The prediction for the state vector is made e.g. using equations (1), (2), (4)–(7), (25), (28) with the corresponding boundary and initial conditions, or by a simpler system of equations. The form of prediction equation for the correlation function of the state vector estimation error is given by the form of the hydrodynamic model used.

The analysis is made upon the arrival of the observations $t = t_1$ and is the optimal interpolation of prediction errors and the optimal correction of the correlation function of the state vector estimation error. In the sequel we will use the field ρ instead of T, S, for the sake of brevity. At the moment $t = t_1$ of a measurement data acquisition the optimal estimates are given by the following relations:

$$\mathbf{U}(\mathbf{x},t_1^+) = \mathbf{U}(\mathbf{x},t_1^-) + A(\mathbf{x},t_1^-)\delta\mathbf{U}(\mathbf{x}_r,t_1^+)\ , \tag{33}$$

where (function arguments are omitted for brevity)

$$A = \left\|\begin{vmatrix} \Delta^{1u} & \Delta^{1v} & \Delta^{1\rho} & \Delta^{1\zeta} \\ \Delta^{2u} & \Delta^{2v} & \Delta^{2\rho} & \Delta^{2\zeta} \\ \Delta^{3u} & \Delta^{3v} & \Delta^{3\rho} & \Delta^{3\zeta} \\ \Delta^{4u} & \Delta^{4v} & \Delta^{4\rho} & \Delta^{4\zeta} \end{vmatrix}\right\|$$

$$\mathbf{U}(\mathbf{x}_r,t_1^+) = \mathbf{Z}(\mathbf{x}_r,t_1) - \mathbf{U}(\mathbf{x}_r,t^-)\ . \tag{34}$$

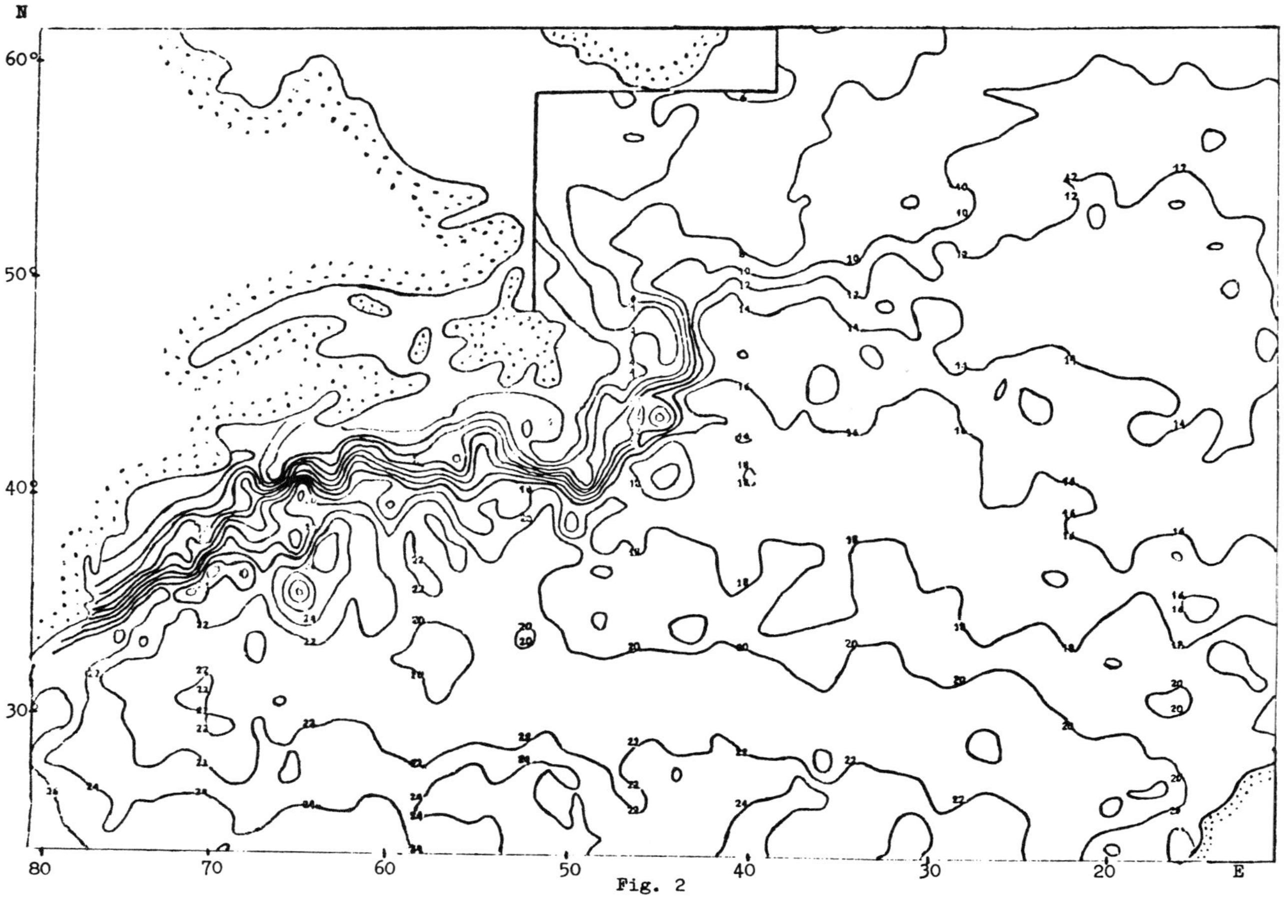

Fig. 2

Fig. 2. Climatic temperature field in the north Atlantic at z = 50 m. in the summer

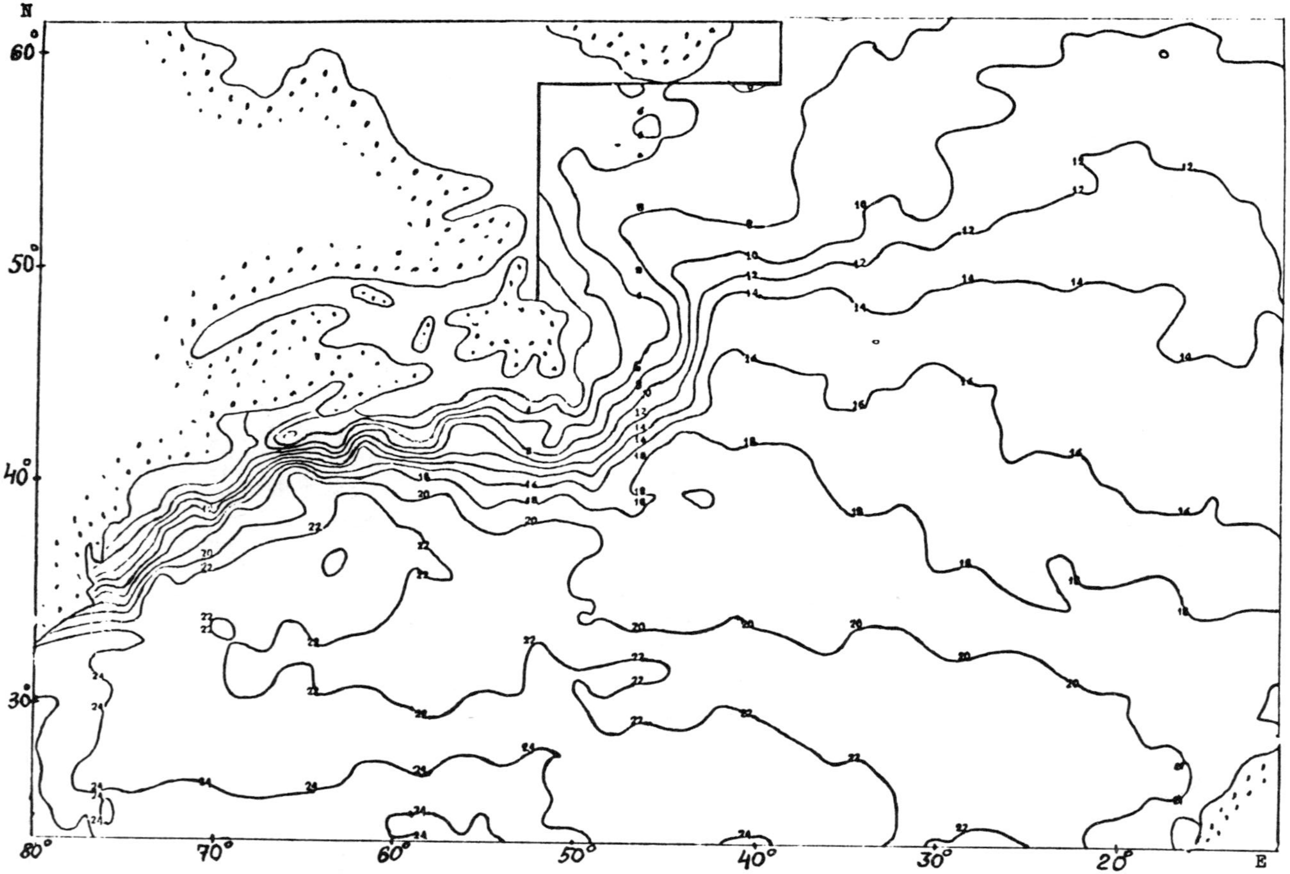

Fig. 3. The same as in fig. 2, but after 10 model days of adaptation

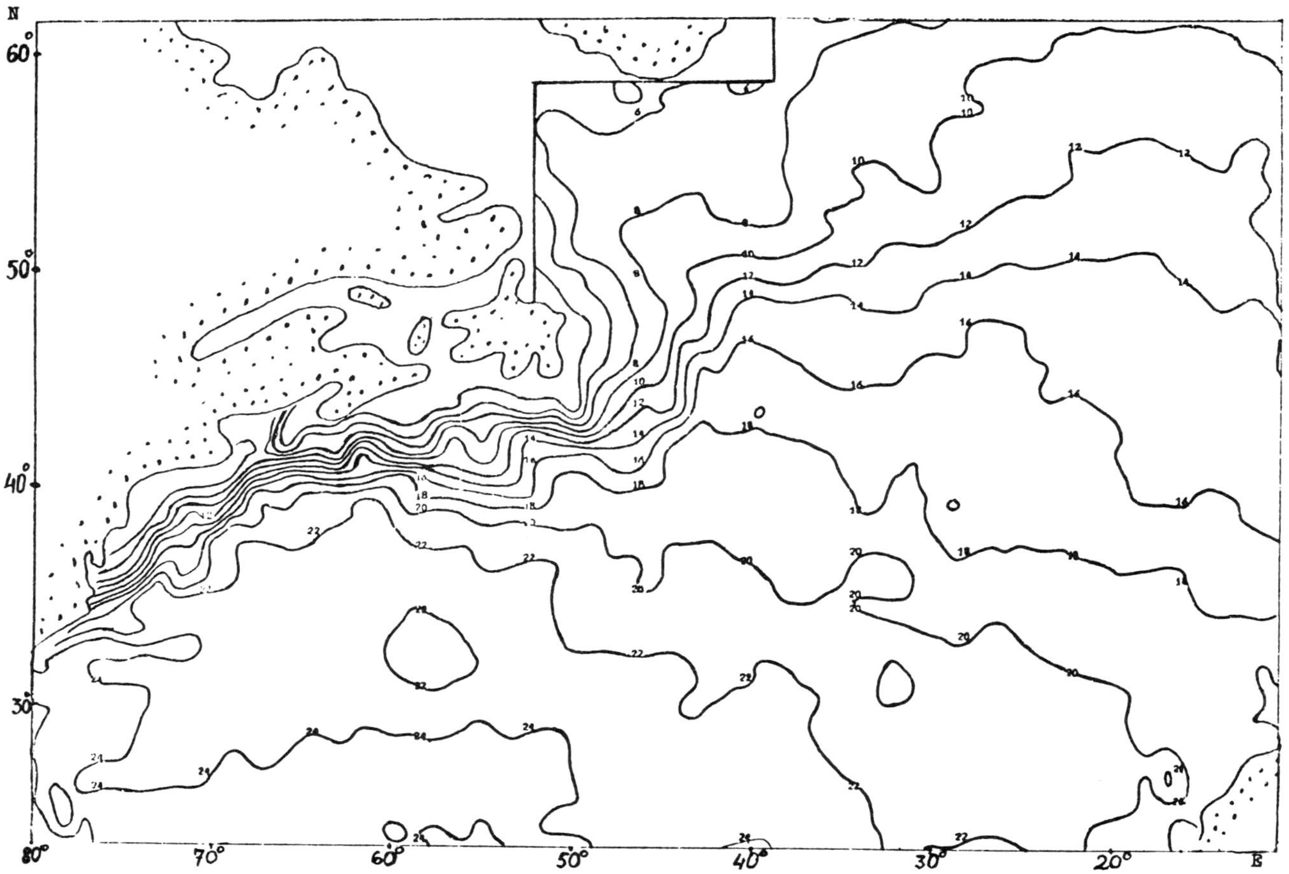

Fig. 4. The same as in fig. 2, but after 45 model days of adaptation

Here $\mathbf{x} = (x,y,z)$; the superscript "–" means that the corresponding functions are calculated disregarding the measurement data acquired at this time; $r = 1,...,N$ are the points of an area where observation data exist at time t_1; $\mathbf{Z}(\mathbf{x}_r,t_1)$ is the state vector of measurements. Δ_r^{iu}, Δ_r^{iv}, $\Delta_r^{i\rho}$, $\Delta_r^{i\zeta}$ are the weight factors calculated by the relations

$(i = 1,...,4;\ r = 1,...,N;\ p = 1,...,N)$:

$$\begin{aligned}
\Delta^{1u}(\mathbf{x},t_{\bar 1}) &= \| P(\mathbf{x}_r,\mathbf{x}_p,t_{\bar 1}) + R(\mathbf{x}_r,\mathbf{x}_p,t_1) \|^{-1} \cdot P_{uu}(\mathbf{x},\mathbf{x}_p,t_{\bar 1}) \,, \\
\Delta^{2u}(\mathbf{x},t_{\bar 1}) &= \| P(\mathbf{x}_r,\mathbf{x}_p,t_{\bar 1}) + R(\mathbf{x}_r,\mathbf{x}_p,t_1) \|^{-1} \cdot P_{vu}(\mathbf{x},\mathbf{x}_p,t_{\bar 1}) \,, \\
\Delta^{3u}(\mathbf{x},t_{\bar 1}) &= \| P(\mathbf{x}_r,\mathbf{x}_p,t_{\bar 1}) + R(\mathbf{x}_r,\mathbf{x}_p,t_1) \|^{-1} \cdot P_{\rho u}(\mathbf{x},\mathbf{x}_p,t_{\bar 1}) \,, \\
\Delta^{4u}(\mathbf{x},t_{\bar 1}) &= \| P(\mathbf{x}_r,\mathbf{x}_p,t_{\bar 1}) + R(\mathbf{x}_r,\mathbf{x}_p,t_1) \|^{-1} \cdot P_{\zeta u}(\mathbf{x},\mathbf{x}_p,t_{\bar 1}) \,,
\end{aligned} \tag{35}$$

where $R(\mathbf{x}_r,\mathbf{x}_p,t_{\bar 1})$ is the covariance error matrix for measurements of state vector (32). Let

$$\begin{aligned}
\Delta^{iu}(\mathbf{x},t_{\bar 1}) &= \| \Delta^{iu}(\mathbf{x},t_{\bar 1})\Delta^{iv}(\mathbf{x},t_{\bar 1})\Delta^{i\rho}(\mathbf{x},t_{\bar 1})\Delta^{i\zeta}(\mathbf{x},t_{\bar 1}) \|^{\mathrm{T}} \,, \\
P_{uu}(x,x_p,t_{\bar 1}) &= \| P_{uu}(\mathbf{x},\mathbf{x}_p,t_{\bar 1})P_{uv}(\mathbf{x},\mathbf{x}_p,t_{\bar 1})P_{u\rho}(\mathbf{x},\mathbf{x}_p,t_{\bar 1})P_{u\zeta}(\mathbf{x},\mathbf{x}_p,t_{\bar 1}) \|^{\mathrm{T}} \,.
\end{aligned} \tag{36}$$

The expressions for P_{vu}, $P_{\rho u}$, $P_{\zeta u}$ have similar forms. The estimate error covariance matrix $P(\mathbf{x}_r,\mathbf{x}_p,t_{\bar x})$ in the general case is of the form

$$P(x_r,x_p,t_{\bar 1}) = \begin{matrix}
P_{uu}(\mathbf{x}_r,\mathbf{x}_p,t_{\bar 1})P_{uv}(\mathbf{x}_r,\mathbf{x}_p,t_{\bar 1})P_{u\rho}(\mathbf{x}_r,\mathbf{x}_p,t_{\bar 1})P_{u\zeta}(\mathbf{x}_r,\mathbf{x}_p,t_{\bar 1}) \\
P_{vu}(\mathbf{x}_r,\mathbf{x}_p,t_{\bar 1})P_{vv}(\mathbf{x}_r,\mathbf{x}_p,t_{\bar 1})P_{v\rho}(\mathbf{x}_r,\mathbf{x}_p,t_{\bar 1})P_{v\zeta}(\mathbf{x}_r,\mathbf{x}_p,t_{\bar 1}) \\
P_{\rho u}(\mathbf{x}_r,\mathbf{x}_p,t_{\bar 1})P_{\rho v}(\mathbf{x}_r,\mathbf{x}_p,t_{\bar 1})P_{\rho\rho}(\mathbf{x}_r,\mathbf{x}_p,t_{\bar 1})P_{\rho\zeta}(\mathbf{x}_r,\mathbf{x}_p,t_{\bar 1}) \\
P_{\zeta u}(\mathbf{x}_r,\mathbf{x}_p,t_{\bar 1})P_{\zeta v}(\mathbf{x}_r,\mathbf{x}_p,t_{\bar 1})P_{\zeta\rho}(\mathbf{x}_r,\mathbf{x}_p,t_{\bar 1})P_{\zeta\zeta}(\mathbf{x}_r,\mathbf{x}_p,t_{\bar 1}) \,.
\end{matrix} \tag{37}$$

The elements of matrix (37) satisfy the corresponding differential equations, and should be calculated by a system of 9 equations [5]. To simplify the calculation of the elements of (37), the approximate calculation by covariance function $P_{\rho\rho}(\mathbf{x}_r,\mathbf{x}_p,t_{\bar 1})$ is usually used [9]. For example, the estimate error covariance matrix for horizontal components of flow velocity vector at arbitrary points of an area $\mathbf{x}$, $\mathbf{x}'$ have the following form:

$$P_{uu}(\mathbf{x},\mathbf{x}',t_{\bar 1}) = \left(\frac{g}{\ell\rho}\right)^2 \frac{\partial^2}{\partial x \partial x'} \int_z^H \int_{z'}^H P_{\rho\rho}(\mathbf{x},\mathbf{x}',t_{\bar \ell})d\mu' d\mu \,,$$

$$P_{uv}(\mathbf{x},\mathbf{x}',t_{\bar{1}}) = -\left(\frac{g}{\ell\rho_0}\right)^2 \frac{\partial^2}{\partial x \partial y'} \int_z^H \int_{z'}^H P_{\rho\rho}(\mathbf{x},\mathbf{x}',t_{\bar{\ell}}) d\mu' d\mu ,$$

$$P_{vu}(\mathbf{x},\mathbf{x}',t_{\bar{1}}) = \left(\frac{g}{\ell\rho}\right) \frac{\partial^2}{\partial x' \partial y} \int_z^H \int_{z'}^H P_{\rho\rho}(\mathbf{x},\mathbf{x}',t_{\bar{\ell}}) d\mu' d\mu ,$$

$$P_{vv}(\mathbf{x},\mathbf{x}',t_{\bar{1}}) = \left(\frac{g}{\ell\rho_0}\right)^2 \frac{\partial^2}{\partial y \partial y'} \int_z^H \int_{z'}^H P_{\rho\rho}(\mathbf{x},\mathbf{x}',t_{\bar{\ell}}) d\mu' d\mu .$$

The expressions for mutual covariance functions of the fields u, v, ρ, ζ errors are of the form

$$P_{u\rho}(\mathbf{x},\mathbf{x}',t_{\bar{1}}) = \frac{g}{\ell\rho_0} \frac{\partial}{\partial y} \int_z^H P_{\rho\rho}(\mathbf{x},\mathbf{x}',t_{\bar{\ell}}) ,$$

$$P_{v\rho}(\mathbf{x},\mathbf{x}',t_{\bar{1}}) = -\frac{g}{\ell\rho_0} \frac{\partial}{\partial x} \int_z^H P_{\rho\rho}(\mathbf{x},\mathbf{x}',t_{\bar{\ell}}) d\mu ,$$

$$P_{u\zeta}(x,y,z;x',y',t_{\bar{1}}) = -\frac{g}{\ell\rho_0^2} \frac{\partial}{\partial y'} \int_0^H P_{\rho\rho}(\mathbf{x},\mathbf{x}',t_{\bar{1}}) d\mu' ,$$

$$P_{\rho\zeta}(x,y,z;x',y',t_{\bar{1}}) = -\frac{1}{\rho_0} \int_0^H P_{\rho\rho}(\mathbf{x},\mathbf{x}',t_{\bar{1}}) d\mu' .$$

Let us note that $P_{u\rho}(\mathbf{x},\mathbf{x}',t_{\bar{1}}) = P_{\rho u}(\mathbf{x},\mathbf{x}',t_{\bar{1}})$, $P_{\rho\zeta}(x,y,z;x',y',t_{\bar{1}}) = P_{\zeta\rho}(x,y;x',y',z',t_{\bar{1}})$, etc. [5].

At the analysis stage, the covariance function $P_{\rho\rho}(\mathbf{x},\mathbf{x}',t_{\bar{1}})$ correction is calculated by the formula

$$P_{\rho\rho}(\mathbf{x},\mathbf{x}',t_1^+) = P_{\rho\rho}(\mathbf{x},\mathbf{x}',t_{\bar{1}}) - \sum_{r=1}^{N} [\Delta_r^{1\rho}(\mathbf{x},t_{\bar{1}}) P_{\rho u}(\mathbf{x},\mathbf{x}',t_{\bar{1}})$$
$$+ \Delta_r^{2\rho}(\mathbf{x},t_{\bar{1}}) P_{\rho v}(\mathbf{x},\mathbf{x}',t_{\bar{1}}) + \Delta_r^{3\rho}(\mathbf{x},t_{\bar{1}}) P_{\rho\rho}(\mathbf{x},\mathbf{x}',t_{\bar{1}})$$
$$+ \Delta_r^{4\rho}(\mathbf{x},t_{\bar{1}}) P_{\rho\zeta}(\mathbf{x},\mathbf{x}',t_{\bar{1}}) .$$

Possible methods for calculating $P_{\rho\rho}(\mathbf{x},\mathbf{x}',t_{\bar{1}})$ at the prediction stage are presented in [9].

A typical four-dimensional analysis of the ocean fields is made in [5], [9], [32]–[34]. In particular, numerical experiments for estimating the influence of the density field and the horizontal components of flow velocities on the optimal estimate value of different components of the state vector have been carried out in [5].

It was experimentally determined that the assimilation of the measurement data concerning only the horizontal components of the velocity field slightly improves the results on hydrophysical fields. The estimation errors are essentially reduced in the case of density and velocity fields. With the same amount of observational data, the efficiency of four-dimensional analysis depends significantly on the appropriate placement of observation stations. Numerical experiments of the model also demonstrated that both inhomogeneity and anisotropy of the correlation function of the density field estimation error should be taken into account.

The four-dimensional analysis of real measurement data obtained with the programs POLYMODE and "Sections" can be found in [9], [32], [34].

Since the quantity of deep-layer measurements is insufficient for proper evaluation of the nonstationary circulation, we used sea-surface temperature measurements made by scientific vessels and specialized satellites. To reduce the probability of unstable stratification which appears in assimilating the surface measurement data, regardless of the correction of the corresponding values at lower layers, we turned from measurements and variance of sea-surface temperature measurement errors to the effective deep-layer measurements and to the effective error variance of deep-layer temperature measurements [32]. To do this, we chose 4 preliminary intervals of the sea-surface temperature variations and plotted the profiles of mean temperature and root mean square deviation of temperature with respect to depth. These dependences were used for constructing the effective vertical profiles on the basis of the surface temperature measurements. This method practically excludes the possibility of the appearance of fictitious heat fluxes. The numerical 4-dimensional analysis using the "Sections" program data was made in the region of North Atlantic current with the coordinates 35°.5 – 55°.5N and 289°.5 – 330°.5 W which includes the Newfoundland energetically active zone [32]. The step in the horizontal direction was 1°; in the vertical direction we considered 16 layers.

We made two numerical experiments, each of them in two stages. The first stage involved (proceeding from diagnostic calculations) an ordinary hydrodynamic prediction for 40 days of model time with the aim of obtaining the adapted fields of density, current velocities and sea-surface topography [31]. We took the fields obtained at the adaptation stage as initial fields for further experiments. In the first version of calculations we performed a hydrodynamic prediction of two months. The second numerical experiment involved a four-dimensional analysis of the fields with the assimilation of surface and deep-layer temperature data. Using results of the second experiment, we plotted a number of charts of sea surface topography, density and current velocities. Figures 5–7 show current fields at the termination of the analysis (the 52nd day) in the layers of 0, 150, and 500 m. Figure 8 is the graph of conventional density (σ_t) corresponding to this moment. A comparison of results of these two experiments shows that the assimilation of measurement data, unlike an ordinary hydrodynamic prediction, increases the velocity in the Gulf Stream upper layers by 5–7 cm s^{-1}, reaching the values of 60–80 cm s^{-1}. The mass flux in quasistationary meander, which is situated on the right of the flow jet, increased. The jet-like flow

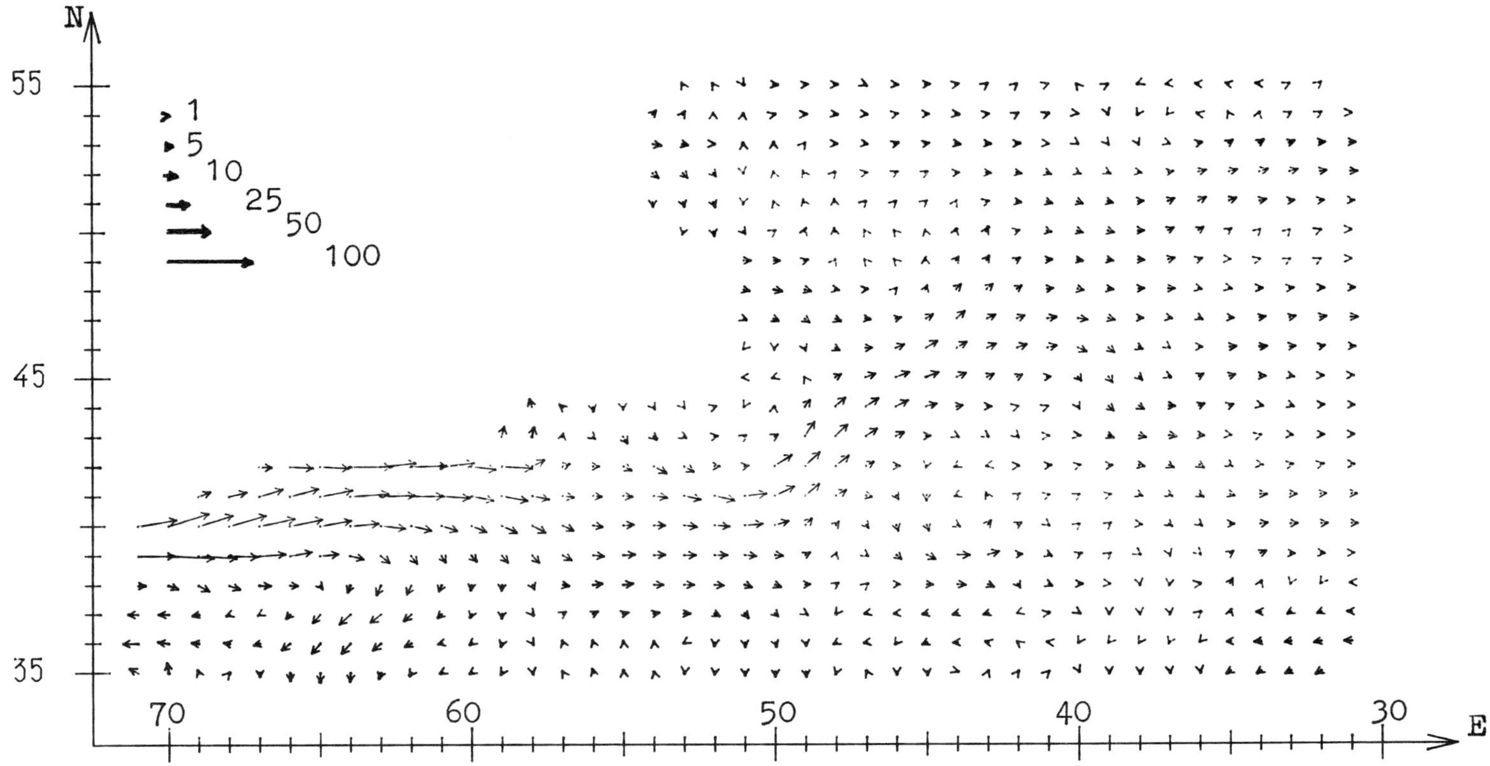

Fig. 5. Surface flow velocity in Gulf Stream region after 52 days of analysis (model prediction with the assimilation of observed data of the "Sections" program)

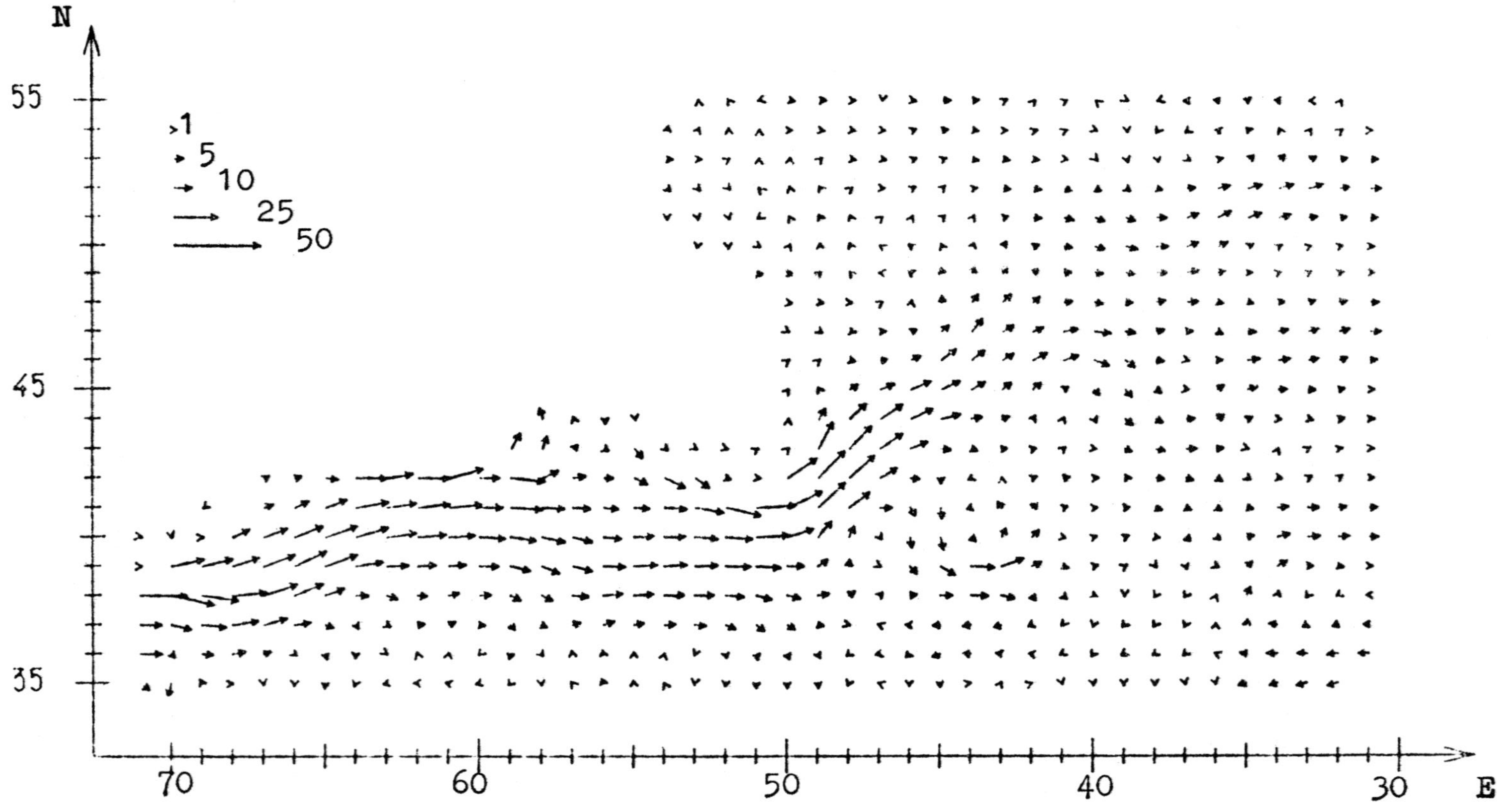

Fig. 6. The same as in fig. 5, but at z = 150 m

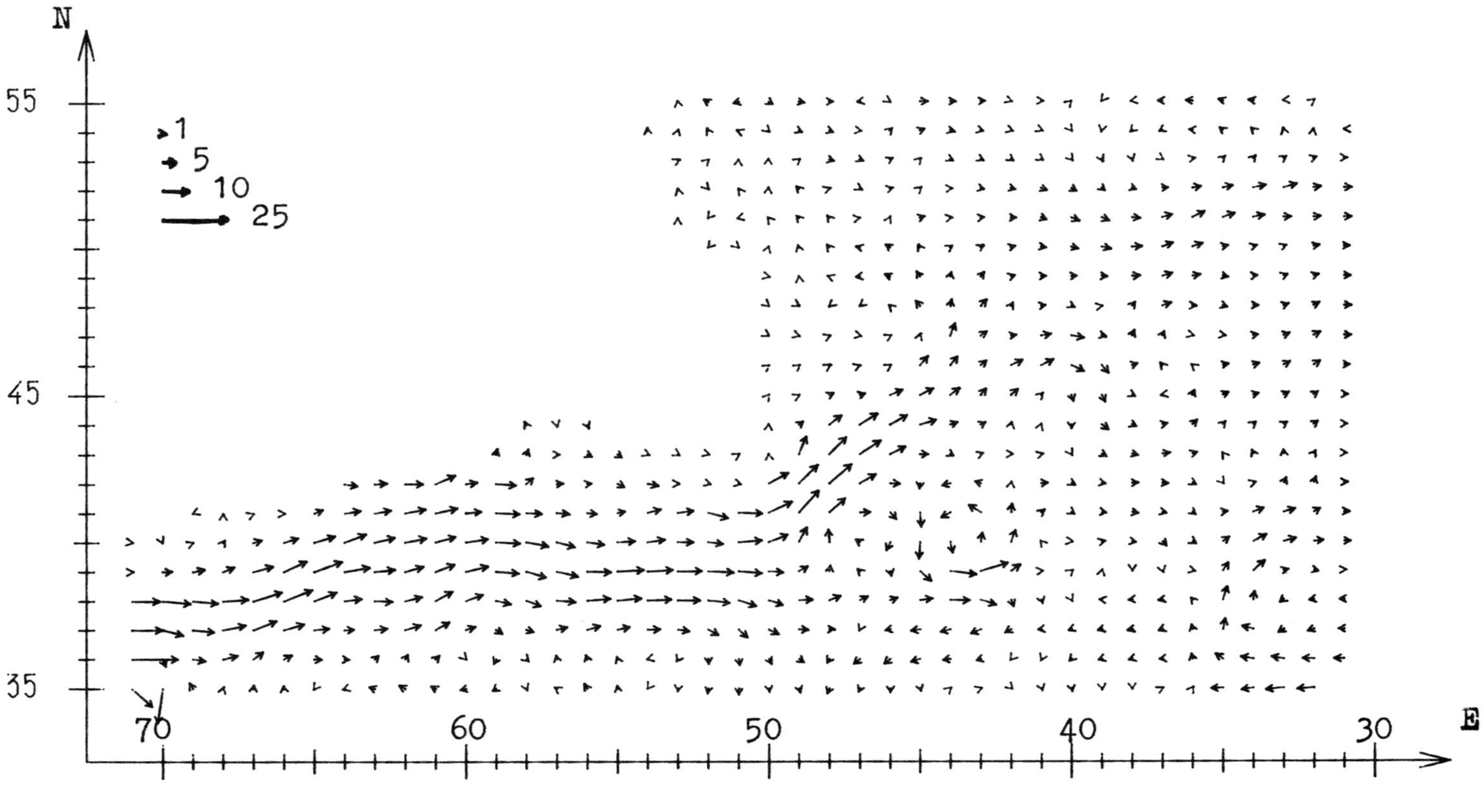

Fig. 7. The same as in fig. 5, but at z = 500 m

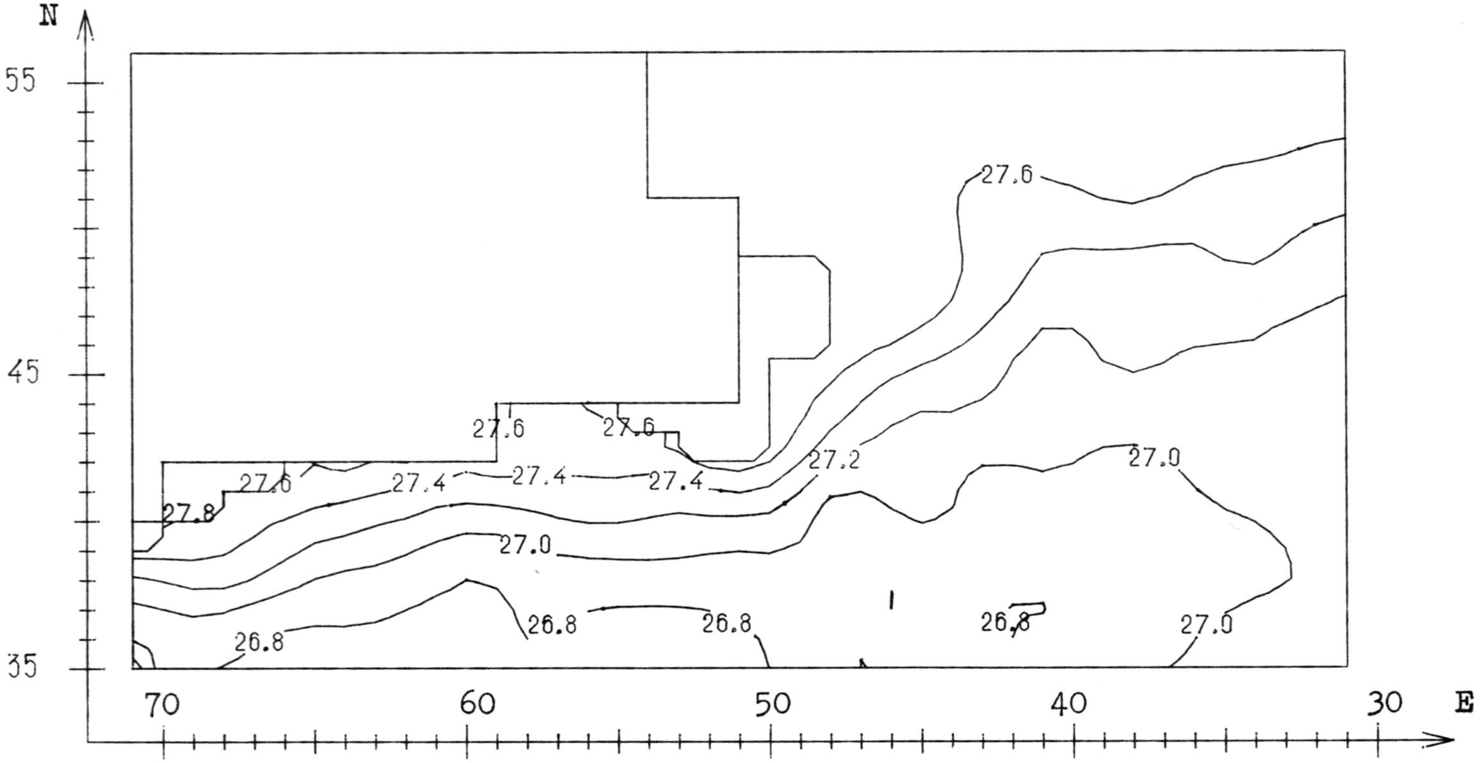

Fig. 8. Conventional density field at z = 500 m after 52 days of analysis (model prediction with the assimilation of the "Sections" program data)

separates into two weak currents in the open ocean, shown in the graphs of kinetic energy (figs. 9, 10); this result agrees with the observational data.

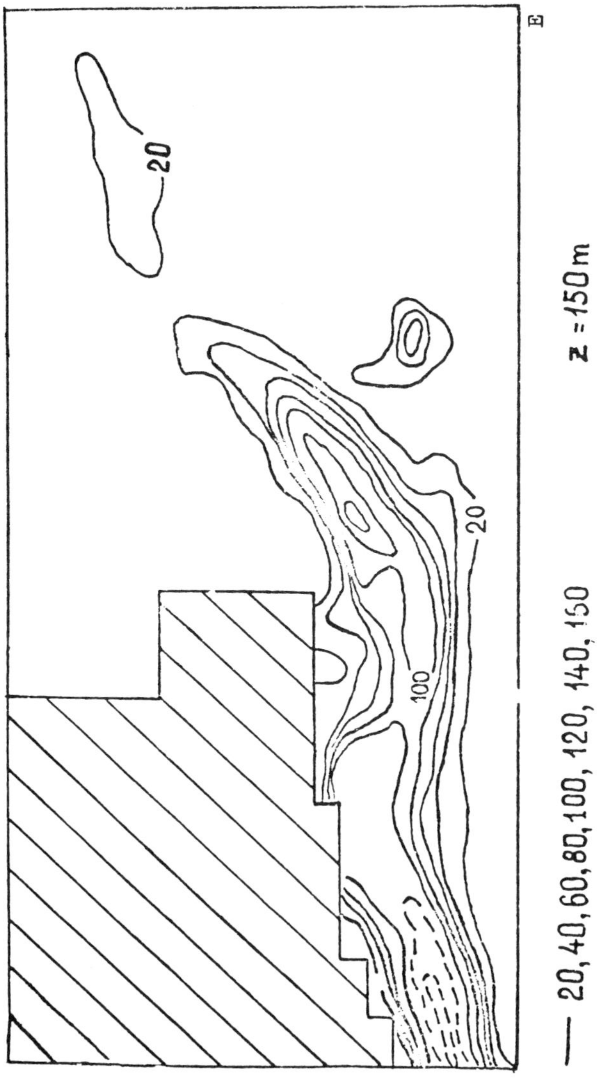

Fig. 9. Kinetic energy at $z = 150$ m after 52 days of model prediction without assimilation of observed data.

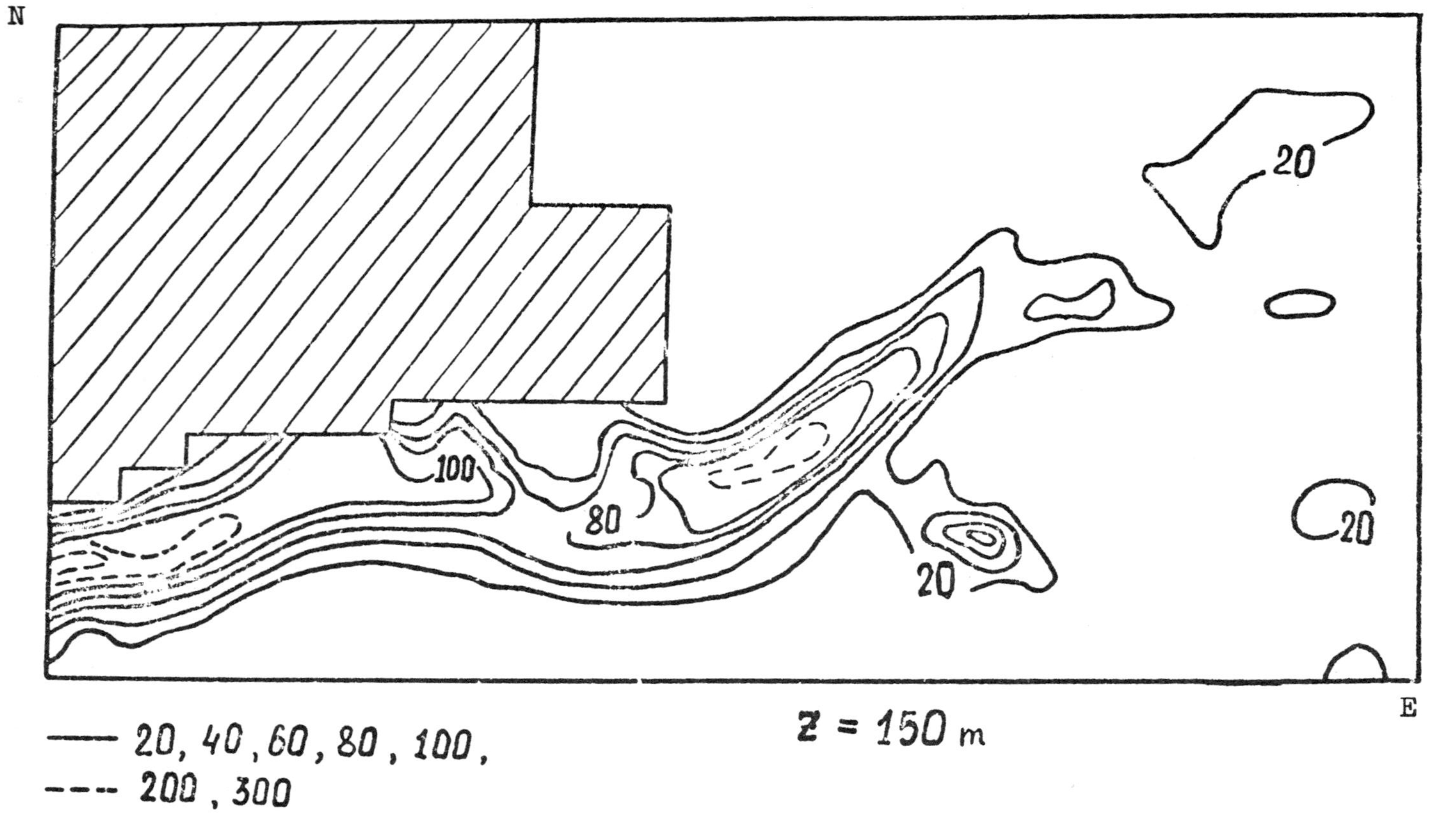

Fig. 10. The same as in fig. 9, but with the assimilation of the "Sections" program observed data.

Conclusion

To summarize, we note that the so–called classical theory of ocean circulation is the most widely used method of investigation of the world ocean surface. The published literature in this area is extensive and growing. However, there is still an essential gap between theory and practice. The reason is manifold: computer limitations, difficulties of subgrid parametrization, among others. The current velocity in the Gulf Stream, obtained by simple diagnostic calculations, is 2–3 times higher than the one obtained by the classical modelling, but perhaps smaller than the actual climatic field. (The measurements of current velocities in the Gulf Stream are still insufficient for obtaining the true large–scale climatic field.) The adaptational process adjusts the diagnostic calculations and, on the whole, smooths them to some extent. The assimilation of temperature field measurements changes only slightly their values, but qualitatively it brings the calculations closer to the general assessment of the hydrophysical ocean fields obtained by observations. The dynamic–stochastic method will be a useful and effective asset in applying the currently available data as well as the rapidly growing satellite data that we may expect during the next decade.

REFERENCES

[1] Balakrishnan, A.V., and Lions, J.L.. 1967. State estimation for infinite–dimensional systems. *J. Comput. and Syst. Sci.* 1:391–403.
[2] Bryan, K. 1969. A numerical method for the study of the circulation of the world ocean. J. *Comput. Phys.* 4, no. 3:347–76.
[3] Cox, M.D. 1975. A baroclinic numerical model of the world ocean: preliminary results. In *Numerical Models of Ocean Circulation*, 107–20. The National Academy of Sciences, Washington, D.C.
[4] Defant, A. 1941. Die absolute Topographie des physikalischen Meeresniveaus und der Druckflächen, sowie die Wasserbewegungen im Atlantischen Ozean. In *Deutsche Atlantische Exped. "Meteor*, 1–25–1–27. *Wiss. Erg*," Bd. 6, 2 Teil, IFR 5.
[5] Demyshev, S.G., and Knysh, V.V. 1981. Model numerical experiments on estimating the reliability of the multivariate four–dimensional analysis of the major physical oceanic fields (in Russian). In *Teoriya Okeanicheskikh Protsessov*, 61–69. Sevastopol: Marine Hydrophysical Institute of the Academy of Sciences of the Ukranian SSR.
[6] Han, Y.J., and Gates, W.L. April 1982. Preliminary analysis of the performance of the OSU six–level oceanic general circulation model. Pt. II: a baroclinic experiment. Report no. 34, Climatic Research Institute.
[7] Haney, R.L. 1980. A numerical case study of the development of large–scale thermal anomalies in the central north Pacific Ocean. *J. of Phys. Oceanogr.* 10, no. 4:222–222.
[8] Kalman, R.E., and Bucy, R.S. 1961. New results in linear prediction and filtering theory. *J. Basic. Eng.* (Trans. ASME, ser. D) 83D:95–108.

[9] Knysh, V.V., Moiseenko, V.A., Sarkisyan, A.S., and Timchenko, I.E. 1980. Complex use of measurement data obtained on hydrophysical oceanic survey areas in the four-dimensional analysis (in Russian). *Doklady Akademii Nauk SSSR*, ser. matem. fiz. 252, no. 4:832–36.

[10] Lamont, G.B., and Kumar, K.S.P. 1972. State estimation in distributed parameter systems via least squares and invariant embedding. *J. Math. Anal. Appl.* 38, no. 3:588–606.

[11] Marchuk, G.I. 1967. On equations of baroclinic ocean dynamics (in Russian). *Doklady Akademii Nauk SSSR*, ser. matem. fiz. 173, no. 6:1317–20.

[12] ————. 1969. On the numerical solution of Poincaré's problem for oceanic circulation (in Russian). *Doklady Akademii Nauk SSSR*, ser. matem. fiz. 185, no. 5:1041–44.

[13] ————. 1972. *Numerical solution of atmospheric and ocean dynamics problem via the splitting method* (in Russian). Baroclinic Institute, Novosibirsk.

[14] ————. 1974. Basic and conjugate equations of atmosphere and ocean dynamics (in Russian). *Meteorologiya i gidrologiya* 2:9–37.

[15] ————. *Numerical Solution of Atmosphere and Ocean Dynamics Problems* (in Russian). Leningrad: Gidrometeoizdat, 1974.

[16] Marchuk, G.I., Dymnikov, V.P., Zalesnyj, V.B., Lykosov, V.N., and Galin, V.Ya. *Mathematical Modelling of the General Atmosphere and Ocean Circulation* (in Russian). Leningrad: Gidrometeoizdat, 1984.

[17] Marchuk, G.I., Zalesnyj, V.B., and Kuzin, V.I. 1979. A numerical model for computing the World ocean thermodynamics (in Russian). Paper presented at the joint IOC/WMO Seminar on Oceanographic Products and the IGOSS Data Processing and Services System, Moscow, 2–6 April 1979.

[18] Marchuk, G.I., Zalesnyj, V.B., and Kuzin, V.I. 1975. On finite-difference and finite-element methods in the global wind-driven ocean circulation problem (in Russian). *Izvestiya Akademii Nauk SSSR, FAiO*, 11, no. 12:1294–1300.

[19] Marchuk, G.I., et al. 1980. Joint atmosphere-ocean circulation modelling (in Russian). In *Matematicheskoe Modelirovanie Dinamiki Atmosfery i Okeana*, pt. 1, 4–46. Novosibirsk: Nauka.

[20] Marchuk, G.I., Kochergin, V.P., and Sarkisyan, A.S. 1973. Calculations of flows in a baroclinic ocean: numerical methods and results. *Geophysical Fluid Dynamics* 5.

[21] ————. 1976. Numerical methods and results of calculations of flows in a baroclinic ocean. In *Matematicheskoe Modelirovanie v Geofizike*, no. 116. Moscow: Izdatel'stvo "IASh–AISh."

[22] Marchuk, G.I., Kochergin, V.P., and Tsvetova, E.A. 1972. On the influence of average density vertical gradient on oceanic currents (in Russian). In *Rezul'taty Issledovanij po Mezhdunarodnym Geofizicheskim Proektam*. Pt. 2: Ocean–atmosphere interaction. Moscow: Nauka.

[23] Marchuk, G.I., and Sarkisyan, A.S., eds. In press. *Mathematical Models of the Ocean Circulation*. New York: Gordon and Breach.

[24] O'Brien, J.J., Clancy, R.M., Clarke, A.J., Crepon, M., Elsberry, R., Gammelsrod, T., MacVean, M., Roed, L.P., and Thompson, J.D. 1977. Updwelling in the ocean: two– and three–dimensional models of upper ocean dynamics and variability. In *Modelling and Prediction of the Upper Layers of the Ocean,* ed. E.B. Kraus, 178–228. Elmsford, New York: Pergamon Press.
[25] Padmanabhan, L., and Colantuoni, G. 1974. Sequential estimation in distributed systems. *Int. J. Syst. Sci.* 5, no. 10:937–86.
[26] Sakawa, J. 1972. Optimal filtering in linear distributed parameter systems. *Int. J. Contr.* 16, no. 1:115–27.
[27] Sandström, I.W., and Helland–Hansen, B. 1903. Über die Berechnung von Meeresströmungen. Res. on Norw. Fish and Mar. Institute.
[28] Sarkisyan, A.S. *Numerical Analysis and Prediction of Sea Currents* (in Russian). Leningrad: Gidrometeoizdat, 1977.
[29] ————. 1977. The diagnostic calculation of a large–scale oceanic circulations. *The Sea* 6:363–458.
[30] ————. 1982. Monitoring large–scale ocean circulation with the aid of time series. *WCRP papers, Time series,* Tokyo, 11–15 May 1981, 13–22.
[31] Sarkisyan, A.S., and Demin, Yu.L. 1983. The semidiagnostic method of sea–current calculation (in Russian). WCRP publ. ser. no. 1. *Large–scale oceangr. exper. in the WCRP* 11:201–14.
[32] Sarkisyan, A.S., Demyshev, S.G., Korotaev, G.K., and Moiseenko, V.A. 1985. Numerical experiments on four–dimensional analysis of POLYMODE and "Sections" programs oceanographic data. *Proceedings of the 16th International Liège Colloqium on Ocean Hydrodynamics.* Forthcoming.
[33] Sarkisyan, A.S., Knysh, V.V., Nelepo, V.A., and Timchenko, I.E. 1979. The dynamic–stochastic approach to the density data analysis in hydrophysical test areas (in Russian). *Izvestiya Akademii Nauk SSSR, ser. FAiO,* 14, no. 10.
[34] ————. 1982. Four–dimensional analysis of the density field at the POLYMODE hydrological survey area. *WCRP papers, Time Series,* Tokyo, 11–15 May 1981, 355–57.
[35] Sarkisyan, A.S., Kochergin, V.P., and Klimok, V.I. 1973. *Calculations of the density and current fields seasonal variations in the north Atlantic* (in Russian). Computing Center of the USSR Academy of Sciences, Siberian Branch, Novosibirsk.
[36] Semtner, A.J., Jr., and Holland, W.R. 1978. Intercomparison of quasi–geostrophic simulations of the western north Atlantic circulation with primitive equation results. *J. Phys. Oceangr.* 8:735–54.
[37] Stommel, H., and Schott, F. 1977. The beta spiral and the determination of the absolute velocity field from hydrographic station data. *Deep Sea Res.* 24:325–29.
[38] Veronis, G. 1976. Model of the world ocean circulation, II. Thermally driven, two layer. *J. Mar. Res.* 34:199–216.

IMMUNOLOGY

A NOTE ON THE MARCHUK–ZUEV IDENTIFICATION PROBLEM *

A.V. Balakrishnan
Department of Electrical Engineering, UCLA
Los Angeles, USA

1. Introduction

Recently, a class of mathematical models for the human immune-response system and for more general disease models have been introduced by G.I. Marchuk in a series of papers. (See the references in his book [1].) Apparently these models have proved successful in interpreting clinical as well as laboratory data so that the problem of identifying model parameters from observed data can now be attempted. Two techniques have been proposed for this purpose, one by Marchuk himself in [1] and the other by S.M. Zuev in [2]. This report presents a review of these techniques, putting them in the context of System Identification problems, providing a level of unification and suggesting yet another variant of the Marchuk–Zuev techniques.

2. Statement of the Problem

We shall of course present only the mathematical statement of the problem. For the essential physiological background the reader should consult the Marchuk monograph [1]. The parametric mathematical model is an ordinary differential equation

$$\dot{x}(t) = f(x(t), \alpha + N(t)), \quad x(\cdot) \in R^m, \quad 0 < t < T < \infty, \tag{2.1}$$

where α is an unknown parameter (in R^n, say) and $N(t)$ represents a high-frequency (relative to $x(\cdot)$) random process. The problem is to identify (estimate) α given m_i independent observations of $x(\cdot)$, at $t = t_i$, $i = 1,\ldots,N$. Also

* Research supported in part by NASA Grant NSG 4015.

$$0 < m_i \ , \qquad m_{i+1} \leq m_i \ .$$

We shall also consider the case where

$$m_i = 1 \ .$$

3. The Marchuk Method of Solution

The technique of estimation proposed by Marchuk [2] follows the paradigms of "inverse" or "ill–posed" problems [3]. We shall elaborate on this from the point of view of maximum–likelihood estimation. One advantage of the latter is that it includes a notion of estimation error.

Let θ denote the set

$$\{t_i\} \ , \qquad i = 1,...,N \ ,$$

and let

$$x(t_i) = \frac{1}{m_i} \sum_{k=1}^{m_i} x^k(t_i) \ ,$$

where the superscript k runs over the available independent observation at t_i. We do include the case where $m_i = 1$. Assume the model

$$\tilde{x}(t_i) = x(t_i,\alpha) + N_i \ , \tag{3.1}$$

where $x(t,\alpha)$ is the solution of

$$\frac{\mathrm{d}}{\mathrm{dt}} x(t,\alpha) = f(x(t), \alpha) \ , \qquad t > 0, \ \ x(0) \text{ given} \tag{3.2}$$

and N_i is Gaussian noise with covariance R_i. Then invoking the principle of maximum likelihood, we may seek to minimize

$$q(\alpha) = \frac{1}{N} \sum_{1}^{N} [\mathrm{R}_i^{-1}(\tilde{x}(t_i) - x(t_i,\alpha)), (\tilde{x}(t_i) - x(t_i,\alpha))] \tag{3.3}$$

for given covariance matrices R_i. And the main point is, we do this by the modified Newton–Raphson method as in [3]. In other words, our algorithm is

$$\alpha_{n+1} = \alpha_n - \mu_n^{-1} g(\alpha_n) \ , \tag{3.4}$$

where

$$M_n = M(\alpha_n) \ ,$$

$$M(\alpha) = \frac{1}{N} \sum_{i=1}^{N} A_i^*(\alpha) \, \mathrm{R}_i^{-1} A_i(\alpha) \ ,$$

$$A_i(\alpha) = A(t_i,\alpha) \ ,$$

$$A(t,\alpha) = \nabla_\alpha x(t,\alpha) \ ,$$

$$\frac{\mathrm{d}}{\mathrm{dx}} A(t,\alpha) = (\nabla_x f(x(t),\alpha))\, A(t,\alpha) + \nabla_\alpha f(x(t),\alpha) \ ,$$

$$(\nabla_\alpha x(t,\alpha))h = \frac{\mathrm{d}}{\mathrm{d}\lambda} x(t,\alpha+\lambda h)\Big|_{\lambda=0} \ ,$$

$$(\nabla_\alpha f(x(t),\alpha))h = \frac{\mathrm{d}}{\mathrm{d}\lambda} f(x(t),\alpha+\lambda h)\Big|_{\lambda=0} \ ,$$

$$g(\alpha) = \frac{1}{N}\sum_1^N A^*(t_i,\alpha)\, \mathrm{R}_i^{-1}\,(x(t_i,\alpha)-\tilde{x}(t_i)) \ .$$

It is assumed that

$$M(\alpha)$$

is nonsingular in the region of α of interest. In particular, $M(\alpha)^{-1}$ at the converged value yields a measure of the estimation error:

$$M(\alpha)^{-1} \approx \mathrm{E}[(\hat{\alpha}-\alpha_{\mathrm{true}})(\hat{\alpha}-\alpha_{\mathrm{true}})^*)] \ .$$

Note that (3.4) is equivalent to solving the linear equations:

$$M_n(\alpha_{n+1} - \alpha_n) = g(\alpha_n) \ .$$

This technique has been successfully used in the flight data reduction; see [4].

4. Zuev's Technique

S.M. Zuev suggests another technique in [2] to meet the special needs of the applications in immunology. Thus he begins with the model

$$\dot{x}_\varepsilon(t) = f(x_\varepsilon(t),\ \alpha+N(t)) \ . \tag{4.1}$$

Let $x(t)$ be the solution of

$$\dot{x}(t) = f(x(t),\alpha) \ . \tag{4.2}$$

Then if we write

$$z(t) = x_\varepsilon(t) - x(t) \tag{4.3}$$

and assume that the noise intensity is small, we can approximate (4.1) to yield:

$$\dot{z}(t) = \nabla_x f(x(t),\alpha)\, z(t) + \nabla_\alpha f(x(t),\alpha)\, N(t) \ , \tag{4.4}$$

where $N(t)$ may be modelled as white Gaussian. Thus we have:

$$\begin{aligned} x_\varepsilon(t) &= x(t) + z(t) \ , \\ \dot{x}(t) &= f(x(t),\alpha) \ , \\ \dot{z}(t) &= A(t,\alpha)z(t) + B(t,\alpha)N(t) \ , \\ z(0) &= 0 \ , \end{aligned} \tag{4.5}$$

where

$$\begin{aligned} A(t,\alpha) &= \nabla_x f(x(t),\alpha) \ , \\ B(t,\alpha) &= \nabla_\alpha f(x(t),\alpha) \ . \end{aligned}$$

We may generalize to partial observation and write

$$v(t) = Cx_\varepsilon(t) + N_o(t) \ , \tag{4.6}$$

where $N_o(t)$ is observation noise and C is a fixed rectangular matrix. Note that we have in this way arrived at a more–or–less "standard" parameter identification model

$$\begin{aligned} \dot{z}(t) &= A(t,\alpha)z(t) + B(t,\alpha)N(t) \ , \\ \dot{x}(t) &= f(x(t),\alpha) \ , \\ v(t) &= C(x(t) + z(t)) + N_o(t) \ . \end{aligned} \tag{4.7}$$

Assuming $N(t)$ and $N_o(t)$ to be independent white noise processes, the continuous–time likelihood ratio formula, following [5], can be expressed as:

$$\exp -\frac{1}{2}\left\{\int_0^T D_o^{-1}[(v(t)-Cx(t)-C\hat{z}(t)),\ (v(t)-Cx(t)-C\hat{z}(t))]\, dt + \int_0^T \text{Tr. } D_o^{-1} CP(t)C^*\, dt\right\} ,$$

where

$$\dot{P}(t) = A(t,\alpha)P(t) + P(t)A(t,\alpha)^* + B(t,\alpha)DB(t,\alpha)^* - P(t)C^*D_o^{-1}CP(t) \ ,$$

$$\dot{\hat{z}}(t) = A(t,\alpha)\hat{z}(t) + P(t)C^*D_o^{-1}[v(t)-Cx(t)-Cz(t)] \ ,$$

$$\hat{z}(0) = 0 \ .$$

We can also construct a discrete–time version corresponding to observing $\{x_\varepsilon(t_i)\}$, $i = 1,...,N$. Let

$$x_\varepsilon(t_i) = x_i^\varepsilon \ ,$$

$$x(t_i) = x_i \ .$$

Then we have

$$z_i = \Phi(t_i)\Phi(t_{i-1})^{-1}z_{i-1} + F_iN_i \ , \tag{4.8}$$

where $\{N_i\}$ is white Gaussian with unit covariance and

$$F_iF_i^* = \int_{t_{i-1}}^{t_i} B(s,\alpha)DB(s,\alpha)^* \, ds \ , \tag{4.9}$$

where D is the spectral density of $N(\cdot)$. Let

$$v_i = v(t_i) \ .$$

Then we have the discrete version of (4.6):

$$v_i = C(x_i + z_i) + N_{o,i} \ .$$

Here we take $\{N_{o,i}\}$, the observation noise, to be white with variance D_o. The likelihood functional is then given by (cf. [6], p. 213)

$$\exp -\frac{1}{2}\Big\{\sum_1^N [J_k^{-1}(v_k - Cx_k - C(A_{k-1}\hat{z}_{k-1})), (v_k - Cx_k - XA_{k-1}\hat{z}_{k-1})] \tag{4.10}$$

$$- \sum_1^N [D_o^{-1}v_k, v_k] + \sum_1^N \log |J_k| + \sum_1^n \log |D_o|\Big\} \ ,$$

where

$$J_n = D_o + CH_{n-1}C^* \ ,$$

$$H_k = A_kP_kA_k^* + F_kF_k^* \ ,$$

$$A_k = \Phi(t_{k+1})\Phi(t_k)^{-1}$$

and

$$P_n = (I + H_{n-1}C^*D_o^{-1}C)^{-1}H_{n-1} \ ,$$

$$\hat{z}_n = A_{n-1}\hat{z}_{n-1} + P_nC^*D_o^{-1}(v_n - CA_{n-1}\hat{z}_{n-1} - Cx_n) \ .$$

Minimization of the likelihood function is a numerical optimization problem, which is amenable to the techniques in [7].

5. An Example

Let us consider a concrete example to clarify some of the issues. Let the basic model be linear, and one–dimensional. Then we have

$$\dot{x}_\varepsilon(t) = (\alpha + N(t))\, x_\varepsilon(t) \ , \tag{5.1}$$

where $N(t)$ is white Gaussian with spectral density d, say. To calculate the statistics, we rewrite it in the equivalent Itô form:

$$\mathrm{d}x_\varepsilon(t) = \left(\alpha + \frac{d}{2}\right)x_\varepsilon(t) + (\sqrt{d})x_\varepsilon(t)(\mathrm{d}W) \ , \tag{5.2}$$

so that in particular

$$\frac{\mathrm{d}}{\mathrm{d}x}\mathrm{E}[x_\varepsilon(t)] = \left(\alpha + \frac{d}{2}\right)\mathrm{E}[x_\varepsilon(t)] \ . \tag{5.3}$$

This yields a measure of how small d must be in relation to α if we want

$$\frac{\mathrm{d}}{\mathrm{d}t}\mathrm{E}[x_\varepsilon(t)] = \alpha\mathrm{E}[x_\varepsilon(t)] \ .$$

Let

$$\dot{x}(t) = \alpha x(t) \tag{5.4}$$

and

$$z(t) = x_\varepsilon(t) - x(t) \ . \tag{5.5}$$

Then

$$\dot{z}(t) = \alpha z(t) + N(t)(x(t) + z(t)) \tag{5.6}$$

or, approximately,

$$\dot{z}(t) = \alpha z(t) + N(t)x(t) \tag{5.7}$$

if we neglect $z(t)$ in comparison to $x(t)$. Let

$$v(t) = \hat{x}_\varepsilon(t) + N_o(t) \ , \tag{5.8}$$

where $N_o(t)$ is the observation noise, whose spectral density is d_o, say. We should note that we cannot obtain the case where there is no state noise by taking the limit as the noise variance goes to zero. To calculate the continuous–time likelihood functional, let

$$\hat{x}_\varepsilon(t) = \mathrm{E}[x_\varepsilon(t) \mid v(s),\ s \le t] \ ,$$

$$p(t) = \mathrm{E}[(x_\varepsilon(t) - \hat{x}_\varepsilon(t))^2] \ .$$

Then the likelihood functional is

$$\exp -\frac{1}{2}\left\{d_o^{-1}\int_0^T (v(t) - \hat{x}_\varepsilon(t))^2\,\mathrm{d}t + \int_0^T \frac{p(t)}{d_o}\,\mathrm{d}t\right\} , \tag{5.9}$$

where

$$\hat{x}_\varepsilon(t) = x(t) - \hat{z}(t) \ ,$$

$$\hat{z}(t) = \mathrm{E}[z(t) \mid v(s),\ s \le t] \ ,$$

$$\dot{\hat{z}}(t) = 2\alpha\hat{z}(t) + \frac{p(t)}{d_o}(v(t) - x(t) - \hat{z}(t)) \ ,$$

where

$$\dot{p}(t) = 2\alpha p(t) + \mathrm{d}x(t)^2 - \frac{p(t)^2}{d_o} \ .$$

We can construct a discrete version of (5.9) following (4.10). We omit the details.

Finally, let us note that if we do not make the small–noise assumption and deal with (5.1) as is, we can still use the likelihood–ratio formula in [5]. However this will involve "non–linear" filtering [8], computer implementation of which is still in its infancy.

REFERENCES

[1] Marchuk, G.I. *Mathematical Models in Immunology.* New York: Optimization Software, Inc., Publications Division, 1983.

[2] Zuev, S.M. "Statistical Estimation of Immune Response Mathematical Models Coefficients." In *Mathematical Modeling in Immunology and Medicine*, ed. G.I. Marchuk and L.N. Belykh, 255–64. Proceedings of the IFIP TC–7 Working Conference on Mathematical Modeling in Immunology and Medicine, Moscow, 5–11 July, 1982. Amsterdam New York Oxford: North–Holland, 1983.

[3] Balakrishnan, A.V. *Stochastic Differential Systems. Filtering and Control.* Lecture Notes in Economics and Math. Systems 84. Berlin New York Heidelberg Tokyo: Springer–Verlag, 1973.

[4] ——————. "Parameter Estimation in Stochastic Differential Systems: Theory and Applications." In *Developments in Statistics,* ed. Paruchuri K. Krishnaiah, 1–32. New York San Francisco London: Academic Press, 1978.
[5] ——————. "Likelihood Ratios for Signals in Additive White Noise." *Lithuanian Math. J.* 18, no. 3 (1978): 320–29. (English transl.)
[6] ——————. *Kalman Filtering Theory.* New York: Optimization Software, Inc., Publications Division, 1984.
[7] Evtushenko, Yu.G. *Numerical Optimization Techniques.* New York: Optimization Software, Inc., Publications Division, 1985.
[8] Liptser, R.S., and A.N. Shiryaev. *Statistics of Random Processes. II. Applications.* New York Berlin Heidelberg Tokyo: Springer–Verlag, 1978.

ON THE SIMPLE MATHEMATICAL MODEL OF INFECTIOUS DISEASE

Leonid N. Belykh

Department of Numerical Mathematics
The USSR Academy of Sciences
Moscow, USSR

1. Introduction

In this paper we discuss some results related to an investigation of the so–called simple mathematical model of infectious disease. This model was developed by Gurij Ivanovich Marchuk in 1975 [1].

In the modern medical literature [2] an infectious disease is conceived in terms of the activity of two interdependent members of biocenosis: by virtue of its pathogenic mechanism, one member is able to live in the other, which, in turn, by virtue of its defense mechanism, is capable of resisting the pathogenic effect produced by its opponent. It is mainly an organism's immune system that defends the body against infection. The essence of immune response to an invasion of genetically different substances (antigen), including the disease stimulants, is to produce specific material substances (antibody molecules of cell–killers) which are capable of neutralizing or destroying this antigen. In these terms, an infectious disease can be interpreted as a confrontation between the population of disease stimulants and the body's immune system.

The model is given by a system of ordinary differential equations with time delay of the following form:

$$\frac{dV}{dt} = (\beta-\gamma F)V ,$$

$$\frac{dF}{dt} = \rho C - \eta\gamma FV - \mu_f F , \tag{1}$$

$$\frac{dC}{dt} = \xi(m)\alpha F_{t-\tau}V_{t-\tau}\theta_{t-\tau} - \mu_c(C-C^*) ,$$

$$\frac{dm}{dt} = \sigma V - \mu_m m$$

with initial conditions at $t = t^0 = 0$

$$V(0) = V^0 \geq 0,\ \ F(0) = F^0 \geq 0\ ,$$
$$C(0) = C^0 \geq 0,\ \ m(0) = m^0 \geq 0\ . \tag{2}$$

The model contains four most essential characteristics of a disease:

1. Concentration (quantity) of viruses $V(t)$. Viruses are treated as multiplying pathogenic (able to damage an organ's cells) antigens. Viruses proper, bacteria, malignant cells, etc. can be regarded as such antigens.

2. Concentration (quantity) of antibodies $F(t)$. The antibodies are regarded as material substrates of the immune system, capable of neutralizing the viruses. Both antibody molecules proper and receptors of immunocompetent cells (e.g., killers) can be regarded as such substrates.

3. Concentration (quantity) of plasma cells $C(t)$. This is a population of antibody carriers and producers. It may be both plasma cells proper and immunocompetent cells, e.g., killer's precursors.

4. Relative characteristic of damaged organ $m(t)$. Let M be a characteristic of a healthy organ (mass or area), and let M' be the same characteristic of the healthy part of the damaged organ. Then $m = 1 - M'/M$. It is apparent that $0 \leq m \leq 1$, and the equality $m = 0$ corresponds to the healthy organ, while $m = 1$ corresponds to the entirely damaged organ. Definitions in the model (1) are the following:

β – the rate of virus multiplication;
γ – the coefficient which allows for the probability of viruses meeting with antibodies and the strength of their interaction;
α – the coefficient of immune-system stimulation which allows for the antigeneity of viruses on the one hand, and the reactive abilities of the immune system on the other hand, e.g., effect of T–B–cooperation or the amount of daughter plasma cells formed by one precursor;
ρ – the rate of antibody production by one plasma cell;
μ_c, μ_f – constants referring to the mean lifetime of plasma cells and antibodies respectively;
η – the amount of antibodies necessary for neutralization of one virus;
σ – the coefficient (rate) of organ injury by viruses;
μ_m – the rate of regeneration of the mass of the damaged organ;
τ – the mean time necessary for division of immunocompetent cells and for formation of plasma–cell clones;

C^* – the constant level of plasma cells (immunocompetent cells) in the healthy body;

$\xi(m)$ – the continuous nonincreasing function which describes the dysfunction of the immune system due to substantial organ damage, $0 \le \xi(m) \le 1$, $\xi(0) = 1$, $\xi(1) = 0$; it is assumed that a threshold level of damage of the organ m^* which does not influence immune-system functioning yet exists (see fig. 1).;

$\theta(t)$ – step function, $\theta(t) = 0$ for $t < 0$, $\theta(t) = 1$ for $t \ge 0$.

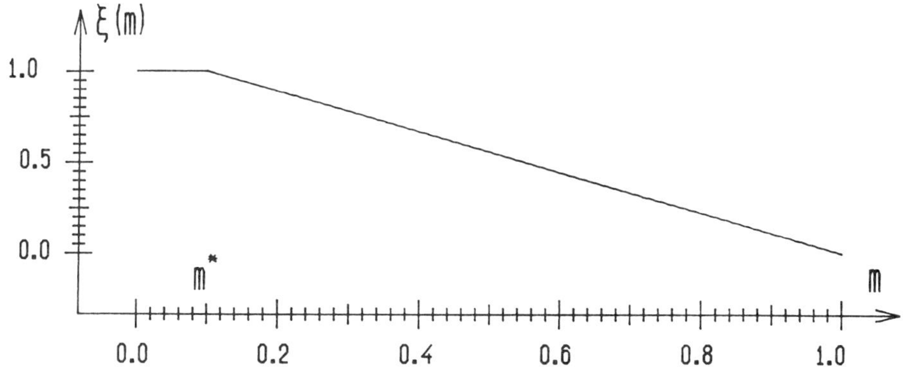

Fig. 1. The possible form of function $\xi(m)$

According to the model (1), the disease process is described as follows. At the moment of infection $t^0 = 0$, a small population of viruses V^0 penetrate into the body and begin to multiply and injure cells of the target organ. Some portion of the viruses bind with the receptors of the immunocompetent cells (with antibodies), and this leads to immune system stimulation resulting in a formation of a large population of plasma cells during the period of time τ. These plasma cells begin to produce antibodies, which neutralize the virus population. An outcome of the disease is determined by the outcome of this competition. If the viruses can damage the organ severely during the formation of the immune response, the general condition of the organism deteriorates and, as a result, the immune response becomes less efficient. The antibody production declines and so does the probability of recovery.

2. The main analytical results

The validity of the following statements has been shown [3], [4] for the model (1).

Theorem 1. *For all* $t \ge 0$ *there exists the unique solution of* (1) *with initial conditions* (2).

Theorem 2. *For all $t \geq 0$ the solutions of system* (1) *with conditions* (2) *is nonnegative.*

Theorem 3. *The stationary solution of system* (1)

$$V_1 = 0, \quad F_1 = \rho C^*/\mu_f = F^*, \quad C_1 = C, \quad m_1 = 0\,, \tag{3}$$

is asymptotically stable if $\beta < \gamma F^*$; in this case at $F^0 = F^*$, $C^0 = C^*$, $m^0 = m^*$ if the inequality

$$0 < V^0 < V^* = \frac{\mu_f(\gamma F^* - \beta)}{\beta\eta\gamma} \tag{4}$$

is valid, then $V(t) < V^0 e^{-at}$ where

$$a = \gamma\rho C^*/(\mu_f - \eta\gamma V^0) - \beta > 0\,.$$

Theorem 4. *The stationary solution of system* (1)

$$V_2 = \frac{\mu_c(\mu_f\beta - \gamma\rho C^*)}{\beta(\alpha\rho - \mu_c\eta\gamma)} > 0, \quad F_2 = \frac{\beta}{\gamma},$$

$$C_2 = \frac{\alpha\mu_f\beta - \eta\mu_c\gamma^2 C^*}{\gamma(\alpha\rho - \mu_c\eta\gamma)}, \quad m_2 = \sigma V_2/\mu_m < m^* \tag{5}$$

is asymptotically stable if

$$\mu_c\tau \leq 1\,,$$

$$0 < \frac{f-d}{a-g\tau} < b - g - f\tau\,, \tag{6}$$

where

$$\alpha = \mu_c + \mu_f + \eta\gamma V_2\,,$$

$$b = \mu_c(\eta\gamma V_2 + \mu_f) - \eta\gamma\beta V_2\,,$$

$$d = \mu_c\eta\gamma\beta V_2\,, \tag{7}$$

$$g = \alpha\rho V_2\,,$$

$$f = \beta\alpha\rho V_2\,.$$

In the case $\alpha \to \infty$ the second condition from (6) *can be reduced to the inequality*

$$0 < \beta - \gamma F^* < \left(\tau + \frac{1}{\mu_c + \mu_f}\right)^{-1}. \tag{8}$$

Theorems 1 and 2 demonstrate the features of the adequacy of the model to real processes. For example, Theorem 1 guarantees no biologically absurd case, i.e., none of the model components reaches infinity during finite time. Theorem 2 emphasizes the biological sense of model variables: they cannot be negative values. Theorem 3 gives the condition of stability of the stationary solution (3), which is interpreted as a healthy body state and estimates the zone of its attraction in the case of infection of the healthy body. This estimate V^* has been called the immunological barrier against given types of viruses. If viruses cannot get over it ($V^0 < V^*$), no disease occurs since the virus population is removed from the body in the course of time.

Theorem 4 defines the stability conditions for the stationary solution (5), which is interpreted as a chronic, or latent form of disease. It is proven that even in the case of a highly sensitive immune response ($\alpha \to \infty$), a stable chronic form of disease is possible.

3. Simulation results

The infection of the healthy body by a small dose of viruses is simulated with appropriate initial conditions:

$$V(0) = V^0 > 0, \quad F(0) = F^*, \quad C(0) = C^*, \quad m(0) = 0 . \tag{9}$$

This simulation shows that there exist four qualitatively different types of solutions, which were interpreted as disease forms: subclinical, acute with recovery, chronic, and lethal outcome. They are diagrammed in fig. 2.

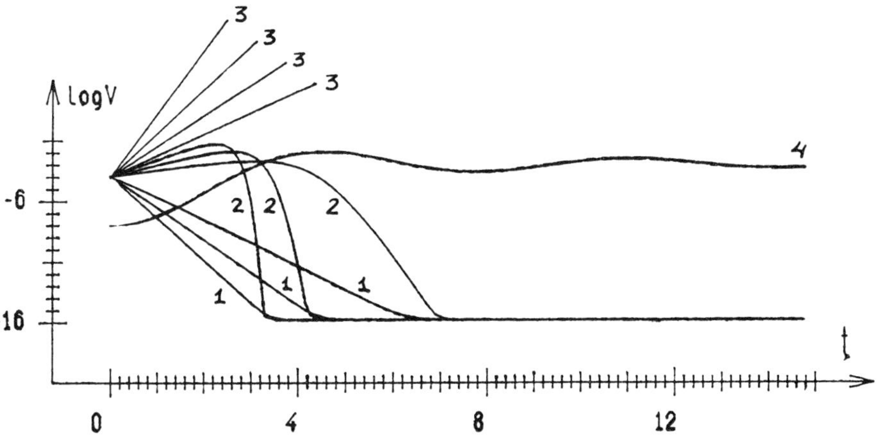

Fig. 2. The possible forms of disease according to model (1):
1 – subclinical form
2 – acute form
3 – lethal outcome
4 – chronic outcome

A subclinical form of disease develops under the conditions of Theorem 3; it is characterized by a stable removal of the viruses from the body (curve 1). The characteristic of the acute form with recovery is a particular dynamic behavior of viruses: first a fast proliferation of viruses during several days and then a drastic contraction, practically to zero, due to a powerful immune response (curves 2). The chronic form of the disease is characterized by a persistent presence of viruses in the body; it arises especially under the conditions of Theorem 4. The unlimited growth of viruses in the body and the entire damage of the organ are characteristic of lethal outcome (curves 3).

We now go on to a more detailed description of numerical experiments simulated for a particular form of the disease. We will also discuss their biological implications.

3.1 SUBCLINICAL FORM OF DISEASE

The simulation results for the case when $\beta < \gamma F^*$ are represented in fig. 3. Here two situations are distinguished: a) $\alpha\rho > \mu_c\eta\gamma$ that corresponds to normal functioning of immune response and b) $\alpha\rho < \mu_c\eta\gamma$ that corresponds to immunodeficiency state. For infection doses smaller than the immunological barrier ($V^0 \leq V^*$), the character of virus removal from the body depends neither on the infection nor the power of the immune response (curves 1,2). This elimination of viruses is possible due to the constant level of antibodies F^*. This situation seems to correspond to daily contact of the body with small doses of antigen which penetrate into the body by respiration or with food.

With an essentially higher dose of infection relative to the immunological barrier, the power of the immune response begins to play a major role. The efficient (normal) immune response is able to prevent an infectious disease (fig. 3(a), curve 4). With a weak immune response, the viruses penetrate through the immunological barrier ($V^0 > V^*$), which leads to death (fig. 3(b), curve 3). Thus the immune resistance of persons with normal immune system ($\alpha\rho > \mu_c\eta\gamma$) is much higher than in immunodeficient patients, who, naturally, are more susceptible to infection.

This case, $\beta < \gamma F^*$, can be interpreted as a vaccination of a healthy body by weakened living antigens. The vaccination is meant to provoke a powerful immune response with the purpose of an essential accumulation of memory cells. According to our model it is equivalent to an increasing level of immunocompetent cells C^* constantly present in healthy body and thereby to a rising immunological barrier V^*. The effect of vaccination is determined by the injected doses of antigen, as well as by the condition of the immune system. The simulation shows that injections of doses smaller than the immunological barrier have only negligible effect because in this case the antigen is removed from the body, stimulating no immune response at all, or only a weak response. In neither situation is there an essential accumulation of memory cells. On the other hand, injections of larger doses ($V^0 > V^*$) into the organism with normal immune system ($\alpha\rho > \mu_c\eta\gamma$) stimulate a strong immune response and lead to desirable results in treatment, whereas the vaccination of immunodeficient patients by high doses can cause a serious form of the disease (fig. 3(b), curve 3).

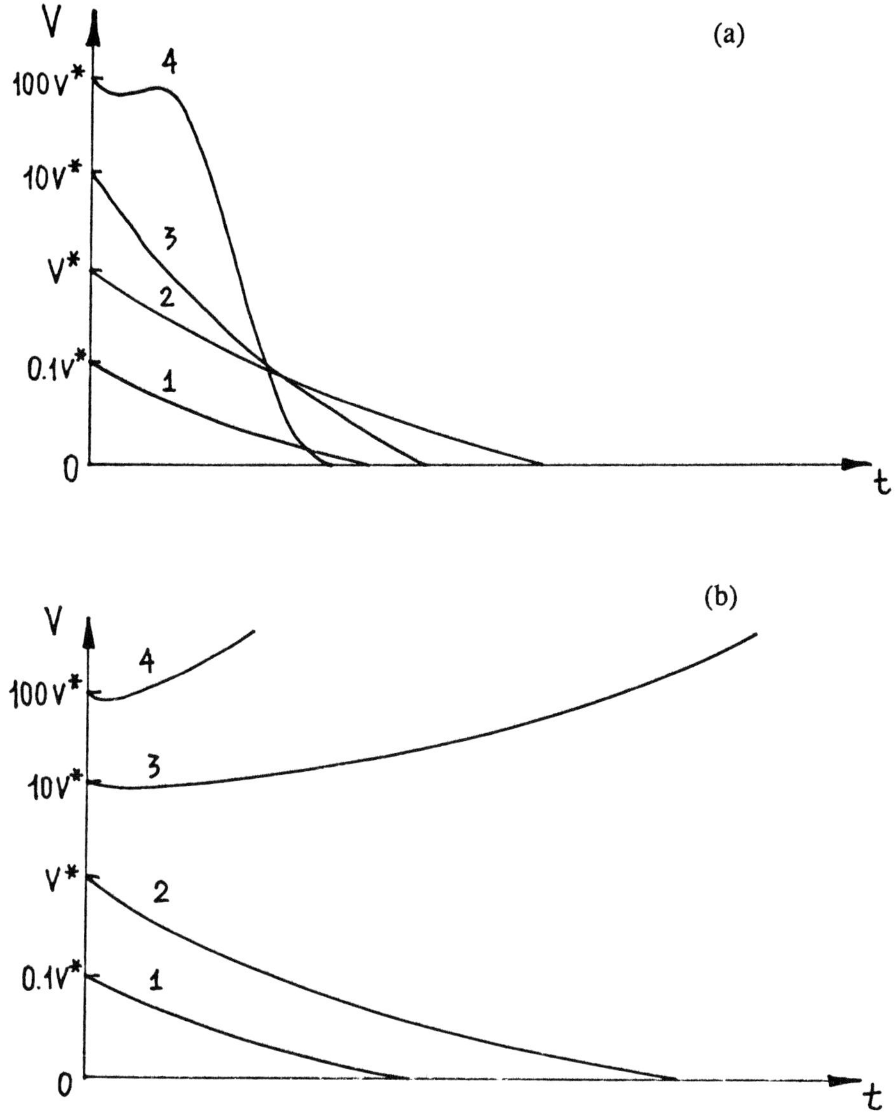

Fig. 3. Subclinical form of disease:
a. normal immune system $\alpha\rho > \mu_c\eta\gamma$
b. immunodeficiency $\alpha\rho < \mu_c\eta\gamma$

Assuming the initial dose of infection V^0 to be the number of tumor cells transplanted, or emerging through mutation, one can interpret these results in the oncological terms.

1. Immune resistance of persons with normal immune system ($\alpha\rho > \mu_c\eta\gamma$) toward sufficiently antigenic tumors is much higher than the immunological barrier toward them, which is not true for persons with immunodeficiency ($\alpha\rho < \mu_c\eta\gamma$). In other words, immunodeficient patients are less protected against tumors.

2. At a quite high natural level of antibodies F^* ($F^* > \beta/\gamma$), in the case of weak antigenic tumors ($\alpha \approx 0$), as well as in the case of immuno–deficiency, the immunological barrier V^* is such that if random mutations do not lead the tumor cells out ($V^0 \leq V^*$), then no cancer process occurs. To simplify, not every weak antigenic tumor leads to cancer and not each immunodeficient patient is expected to develop cancer.

3. If the initial population of tumor cells is sufficiently large, then even a normal immune system cannot prevent a further growth of a tumor. In this case, only external influence—such as a decrease in the population of cancer cells to the value of the immunological barrier—can lead to recovery, provided that the formation of a large initial population of cancer cells is an unlikely random event rather than a manifestation of some regularity, e.g., a genetic one.

Moreover, one can notice that, first, the tumor behavior for $\alpha\rho > \mu_c\eta\gamma$ (fig. 3(a)) is qualitatively similar to the experiments with tumor transplantation cited in the literature in immunology: small tumors disappear; average–size tumors progress initially and then are rejected; large tumors lead to death of the organism. Secondly, physicians know cases when the well–diagnosed tumors have disappeared. Thirdly, it is possible to explain the well–known immunological paradox—very seldom do tumors devel–op in mice with no thymus in spite of the absence of antitumor response to tumors transplanted. These mice appear to have a high immunological barrier against "self" tumors, which is determined by a natural level of "antibodies" F^*. It means that the probability of leading the population of tumor cells out of it is very small. For "non–self" tumors due to the absence of T–system immunity ($\alpha \approx 0$) there is no such barrier, and these organisms are not protected against tumor transplantation.

3.2 ACUTE FORM OF DISEASE

Simulation results of an acute form of disease with recovery in the case of a normal immune system ($\alpha\rho < \mu_c\eta\gamma$) are presented in fig. 4(a). This form of disease occurs when $\beta > \gamma F^*$ and hence there is no immunological barrier to the stimulant of disease. As we noted earlier, the characteristics of this course of illness are: very fast (during several days) growth of viruses in the body until their number substantially exceeds the value of the infective dose, and very fast elimination of antigens from the body. The reason is twofold:

(1) a high rate of virus multiplication leading to fast accumulation of them in the body and (2) the effective immune response caused by the accumulated antigenic mass.

Fig. 4(a) illustrates the course of an acute form of disease depending on the rate of virus multiplication β and infective dose V^0. The higher the multiplication rate at a given infective dose, the higher the maximum quantity of viruses, the faster they reach it, and the faster the process terminates. This is explained by the fact that high infective dose or high rate of multiplication enable the viruses to reach the amounts which effectively stimulate the immune system in a short period of time, and as a result, the powerful immune system becomes capable of resisting the infection.

It appears that under other equivalent circumstances the maximum level of viruses depends very little (practically independent) on infective dose (see fig. 4(b)). We obtained the estimate of this maximum V_{max}, which is independent of V^0 [3], [4]:

$$V_{max} = \frac{(\beta-\gamma F^*)(\mu_f+a)}{\gamma(\rho g-\eta\gamma f)}, \tag{10}$$

where

$$f \in (F^*,\beta/\gamma), \quad a = \beta-\gamma f, \quad g = afe^{-a\tau}(\mu_c+a)^{-1} .$$

In fig. 4(b) we choose $f = (F^*+\beta/\gamma)/2$. Hence in the case of an acute form of disease the value of the "peak of the disease" is independent of infective dose but determined by the immune characteristics of the organism with respect to viruses of a given type (the set of model parameters). The infective dose influences the moment of reaching the peak: the smaller the V^0, the later the peak is reached.

Fig. 4(c) demonstrates possible changes in the acute form with increasing coefficient of organ damage σ. As a result of the organ damage the acute form can turn into a chronic one (curve 2), into a chronic form with unpredictable outcome (curve 3), or chronic form with lethal outcome (curve 4). The possibility of such transition is due to the fact that because of damage the general condition of the body deteriorates, which makes the efficiency of the immune response decrease and the antibody production fall. Therefore, to prevent transition of the acute form into the more serious form, the treatment is to be aimed at either lowering the virus pathogeny or to protect the organ against damage.

3.3 CHRONIC FORM OF DISEASE

We have already noted the possibility of the occurrence of chronic form from acute infection, with serious organ damage (fig. 4(c), curve 2). Now we deal with other kinds of stable chronic forms occurring especially under the conditions of Theorem 4. Characteristic of such typical chronic form is the

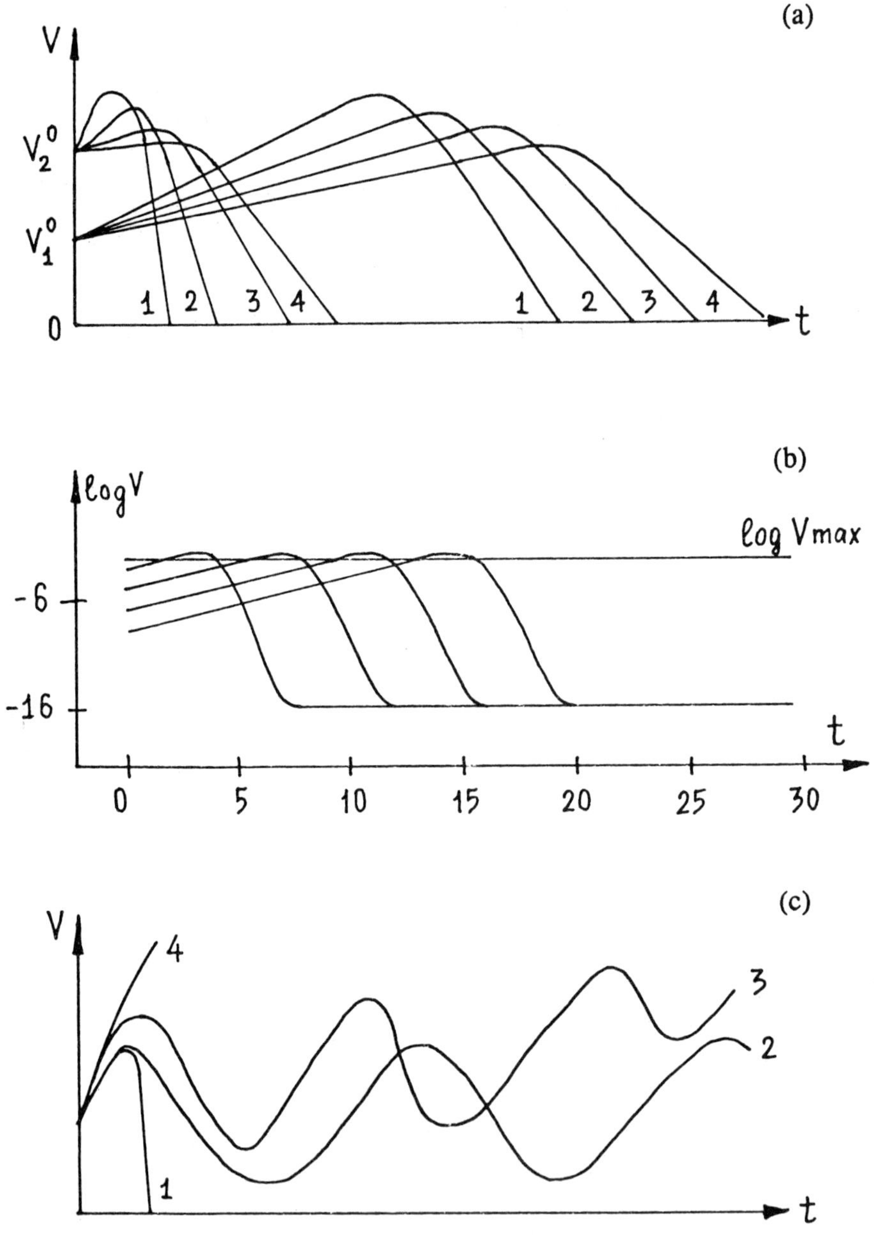

Fig. 4. Acute form of disease:

a. dependences on infection dose V^0 and virus reproduction rate β

b. independence of maximal virus concentration on infection dose

c. dependence on the coefficient of organ damage σ

flaccid dynamics of viruses relative to the acute form. In this case the passive virus dynamics leads in time to equilibrium between amounts of newborn viruses and those neutralized by disease stimulants. Their concentration tends to a stationary level V_2. With an increase of infective dose above V_2, the dynamics of disease stimulants is more expressed and the transition into the acute form with recovery becomes possible (fig. 5(a), curve 3). The efficiency of the immune response can be enhanced by injecting higher infective doses. An analysis of the dependence between the course of the chronic form of disease and the infective dose of weakly pathogenic viruses has brought us to the following conclusions:

1. It is possible to treat a chronic form of disease by exacerbation (essentially increasing the number of viruses in the body).

2. It is not reasonable for the immune system to react to small doses of virus in order to prevent a chronic form of disease.

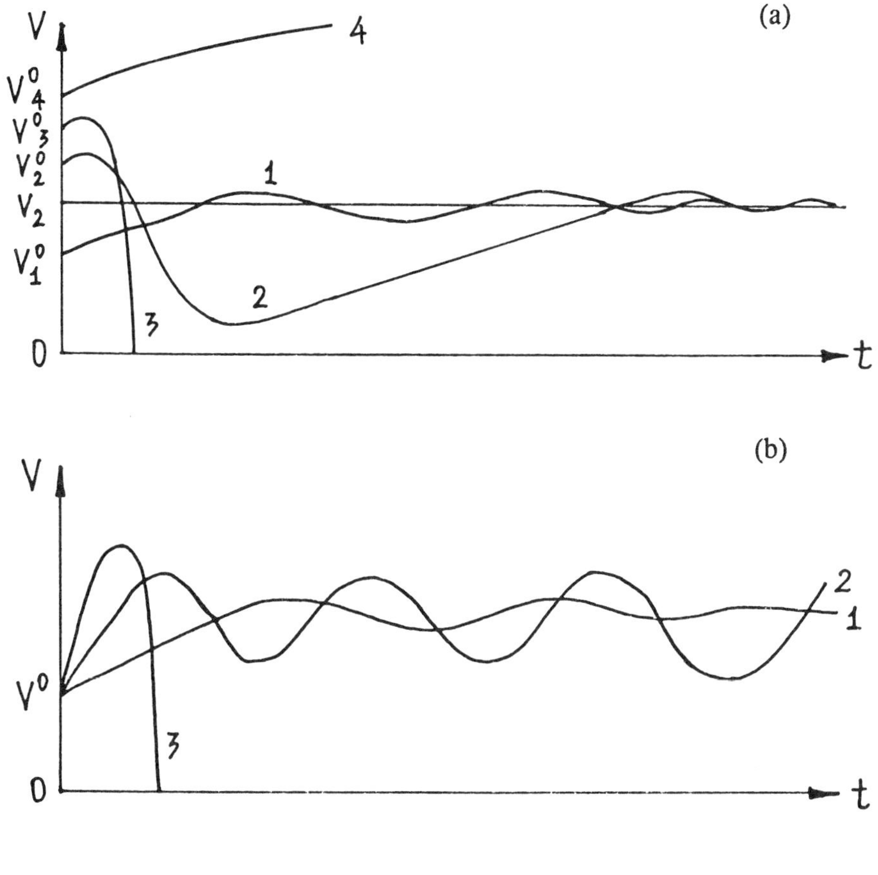

Fig. 5. Chronic form of disease:
a. dependence on infection dose V^0
b. dependence on virus reproduction rate β: $\beta_1 < \beta_2 < \beta_3$

A study of dependence of the course of chronic form on a virus multiplication rate β (see fig. 5(b)) proves the existence of a stable periodic solution (curve 2) and establishes that the treatment of the acute form using drugs, to decrease the multiplication rate, promotes chronization of the disease process. It should be noted that the existence of periodic solutions is proved theoretically in [5].

The existence and stability of the so-called hypertoxic chronic form of disease when the damage level m_2 is higher than the limiting value m^* is shown in [6].

4. The origin of chronic forms of disease and their possible treatment

In [3], [4] a hypothesis on the immunological origin of chronic forms has been propounded: chronic forms of disease are due to weak stimulation of the immune response. This hypothesis is based on the following premises. In the framework of the model, the disease outcome (chronization or recovery) depends on the width of an interval (t_1,t_2) at which the concentration of viruses is decreasing and consequently $dV/dt < 0$. If this interval is sufficiently wide (see fig. 6, solid line), then the number of viruses decreases until the values close to zero are taken as the recovery. Otherwise, i.e., in a sufficiently narrow interval (t_1,t_2) the amount of viruses fails to approach zero, but for $t = t_2$ it reaches the minimum and begins to grow again at $t > t_2$. Then the process is repeated. This is the way the chronic form develops. Since $dV/dt < 0$ means $F(t) > \beta/\gamma$, the width of the interval (t_1,t_2) is determined by how long the latter inequality holds. Apparently the more antibodies produced and the higher their maximum, the wider the interval (t_1,t_2). If we allow for the fact that antibody production is essentially determined by the efficiency of the immune-system stimulation, then the competence of the suggested hypothesis is obvious.

This hypothesis explains the simulation results obtained, namely the transition of acute form to chronic one with serious organ damage and transition of chronic form to acute with high infective dose. In the first case organ damage reduces the efficiency of immune system stimulation that leads to a narrower interval (t_1,t_2) and thus to a chronic process. In the second case there is an inverse effect: high dose of infection enhances the stimulation thus leading to a wider interval (t_1,t_2).

It became theoretically obvious that the treatment of the chronic form should promote widening the interval (t_1,t_2). In practice, the stimulant of antibody production (SAP) and disease exacerbation (biostimulation) have been used [3], [4].

The action of SAP factor is demonstrated by a threefold increase of the quantity of antibodies when the SAP factor has been injected at the peak of immune response. This apparently makes the interval (t_1,t_2) wider. The simulation of SAP-factor action shows its possible, successful application to treating chronic forms of disease [3].

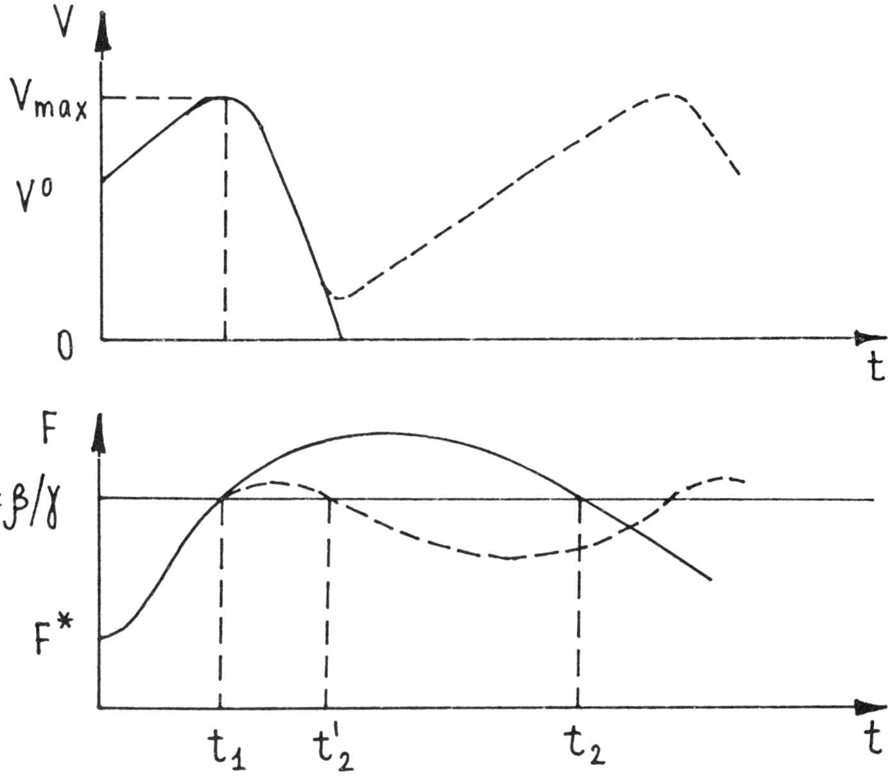

Fig. 6. The rise of chronic form from acute as a consequence of narrowing the interval (t_1, t_2).

In the case of exacerbation, the so-called biostimulation theory was propounded and its mathematical model was constructed [7], [8]. The basic notion of this theory is the following. In the body subject to a stable chronic form of disease, a new nonpathogenic, nonmultiplying antigen (biostimulator) is injected, beginning from some instant of time. The injections are repeated over some discrete interval of time, and the dose of injection grows with time. This leads to the situation that due to the concurrence of microphages between the two antigens (biostimulators and disease stimulants) the immune response to viruses is blocked. So, the immune system "forgets" the disease stimulants and this enables the viruses to increase their antigenic mass. Some time later the biostimulator injections are terminated and then removed quickly from the body. The organism is again face-to-face with the disease stimulants. But the situation has essentially changed. During the interval when biostimulators were in the body, the amount of viruses in the body has reached the values which stimulate effectively the immune system. As a result, a powerful immune response is formed and this leads to complete elimination of the viruses from the body. Recovery follows.

The model corresponding to this theory has the following form:

$$\frac{dV}{dt} = (\beta - \gamma F)V ,$$

$$\frac{dF}{dt} = \rho C - \eta\gamma FV - \mu_f F ,$$

$$\frac{dC}{dt} = p_S(V)\xi(m)\alpha F_{t-\tau}V_{t-\tau} - \mu_c(C - C^*) ,$$

$$\frac{dm}{dt} = \sigma V - \mu_m m , \tag{11}$$

$$\frac{dB}{dt} = -\gamma_B \varphi B + f(t) ,$$

$$\frac{d\varphi}{dt} = \rho S - \eta_B \gamma_B \varphi B - \mu_\varphi \varphi ,$$

$$\frac{dS}{dt} = p_S(B)\alpha_B \varphi_{t-\tau} B_{t-\tau} - \mu_S(S - S^*) .$$

Here, except for previous notations which are relevant to the infectious process, new variables are introduced:

$B(t)$ – concentration of biostimulators

$\varphi(t)$ – concentration of antibodies specific to biostimulators;

$S(t)$ – concentration of plasma cells producing the antibodies against biostimulators.

The function $f(t)$ describes the biostimulator injection and has the form

$$f(t) = Q(n)\delta(t - n\Delta t) ,$$

where $Q(n) = Q_0 + an$; $Q_0 > 0$; $a > 0$; $n = 1,\ldots,M$; M is the amount of injections; Δt is the time interval between consecutive injections. The functions $p_S(V)$ and $p_S(B)$ describe the probabilities of stimulation of the immune system by the antigens V and B, respectively. They have the form

$$p_S(V) = \frac{FV}{FV + \varphi B}, \quad p_S = \frac{TB}{FV + \varphi B} .$$

Using inequality (8), we arrive at the conclusion that for successful treatment (complete elimination of viruses from the body) it is necessary to continue injecting biostimulators during three to four weeks [7], [8]. Figure 7 shows the simulation of treatment of a typical chronic form by exacerbation.

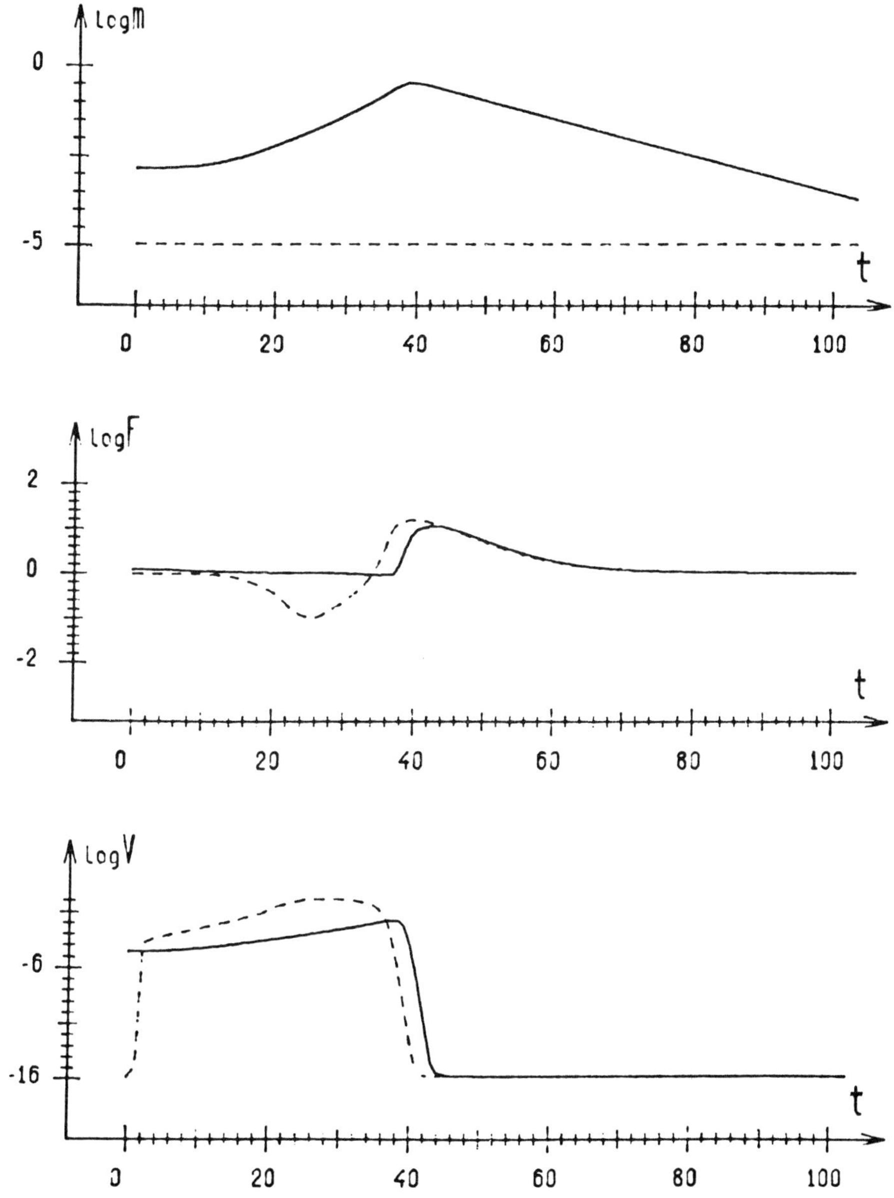

Fig. 7. The treatment of chronic form by aggravation.

dynamics of components of an infectious disease process are depicted by a solid line and those of the treatment dynamics by a broken line. Biostimulators have been injected during 23 days at an interval $\Delta t = 1$. As is easily seen, the exacerbation results in a considerable damage of the organ and therefore biostimulators need to be combined with an antipathogenic therapy.

Concerning the biostimulation which results in a powerful immune response, it is assumed [3], [4] that a sufficient number of memory cells have formed to create an immunological barrier to viruses of a given type. Then, subsequent contacts of the body with the same viruses do not result in the infection of the organism. Other methods of treating the patient, for example by antibiotics even when the viruses have been completely eliminated from the body, do not provide an immunological barrier and subsequent contacts with these viruses lead to the occurrence of a chronic form of the disease.

Elaborating the idea of weak stimulation of the immune system, we point out that the failure of T–B–cooperation is possibly involved. The reason for such failure may be T–immunodeficiency, which may entail: (a) production of IgM antibodies only, rather than the chain IgM–IgG–IgA as usual and (b) the failure of low–dose tolerance. The first factor narrows the interval (t_1,t_2) (see fig. 8) and the second will force the immune system to react to small doses of viruses. This, in turn, may lead to chronization of the process. Thus, both low–dose tolerance and the chain IgM–IgG–IgA of antibody production are reasonable methods to prevent the development of chronic forms.

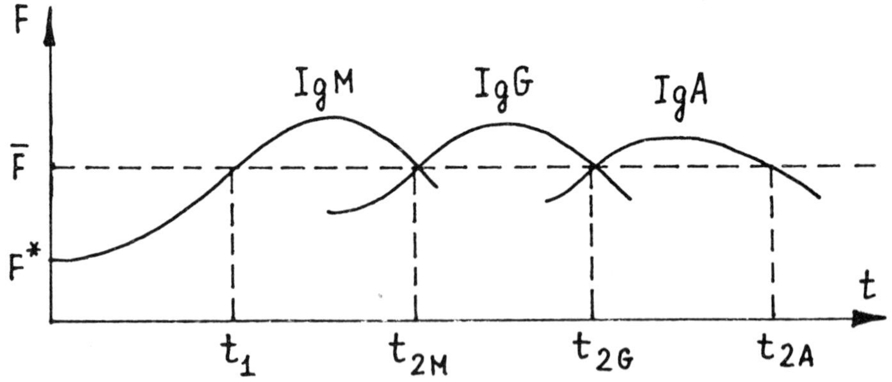

Fig. 8. The chain IgM–IgG–IgA production as widening the interval (t_1,t_2).

Finally, the simple mathematical model of an infectious disease enables one to study, from a single immunological viewpoint, properties of the four main forms of disease. The conclusion is that the occurrence of any particular form of disease originated by a small infective dose, is not directly related to this dose. Rather, it is determined by the immunological status of the body with respect to virus of a given type (the set of model parameters).

The simple mathematical model of an infectious disease developed by Gurij Ivanovich Marchuk opened a new vista in science—mathematical modelling of an infectious disease. The original model was modified in order to describe biinfection, to investigate a role of the immunological memory [9] and organism temperature reaction [10] in the pathological process, as well as to describe and interpret the experimental data on viral hepatitis [11]. Using this model, the practical immunological problem of the SAP–action mechanism was solved [12]. The mathematical model of antiviral immune response recently constructed by Marchuk and Petrov [13] is an elaboration and generalization of the original simple model. Moreover, new techniques for constructing methods simplifying the analysis of stationary–solution stability in time–delay systems [14], and their numerical integration [15] and identification [16] have been proposed.

REFERENCES

[1] Marchuk, G.I. 1975. *The Simple Mathematical Model of a Viral Disease* (in Russian). Preprint of the Computing Center of the USSR Academy of Sciences, Siberian Branch, Novosibirsk.

[2] Baroyan, O.V., and Porter, J.R. *Mezhdunarodnye i Natsional'nye Aspekty Sovremennoj Epidemiologii i Mikrobiologii* (International and National Aspects of Modern Epidemiology and Microbiology). Moscow: Izdatel'stvo "Meditsina," 1975.

[3] Belykh, L.N., and Marchuk, G.I. 1983. Qualitative analysis of the simple mathematical model of an infectious disease (in Russian). In *Matematicheskoe Modelirovanie v Immunologii i Meditsine*, ed. G.I. Marchuk, 5–27. Novosibirsk: Nauka.

[4] Marchuk, G.I. *Mathematical Models in Immunology*. New York: Optimization Software, Inc., Publications Division, 1983.

[5] Skalko, Yu.I. 1983. The analysis of periodic solutions of mathematical models of a disease (in Russian). Preprint no. 68, Department of Numerical Mathematics, the USSR Academy of Sciences, Moscow.

[6] Belykh, L.N., and Kalyaev, D.B. 1985. The analysis of hypertoxic chronic forms of disease in the framework of a mathematical model (in Russian). In *Vychislitel'nye Protsessy i Sistemy*, ed. G.I. Marchuk, 180–87. Moscow: Nauka.

[7] Belykh, L.N., and Marchuk, G.I. 1978. Chronic forms of a disease and their treatment according to mathematical immune–response models. In *Modelling and Optimization of Complex Systems*, 79–86. Proceedings of the IFIP Working Conference on Complex Systems and Optimization, Novosibirsk, USSR, July 1978. Berlin New York Heidelberg Tokyo: Springer–Verlag, 1979.

[8] Belykh, L.N. 1982. A mathematical model of biinfection and the treatment of chronic forms of a disease (in Russian). In *Matematicheskoe Modelirovanie v Immunologii i Meditsine*, ed. G.I. Marchuk, 33–40. Novosibirsk: Nauka.
[9] Skalko, Yu.I. 1983. The onset and development of a disease with decreasing efficiency of the immune–system functioning (in Russian). Preprint no. 69, Department of Numerical Mathematics of the USSR Academy of Sciences, Moscow.
[10] Asachenkov, A.L. 1982. A simple model of temperature–reaction influence on the immune–response dynamics. In *Matematicheskoe Modelirovanie v Immunologii i Meditsine*, ed. G.I. Marchuk, 41–47. Novosibirsk: Nauka.
[11] Romanyukha, A.A. Comparative analysis of the mathematical model of a disease and clinical data. Ibid., 27–32.
[12] Stepanenko, R.N., and Skalko, Yu.I. 1983. On the mechanisms of stimulator of antibody production action. In *Mathematical Modelling in Immunology and Medicine*, ed. Marchuk, G.I., and L.N. Belykh, 225–36. Proceedings of the IFIP TC–7 Working Conference on Mathematical Modeling in Immunology and Medicine, Moscow, 5–11 July 1982. Amsterdam New York Oxford: North–Holland Publ. Co.
[13] Marchuk, G.I., and Petrov, R.V. 1983. Mathematical model of antiviral immune response (in Russian). In *Vychislitel'nye Protsessy i Sistemy*, ed. G.I. Marchuk, 5–19. Moscow: Nauka.
[14] Belykh, L.N. *Analiz Nekotorykh Matematicheskikh Modelej v Immunologii* (Analysis of Some Mathematical Models in Immunology). Moscow: Nauka. In press.
[15] ——————. 1983. On the computational methods in disease models. In *Mathematical Modeling in Immunology and Medicine*, ed. G.I. Marchuk and L.N. Belykh, 79–84. Proceedings of the IFIP TC–7 Working Conference on Mathematical Modeling in Immunology and Medicine, Moscow, 5–11 July 1982. Amsterdam New York Oxford: North–Holland Publ. Co.
[16] Zuev, S.M. 1983. Statistical estimation of immune–response mathematical model coefficients. Ibid., 255–65.
[17] Marchuk, G.I., ed. *Matematicheskoe Modelirovanie v Immunologii i Meditsine* (Mathematical Modelling in Immunology and Medicine). Novosibirsk: Nauka, 1982.
[18] Marchuk, G.I., and Belykh, L.N., eds. *Mathematical Modeling in Immunology and Medicine*. Proceedings of the IFIP TC–7 Working Conference on Mathematical Modeling in Immunology and Medicine, Moscow, 5–11 July 1982. Amsterdam New York Oxford: North–Holland Publ. Co., 1983.

LYMPHOCYTE DISTRIBUTION AND LYMPHATIC DYNAMICS

R.R. Mohler††, Z. Farooqi, and T. Heilig

Department of Computer and Electrical Engineering
Oregon State University
Corvallis, Oregon, USA

Abstract

Linear time–delay models are developed for the circulation of lymphocytes throughout the immune system. A building–block synthesis of the lymphatic system is presented. The models mimic experimental tracer data for rats, but more extensive data is needed to do a good job of parameter estimation.

1. Introduction

This paper attempts to describe the dynamic behavior of circulating lymphocytes as a base for the understanding of the organ–distributed immune function. In particular, new mathematical models are presented, simulated and compared to other models in their ability to mimic experimental tracer data for rats.

It is intended that the development of such a model will be used for predictive purposes in experimental planning. Eventually such modelling, analysis and experimentation may have an impact on tumor control, cancer and immunology in general. In the long run, such research could relate system control theory to effective immunotherapy and chemotherapy. Radiation and chemotherapy adversely affect the immune response in a manner which may be similar to pollutant effect. Systemic immune research could help explain such effects and provide a base for improved treatment.

---

† Research sponsored by NSF Grant No. ECS–8215724.

†† NAVELEX Professor of Electrical and Computer Engineering, Naval Postgraduate School, Monterey, CA 93943. (1984–85)

An excellent introduction to immunology is given by Roitt [1]; a treatment of more detailed aspects of its theory is edited by Bell, et al. [2]. An overview of mathematical system theory in immunology and in disease control is given by Mohler, Bruni and Gandolfi [3] and by Marchuk [4] and [5], respectively.

Experiments have been done to look at the quantitative aspects of this recirculating pool. The data for the present paper was obtained from one such experiment, Smith and Ford [7].

Apparently, there is a need to better understand migratory patterns of immune mechanisms. A preliminary, three–compartment, humoral model is studied by Mohler, et al. [3],[8],[9]. The present analysis studies only lymphocyte migration which is basic to the humoral process but includes mostly thymus–derived T–cells. Also included here are twelve compartments and extensive experimental data.

2. Experimental summary

Details of the experiment from which the data are derived are given by Smith and Ford [7]. Briefly, the data were taken from a uniform strain of rats as near to the natural physiological state as possible. Lymphocytes were taken from the thoracic duct of a donor, radioactively labelled in vitro, passaged from blood to lymph in an intermediate rat and finally injected into a series of recipients for examination at thirteen time points from one minute to one day. Thirteen tissues were examined from sacrificed rats at each time.

To better understand the system dimensions, it is interesting to note that 180 rats (AO female) were used in the experiment with blood sampled and cells injected on the venous side of the right heart. The total pool of recirculating lymphocytes number about $1.2(10)^9$ with about $40(10)^6$/hour circulating through the thoracic duct and other efferent lymphatics each (see fig. 1). The coeliac LN weigh only about 8 mg out of a total LN weight of 700 to 800 mg.

At 1, 2 and 5 minutes after injection most of the labelled cells are in blood, lungs, and liver [7]. Concentrations in these compartments subsided during the ensuing 25 minutes as more cells entered the spleen, lymph nodes, and Peyer's patches, where they peaked between 1 and 18 hours. The migratory pattern of lymphocytes is summarized in fig. 1 with experimental data compared to model–simulated data in figs. 2 to 4 for the spleen, bone marrow and lungs, which exemplify the other organs.

3. Circulatory lymphocyte

The models studied here consist of separate compartments and states for the blood, bone marrow, lungs, liver, spleen, lymph nodes, Peyer's patches, gut and miscellaneous tissues. The lymph nodes were further broken down into mesenteric, coeliac, subcutaneous, right and left popliteal, and deep and superficial cervical lymph nodes for certain data collection.

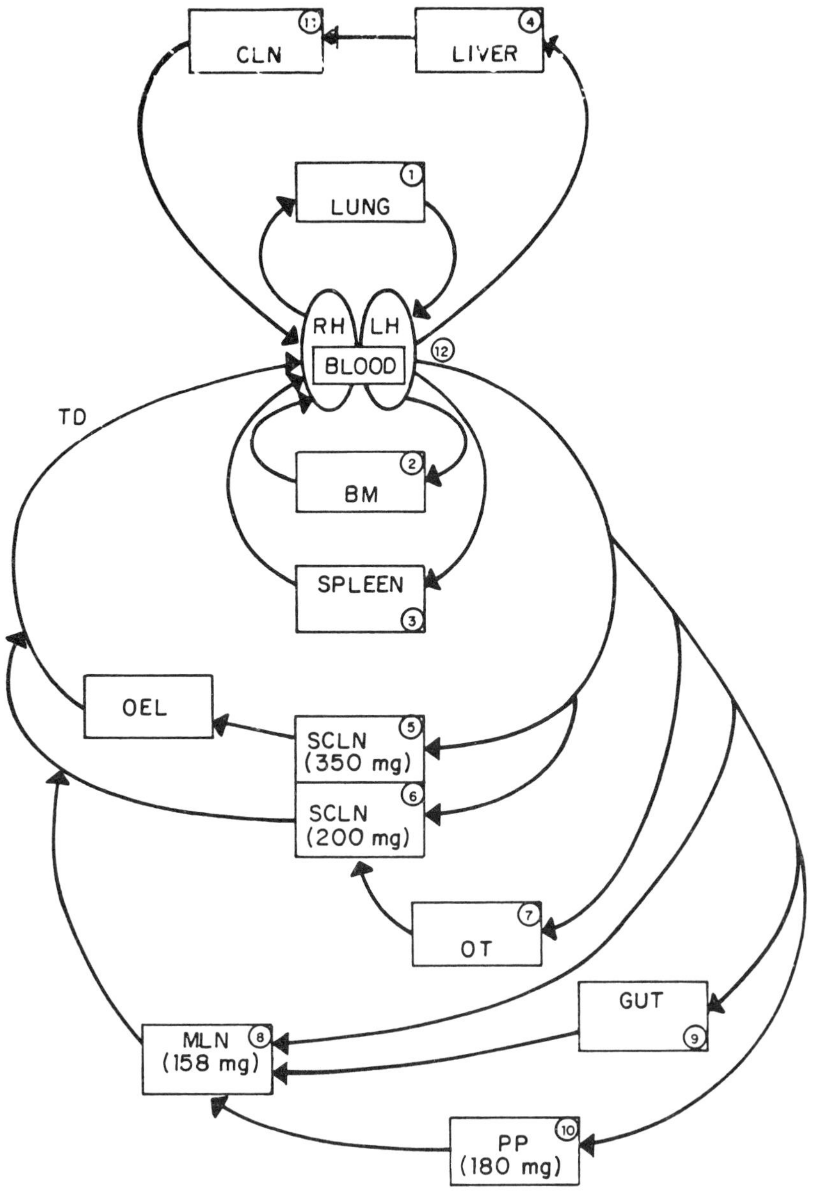

Fig. 1. Lymphocyte circulation

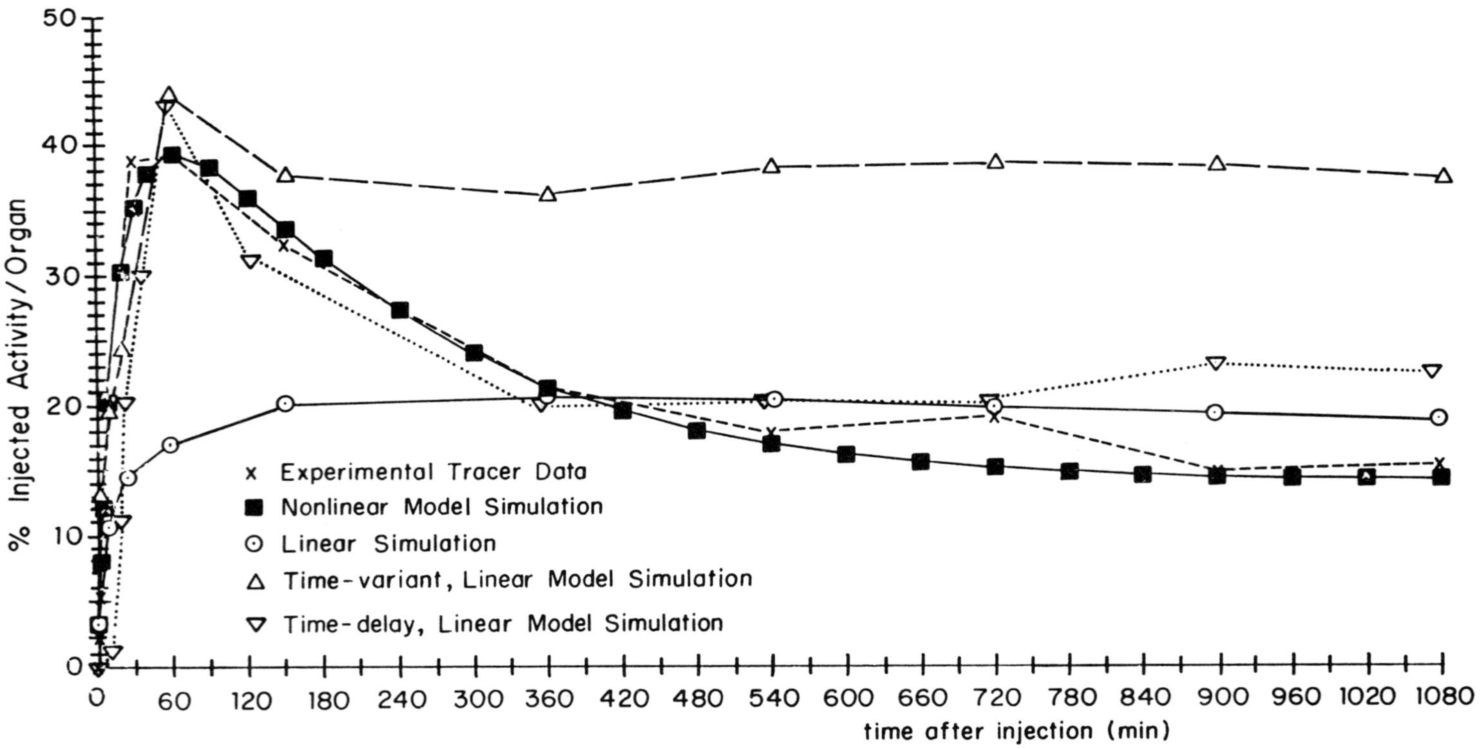

Fig. 2. Rat spleen lymphocyte response

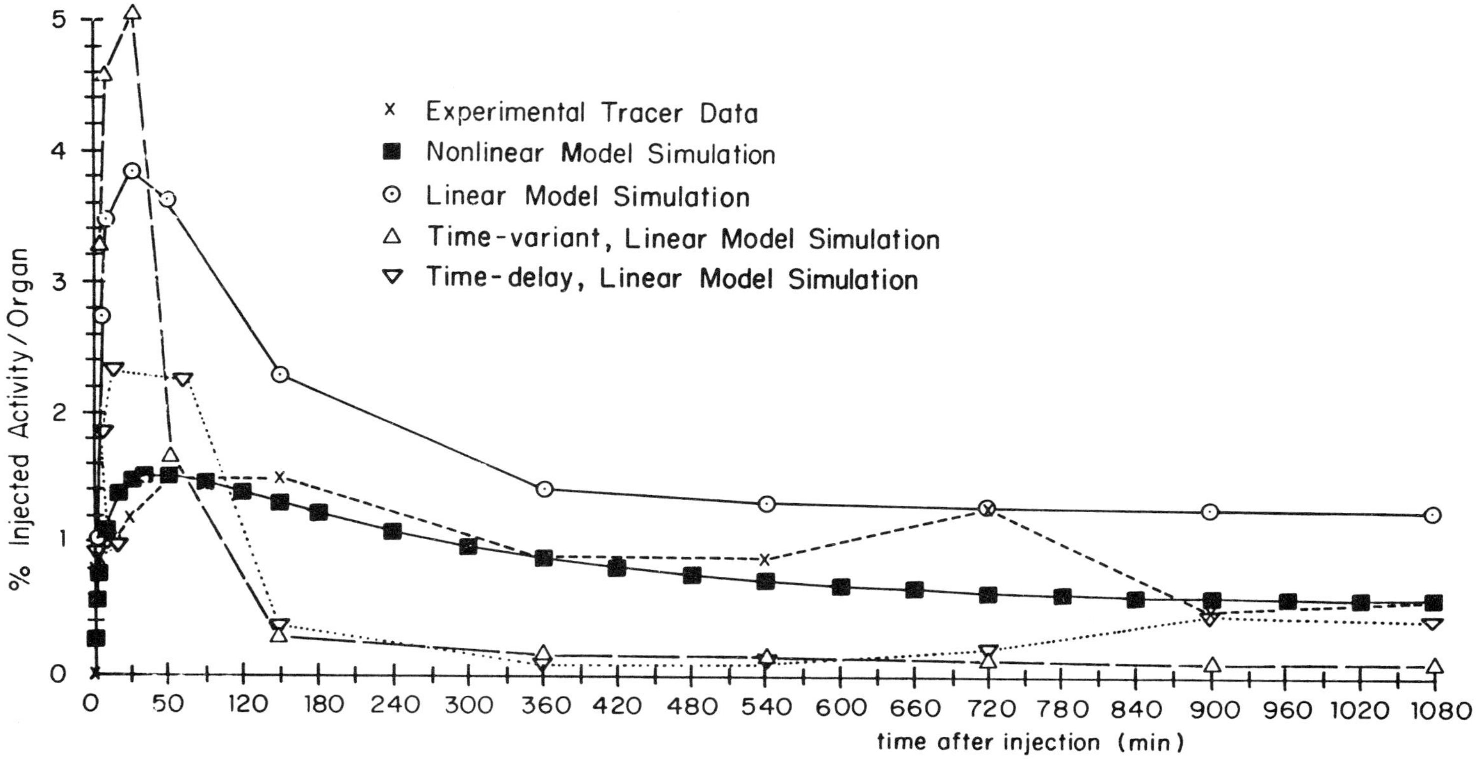

Fig. 3. Rat bone–marrow, lymphocyte response

Each of these organs can be treated as separate compartments with a percent of lymphocytes in that organ as its state. Many of the lymph nodes serve very similar functions and bear the same relation to blood and other organs so that they can be lumped together into a single compartment labeled subcutaneous lymph nodes. This was done with popliteal LN, deep and superficial cervial LN. They form the SCLN, in fig. 1. This compartment has been divided into two subcompartments, one of which drains the miscellaneous tissues while the other does not.

The most common approach to compartmental models assumes lumped time-invariant linearity with diffusions proportional to the concentration differences between the compartments. A slight generalization of this leads to the nonlinear, time-variant linear and time-invariant models derived from Mohler, Farooqi, and Heilig [8].

Here a new linear model is presented which considers time delays in the transport of lymphocytes between certain compartments. The state equations which evolve are given as follows:

$$\dot{x}_1(t) = \alpha_{12}x_{12}(t) - \beta_{12}(t) ,$$

$$\dot{x}_2(t) = \alpha_2 x_{12}(t) - \beta_2 x_2(t) - \gamma_2 x_2(t-\tau_2) ,$$

$$\dot{x}_3(t) = \alpha_3 x_{12}(t) - \beta_3 x_3(t) - \gamma_3 x_3(t-\tau_3) ,$$

$$\dot{x}_4(t) = \alpha_4 x_{12}(t) - \beta_4 x_4(t) - \gamma_4 x_4(t-\tau_4) ,$$

$$\dot{x}_5(t) = \alpha_5 x_{12}(t) - \beta_5 x_5(t) - \gamma_5 x_5(t-\tau_5) ,$$

$$\dot{x}_6(t) = \alpha_6 x_{12}(t) - \beta_7 x_7(t) - \gamma_7 x_7(t-\tau_7) - \beta_6 x_6(t) - \gamma_6 x_6(t-\tau_6) ,$$

$$\dot{x}_7(t) = \alpha_7 x_{12}(t) - \beta_7 x_7(t) - \gamma_7 x_7(t-\tau_7) ,$$

$$\dot{x}_8(t) = \alpha_8 x_{12}(t) - \beta_9 x_9(t) - \gamma_9 x_9(t-\tau_9) + \beta_{10} x_{10}(t) + \gamma_{10} x_{10}(t-\tau_{10}) - \beta_8 x_8(t) - \gamma_8 x_8(t-\tau_8) ,$$

$$\dot{x}_9(t) = \alpha_9 x_{12}(t) - \beta_9 x_9(t) - \gamma_9 x_9(t-\tau_9) ,$$

$$\dot{x}_{10}(t) = \alpha_{10} x_{12}(t) - \beta_{10} x_{10}(t) - \gamma_{10} x_{10}(t-\tau_{10}) ,$$

$$\dot{x}_{11}(t) = \beta_4 x_4(t) - \gamma_4 x_4(t-\tau_4) - \beta_{11} x_{11}(t) - \gamma_{11} x_{11}(t-\tau_{11}) ,$$

$$\dot{x}_{12}(t) = -(\dot{x}_1(t)+\dot{x}_2(t)+\dot{x}_3(t)+\dot{x}_5(t)) - (\alpha_4+\alpha_6+\alpha_7+\alpha_8+\alpha_9+\alpha_{10})x_{12}(t) + \beta_6 x_6(t) + \beta_8 x_8(t) + \beta_{11} x_{11}(t) + \gamma_8 x_8(t-\tau_8) + \gamma_{11} x_{11}(t-\tau_{11}) ,$$

$$\dot{x}_{13}(t) = x_5(t) + x_6(t) .$$

The subscripts refer to the following:

1 = lungs	7 = miscellaneous tissues
2 = bone marrow	8 = mesenteric LN
3 = spleen	9 = gut
4 = liver	10 = Peyer's patches
5 = SCLN with efferent lymphatics	11 = coeliac LN
	12 = blood
6 = SCLN with other tissues	13 = SCLN, total

The parameters α_i, β_i, γ_i ($i = 1, 12$) represent directional permeabilities that are proportional to flow rates in the various circulatory vessels and organs in different regions of the body. τ_i ($i = 2,...,11$) represent discrete-time delays in different organs. In all compartments other than the lungs and the blood there are two components to the output, one consisting of those lympho-cytes that enter the compartment and are just "flushed out" and the other consisting of those that stay in the compartment for some time before leaving it. The average period of this sojourn is the basis of time delays in this model.

TABLE 1
Model Parametric Values

i	1	2	3	4	5	6
α_i	1.0	0.01	0.1	0.3	0.016	0.005
β_i	0.8	0.015	0.0007	0.3	0.0001	0.008
γ_i	–	0.004	0.0075	0.0005	0.0027	0.0065
τ_i	–	250	60	60	180	150

i	7	8	9	10	11
α_i	0.05	0.006	0.02	0.012	
β_i	0.002	0.0006	0.03	0.001	0.7
γ_i	0.0004	0.0035	0.0005	0.0023	0.001
τ_i	300	150	150	180	180

The simulation results for the spleen, bone marrow, lungs and liver are compared with the experimental data in figs. 2–5. In general the fit of the model is quite close to the data. The state equations used here are time–invariant, linear, delay differential equations. It is interesting to compare the results obtained here with those in [8], which are reproduced here for the sake of convenience. The present model gives a better approximation to the real system than the two previous linear models.

Because of the nature of the radiolabeling process, mostly T–cells were studied in the experiment by Smith and Ford [7]. B–cells and T–cells do not experience the same time delays in different compartments. For example, the time delays for B–cells are much larger for B–cells than T–cells in the lymph nodes. In this paper lymphocytes have been treated as one broad category of cells and have not been separated into T– and B–cells. Time–delays in the model are thus approximations for the broad category and not for one of the sub–categories. This will have to wait until data is available on T–cells and B–cells separately. That will also result in a better fit to the real system. For example, then two time–delay terms could be used in the equations for SCLN, one term for the T–cells and one for B–cells. Thus more statistical data needs to be collected for a more complete model of lymphocyte recirculation.

While the nonlinear model seems to mimic lymphocyte circulation most accurately, the time–delay linear model does approximate the following experimental results. After a rapid lymphocyte exchange with the *lungs* during the first couple of minutes after injection, the level of blood lymphocytes decreases for the next hour with a half life of approximately 16 minutes. As lymphocytes return to *blood* (particularly from spleen), the exponential decay ceases 1 and 2.5 hours after injection followed by a slow rise to near equilibrium at 6 hours onward. Localization of lymphocytes in the *liver* is somewhat similar to blood in its time response, but has a slower terminal decay of approximately a 24–minute half life. Approximately 40 percent of the injected lymphocytes are found in the spleen at the 30 minute mark. This is followed by a decay mode of approximately 300–minute half life. *LN lymphocytes* gradually build up to almost 60 percent in about 18 hours. *MLN* and *SCLN* responses have a similar shape. *Peyer's patch level* builds up to about 7 percent in about 1.5 hours. Modeling of the liver is particularly complicated due apparently to three independent phenomena involving the lymphocyte migration. First, there is intravascular pooling similar to lungs, which results in rapid initial response. Then there is genuine recirculation blood to liver, to coeliac LN, to thoracic duct and back to blood again. Finally, there is an accumulation of dying cells in liver which involves only about 1% to 2% of the total population per day. Still, the latter can be a substantial part of the liver response itself. This may very well account for the long–term error which was found between the model simulation and certain other compartments—such as liver.

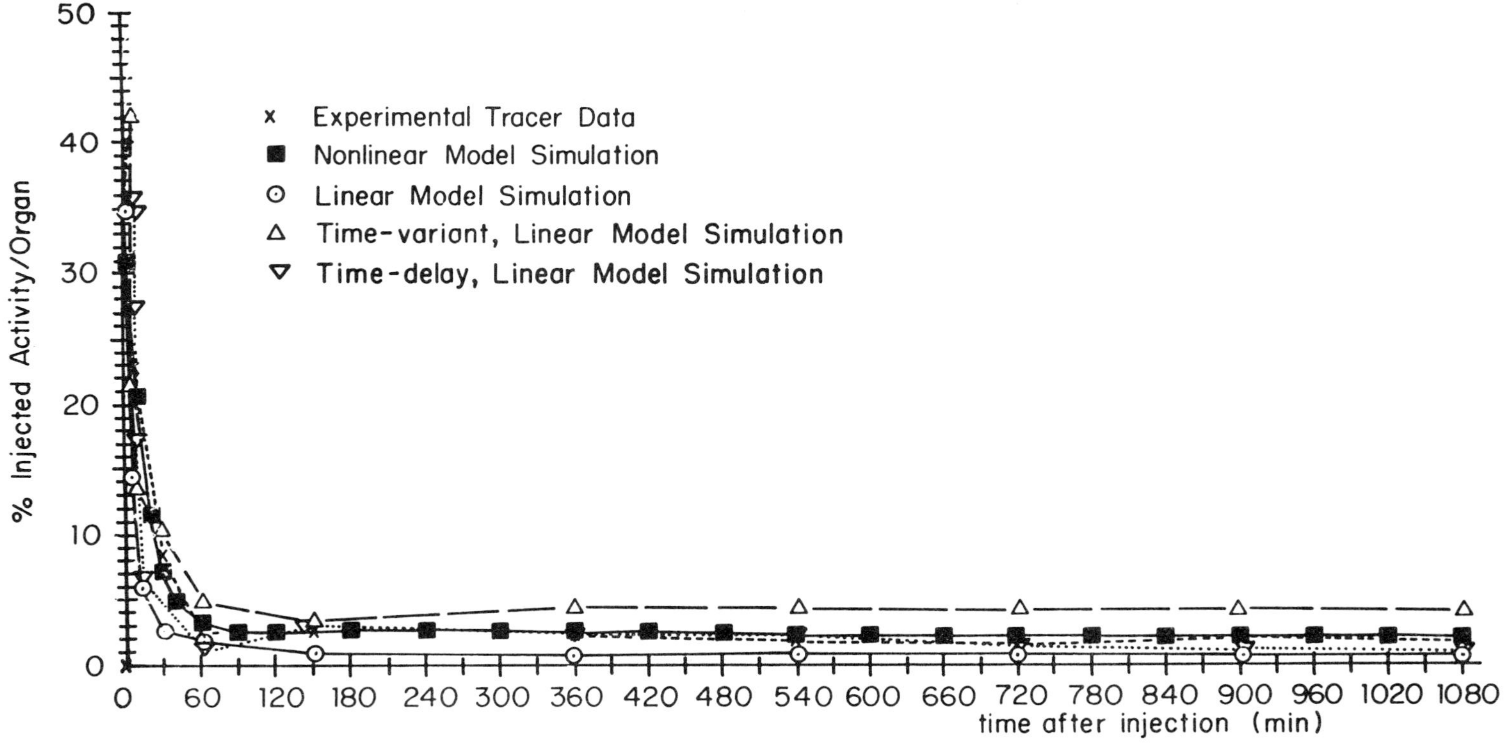

Fig. 4. Rat lungs, lymphocyte response

4. Lymph node model

Lymph nodes are the only lymphoid organs placed in the course of lymphatic vessels. While tonsils, spleen and thymus have only efferent lymphatics, lymph nodes are the entrance port for lymphocytes crossing from blood to lymph. As shown in fig. 1, lymphatic vessels collect cells which leave the blood in tissue. Consequently, these cells are passed through a chain of lymph nodes prior to their return to blood via the thoracic duct. In some cases, lymphocytes seem to find their way into lymph by direct entry to lymph nodes.

Based on information available in the literature [11], [12], lymph node lymphocyte pathways may be represented by fig. 5. While lymph nodes are conventionally divided into superficial cortex, deep cortex and medulla, these regions merge with no clear boundaries. Thus, they are inappropriate compartments for studies which rely on tracer measurements. Both T– and B–cells enter the lymph mode by crossing walls of the high endothelial venules, HEV. T–cells either remain in the paracortex surrounding the HEV or move to nearby paracortical nodules. Meanwhile, B–cells (of the lymphocyte population) migrate to primary follicles and to lymphocyte corona in the superficial cortex [12].

A detailed derivation of the lymph node model will be given in another publication. Briefly, however, the model is of the form identical to that above comprising a time–delay set of ordinary differential equations. For each node (whether subcutaneous, mesenteric, coeliac or whatever), the basic model takes the following form:

$$
\begin{aligned}
\dot{x}_h(t) &= \alpha_h x_{12}(t) - \beta_h x_h(t) \,, \\
\dot{x}_s(t) &= \alpha_s x_{12}(t) - \beta_s x_s(t) \,, \\
\dot{x}_{i1}(t) &= \alpha_i [x_h(t-\tau_i)] \,, \\
\dot{x}_{i2}(t) &= \alpha_i x_h(t-\tau_i) - \beta_{i2} x_{i2}(t) \,, \\
\dot{x}_{p1}(t) &= (1-f_p)\alpha_p x_{i2}(t) + f_q \alpha_p x_{i2}(t-\tau_p) - \beta_p x_{p1}(t) \,, \\
\dot{x}_{p2}(t) &= f_p \alpha_p [x_{i2}(t) - x_{i2}(t-\tau_p)] \,, \\
\dot{x}_{f1}(t) &= (1-f_p)\alpha_f [x_i(t) - x_i(t-\tau_f)] \,, \\
\dot{x}_{f2}(t) &= f_p \alpha_f [x_i(t) - x_i(t-\tau_f)] \,, \\
\dot{x}_m(t) &= \alpha_m x_{p1}(t) - \beta_m x_m(t) \,.
\end{aligned}
$$

Here, the subscripts refer to the following:

h = high endothelial walls,
s = superficial sinuses,
i = interfollicular interstitum,
p = paracortical nodules,
f = follicular nodules,
m = medullary sinuses.

f_p is the fraction of delayed cells in paracortical nodules and follicular nodes. As before, the parameters depend on appropriate lymph or blood flow rates, compartmental volumes and resistances.

While a few of the parameters such as for high endothelial walls (HEW) and medullary sinuses are reasonably well determined, the same is not true for cortex parameters. Unfortunately, experimental results are extremely limited.

Fig. 6 shows a comparison of the model simulation, with the various compartmental populations summed up relative to the previous experimental results of Smith and Ford [7]. It was found that this total lymph node response in very insensitive with respect to changes in the time delays τ_i, τ_p, τ_f. The corresponding simulated response for the various lymphocyte population was broken down in T– and B–cells for the medullary sinuses, since separate relative values of α_m and β_m are available for T– and B–cells.

After injection of labelled thoracic–duct cells, there is a steep rise in population during the first sixty minutes, corresponding to the exponential fall in blood. When the concentration in blood reaches equilibrium, the rise slows significantly, but it is maintained until 12 hours after injection. The simulation matches the data quite accurately.

The population of HEW cells rises sharply after injection to reach a peak only 20 minutes later. Then a steep decline results in an approximate equilibrium value of 1% after only 2 hours. This is consistent with qualitative descriptions [12]. The peak in the paracortex is reached only slightly before that of the total lymph node projection—about ten hours after injection. It would be expected to be similar since a majority reside in the paracortex. Inspecting the interfollicular–intestitium region of the cortex an initial sharp rise to a peak at 90 minutes is observed which is followed by an exponential decay toward equilibrium after about three hours. The uptake in paracortical nodules and follicular nodes does not begin until about 90 minutes after injection—reaching maxima at 11 and 20 hours, respectively.

Medullar sinuses show a small population increase at about two hours after injection, reaching a peak at four hours, followed by a second peak about eight hours later. The latter is due to the release of cells from the paracortical nodes.

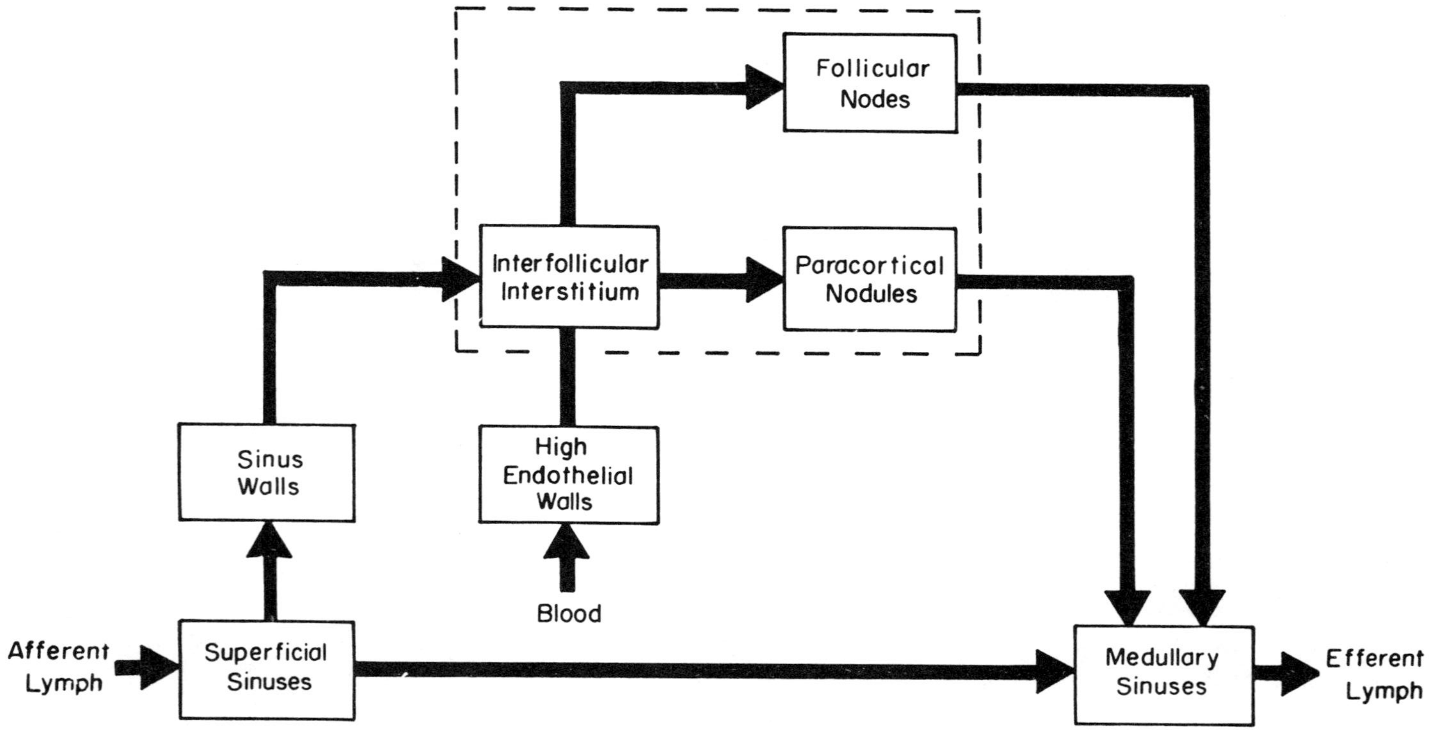

Fig. 5. Lymphocyte pathway through a lymph node

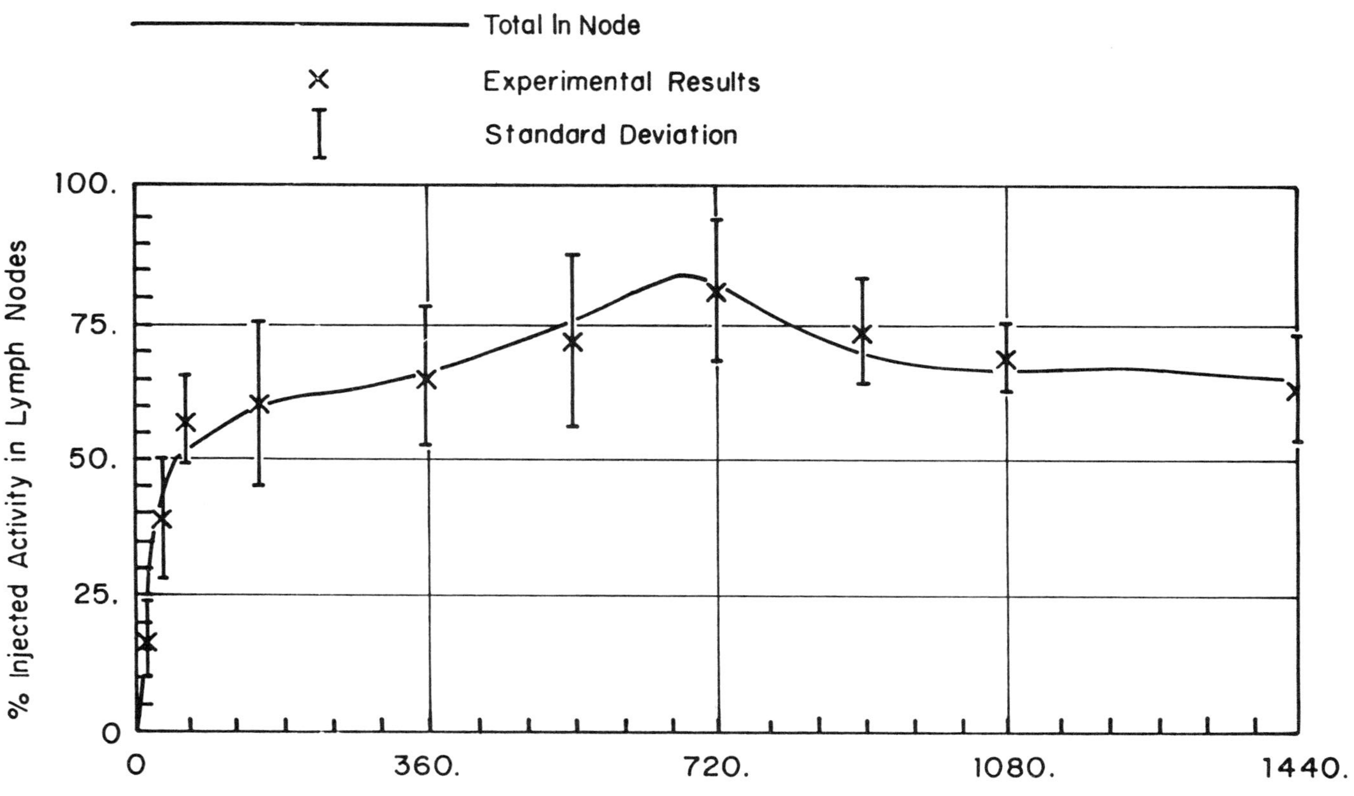

Fig. 6. Comparison of lymph node experimental data and simulation

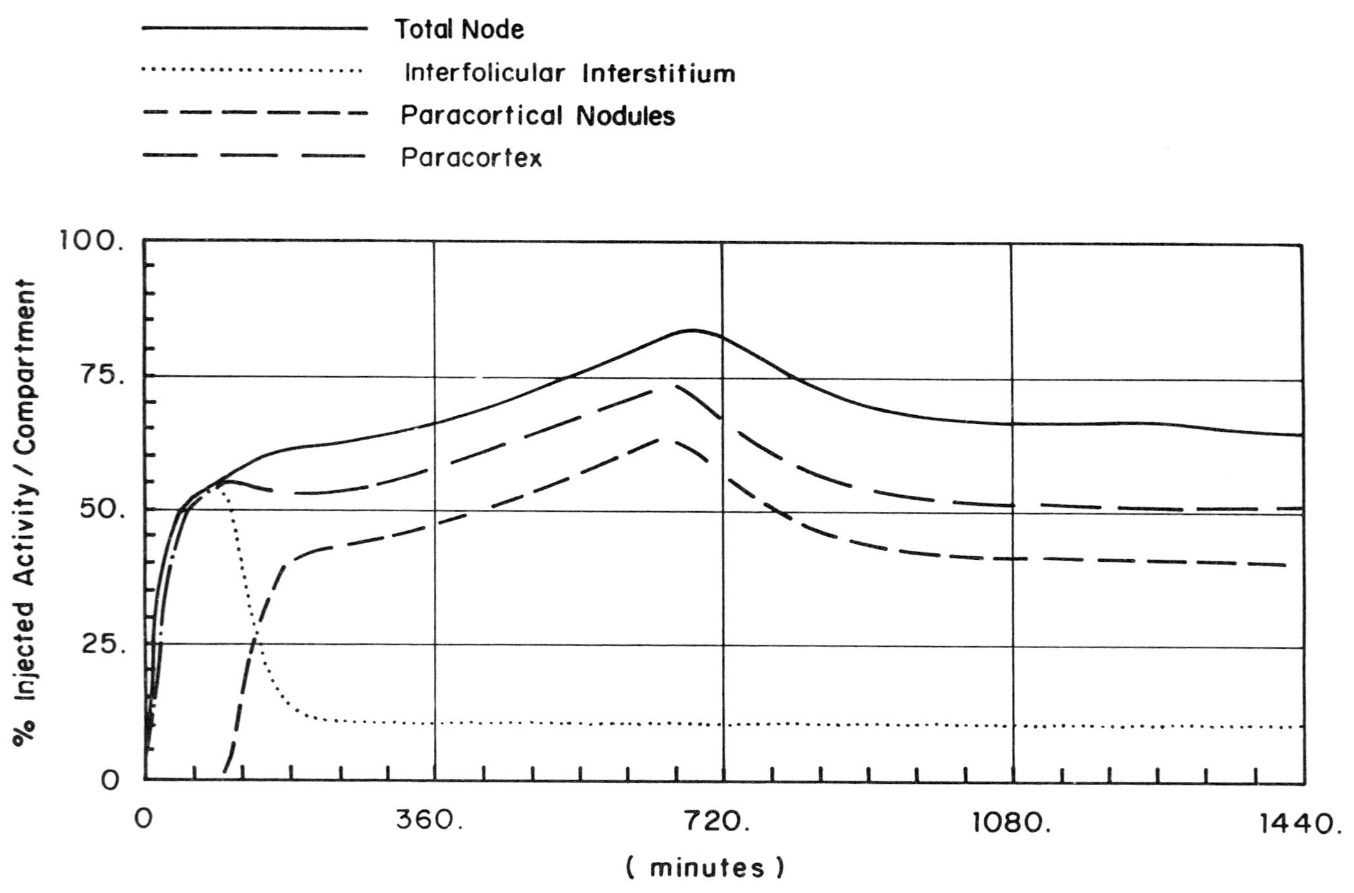

Fig. 7. Simulation of lymphocyte response in node compartment

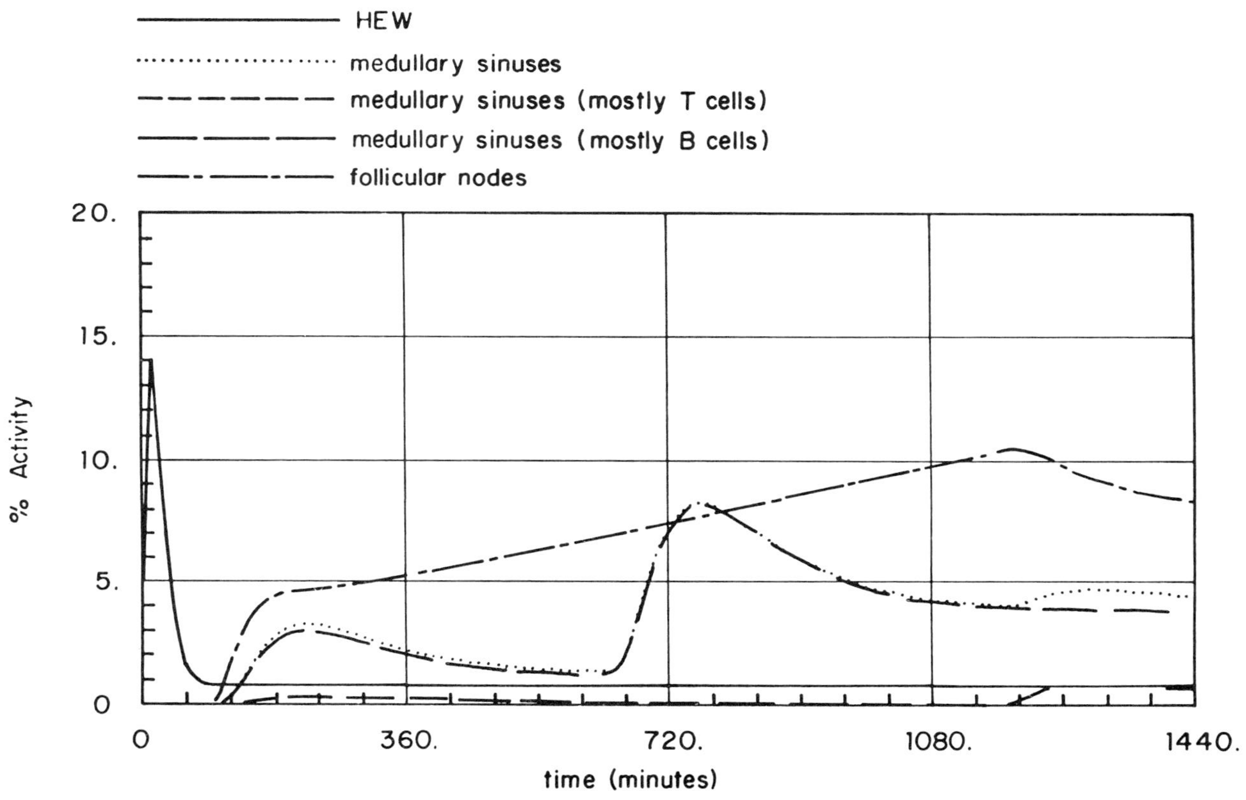

Fig. 8. Simulation particular nodes

Conclusion

It is seen that linear time–delay differential equations mimic the experimental data for lymphocyte distribution of rats within the accuracy of the data available. Unfortunately, more extensive data is required to do an adequate job of parameter estimation, and such data is not readily obtained. This is particularly true for the lymph–node compartments presented here as a building–block synthesis of the lymphatic system. Eventually, it is hoped that data will be available to check models for dynamic behavior of antibodies and antigen as well as T– and B–lymphocytes.

Acknowledgement

The authors are grateful for the collaboration of Academician G.I. Marchuk and his associates and their encouragement of our research by their ability to apply such results to health care delivery. The authors wish to express their gratitude for the experimental cooperation of Professor Bill Ford (University of Manchester Medical School) and his associates, and, at the same time, to express our bereavement at the recent sudden death of Professor Ford. The profession has lost a great man.

REFERENCES

[1] Roitt, I. *Essential Immunology*. London Oxford: Blackwell Scientific, 1974.

[2] Bell, G.I., A.S. Perelson, and G.H. Pimbley, Jr., eds. *Theoretical Immunology*. New York: Marcel Dekker, 1978.

[3] Mohler, R.R., C. Bruni, and A. Gondolfi. 1980. A systems approach to immunology. *IEEE Proc*. 68:964-90.

[4] Marchuk, G.I. *Mathematical Models in Immunology*. New York: Optimization Software, Inc., Publications Division, 1984. (English transl.)

[5] Marchuk, G.I., and L.N. Belykh, eds. *Mathematical Modelling in Immunology and Medicine. Proceedings of the IFIP TC-7 Working Conference on Mathematical Modelling in Immunology and Medicine*, Moscow, USSR, 5-11 July, 1982. Amsterdam New York Oxford: North-Holland Publ. Co., 1983.

[6] DeSousa, M. *Lymphocyte Circulation*. Chicester, U.K.: John Wiley & Sons Publ. Co., 1981.

[7] Smith, M.E., and W.L. Ford. 1983. The recirculating lymphocyte pool of the rat: a systematic description of the migratory behavior of recirculating lymphocytes. *Immunology* 49:83-94.

[8] Mohler, R.R., Z. Farooqi, and T. Heilig. 1978. An immune lymphocyte circulation model. In *System Modelling and Optimization.* Proceedings of the 11th IFIP Conference, Copenhagen, Denmark, July 25-29, 1983, ed. P. Thoft-Christensen, 694-702. Lecture Notes in Control and Information Sciences 59. Berlin New York Heidelberg Tokyo: Springer-Verlag, 1984.

[9] Mohler, R.R., and C.F. Barton. 1978. Compartmental control model of the immune process. *Optimization Techniques*, ed. J. Stoer, part 1, 421-30. *Proceedings of the 8th IFIP Conference on Optimization Techniques,* Wurzburg, September 5-9, 1977. Lecture Notes in Control and Information Sciences 6. Berlin New York Heidelberg Tokyo: Springer-Verlag, 1978.

[10] Yoffey, J.M., and F.C. Courtice. *Lymphatics, Lymph and the Lymphomyeloid Complex.* London: Academic Press, 1970.

[11] Fossum, S., M.E. Smith, and W.l. Ford. 1983. The recirculation of T- and B-lymphocytes in the athymic nude rat. *Scand. J. Immunology* 17:551-57.

[12] Nieuwenhuis, P., and W.L. Ford. 1976. Comparative migration of B- and T-lymphocytes in the rat spleen and lymph nodes. *Cell. Immunology* 23:254-67.

MATHEMATICAL METHODS FOR DATA PROCESSING AND MODEL CONSTRUCTION FOR VIRAL HEPATITIS

N.I. Nisevich+, I.I. Zubikova+, I.B. Pogozhev, A.A. Romanyukha

+ Department of Infantile Infectious Diseases of the
Second Moscow State Medical Institute

Department of Numerical Mathematics of the USSR
Academy of Sciences

A great number of methods for evaluating the functional state of the liver in patients with viral hepatitis have been developed and are now being introduced into clinical practice for assessing the gravity of the pathological process. The aim of the clinician is to find an appropriate combination of biochemical indicators, which together with the clinical data would accurately determine the functioning of the liver, minimizing however the number of these indicators. Since the degree of the functional damage to the liver does not always correspond to the gravity of disease and no test can accurately demonstrate all of the hepatic functions, clinicians have to use a great wealth of clinical and laboratory indices in order to accurately evaluate the gravity of the disease as well as the extent of the liver damage and the dynamics of the functional restoration of the organ. To thoroughly analyze the disease pathogenesis and, in turn, appropriately prescribe a therapy and evaluate the outcome in each individual case, one needs to employ a wide spectrum of methods. It is difficult, if not practically impossible, to correctly interpret the available information concerning the condition of each individual patient with viral hepatitis, or any other disease. The constructing of mathematical models for computer processing of clinical and laboratory data requires the joint effort of clinicians and mathematicians, as an interdisciplinary team.

1. Application of mathematical models for clinical and laboratory data processing

As is well known, it is the liver which is the main victim of viral hepatitis. An estimation of the degree of hepatic damage requires numerous laboratory tests.

The welter of biochemical indices, their inconsistent changes with respect to the degree of the organ's damage, as well as the lack of correspondence between the clinical manifestation of the disease and the degree of functional damage of the liver—all this makes the interpretation of the data and the estimation of the severity of viral hepatitis a difficult task. Therefore, the clinician needs to find a general technique for the combined analysis of the clinical symptoms and biochemical indices, keeping the number of biochemical tests for each patient within reasonable bounds.

It has been established that among 72 biochemical tests which reflect the various functional disorders in the liver only five tests provide sufficient information and at the same time are easy to use: the content of bilirubin and its fractions which reflect the hepatic pigmental dysfunctioning; the activity of fructose–1–phosphataldolase which characterizes the intensity of cytolytic processes of the hepatocyte; and one of the indicators of the protein—synthetic liver function—the content of β–lipoproteins. Among biochemical indices, the most typical for viral hepatitis are: flaccidity, loss of appetite, vomiting, ictericity of the skin and sclera, enlarged liver, a hemorrhagic syndrome and agitation.

We introduce a clinical index (φ_c) and a biochemical index (φ_b) in the formula for estimating the gravity of viral hepatitis (gravity index φ_s). The clinical index φ_c accounts for the above–mentioned symptoms: flaccidity (A), loss of appetite (Ar), vomiting (V), ictericity of the skin and sclera (I), enlarged liver (S), hemorrhagic syndrome (H), and agitation (R). We estimate the degree of each symptom by 1, 2, 3 (1093 case histories). The clinical index is given by the formula

$$\varphi_c = 0.25(A + Ar + V + I + S + H + R) .$$

Substituting the corresponding value for the degree of each symptom gives us the clinical index for an individual patient.

To calculate the biochemical index (φ_b), we have used Todorov's hypothesis concerning the mechanism of liver pigmental dysfunctioning and the notion of a mechanism of hyperfermentemia and bilirubin–protein dissociation suggested by Bluger. The formula for the biochemical index is:

$$\begin{aligned}\varphi_b &= K_1(p)[0.1(p - 1.5) + 0.02(f - 1.2) + 0.005(\beta - 40)] \\ &\quad + K_2(p)\left[\frac{20}{\beta} + \frac{b+B}{5f}\right] ,\end{aligned}$$

where b is the content of free bilirubin (mg%), B is the content of conjugated bilirubin (mg%), f is the activity of fructose–1–phosphataldolase (units), β is the content of β–lipoproteins (units). The disorder of the liver pigmental function is expressed in terms of free bilirubin $p = b + 3B$. The coefficients are $K_1 = 2.2 - 0.12p$ and $K_2 = 2 - K_1$ [1].

To calculate the clinical and biochemical indices we used a mathematical formalization: the values of the indices equal to 1, 2, and 3 correspond to the light, medium–severe and severe forms of viral hepatitis, those in the range of 2.5 to 3.0 correspond to the medium–severe form with transition to the severe form, and those in the range of 1.5 to 2.0 to the light form with transition to the medium–severe form.

The gravity index (φ_s) accounts for the set of various clinical symptoms, denoted by φ_c, as well as the gravity of the liver functional state (φ_b)

$$\varphi_s = 0.25\varphi_c + 0.75\varphi_b .$$

Thus, the formula for estimating the gravity of the pathological process accounts for 12 various clinical and biochemical indices, allowing for each index. The weight coefficients in this formula are obtained by a statistical analysis.

The quantitative values of the biochemical and clinical indices for estimating the severity of the disease have been determined during the peak of the disease.

In some cases there may be a lack of correspondence between the clinical condition of the patient and the degree of functional disorder. This has been observed, as a rule, in children in the first year of life, when strongly pronounced clinical manifestations combine with relatively small functional disturbance, and also when the disease is accompanied by pronounced cholestasia.

Compared with the estimation of the gravity of the desease in children with viral hepatitis via the most commonly used clinical methods, the estimation via the gravity–index method proved accurate in 97% of 398 patients examined. The quantitative methods significantly contribute to the accurate estimation of the gravity of viral hepatitis in children.

In our attempt to do without the quantitative method in estimating the liver functional capacity—the biochemical index—we studied this method in the disease dynamics in order to determine the hepatic functional–recovery rate, using the following normalization method. The values of the biochemical index in the disease dynamics (in an individual patient) are divided by the value of the index during the peak of the disease (i.e., the period of the highest gravity of the disease). We call this index the "relative biochemical index." Its dynamics, independent of the disease gravity, gives a good picture of the liver functional–recovery rate with respect to the greatest functional disorder during the peak of the disease.

Since the greatest functional disorder (the peak of the viral hepatitis) occurs randomly, in a different number of days after the onset of the disease, we examined the dynamics of the liver functional recovery beginning from the peak of the disease. For an individual patient, we marked the values of the relative biochemical index on a particular day (beginning with the peak of the disease) on a diagram, and then drew a straight line to connect these points, obtaining thus the dynamics of the liver functional recovery in each patient.

The analysis of the functional–recovery process in a large group of patients having a smooth course of illness showed that in 88% of the children the dynamic processes lie in an area with confidence intervals depending neither on the gravity of the disease nor on age. It turned out that, in general, the process of recovery in this area can be described by an exponential curve, which we call the universal curve of liver functional recovery (figure 1). We found out that the liver functional recovery in the majority of patients occurs at a fixed rate of 12% a day. Moreover, in 6% of the patients, the liver functional recovery was slower and its dynamics went beyond the upper boundary of the confidence interval.

Taking into account the fact that the dynamics of the liver functional recovery in the overwhelming majority of patients with smooth course of the disease (88%) remains within the universal curve, it is appropriate to use the dynamics as the criterion for estimating the process of the liver functional recovery of each individual patient during hospitalization.

The data on the rate of the liver functional recovery of each patient is entered under the heading "the liver functional recovery." The space under the heading "Norm," bounded by the upper and lower confidence intervals, corresponds to the normal or universal rate of recovery. Other two areas are: slow functional recovery—above the universal curve, and fast recovery—below the curve. Marking the values of the relative biochemical index after each subsequent biochemical test and connecting the points by straight line, the clinician can compare the rate of the liver functional recovery in a particular patient with the universal curve between two biochemical tests. There is no other, more reliable method in clinical practice for estimating the rate of functional recovery of the liver. The comparison of the results of each subsequent blood test with the previous results allows the clinician, in addition to his or her own experience, to classify the dynamics of functional recovery only generally as "satisfactory," "good" and "slow." Therefore, the "universal curve" is a valuable supplement to the usual clinical observation of the disease dynamics.

Let us give an example. A child of 14 has a disease which starts in acute form: temperature elevating to 39.0°C, flaccidity, loss of appetite. The next day, the temperature falls to 37.8°C, but flaccidity and poor appetite remain. On the 3rd and 4th days, temperature returns to normal but vomiting appears. In a few days, the child's condition slightly improves but poor appetite still remains. On the 10th day of the illness the abdominal pain develops and the skin and sclera become icteric and the urine dark.

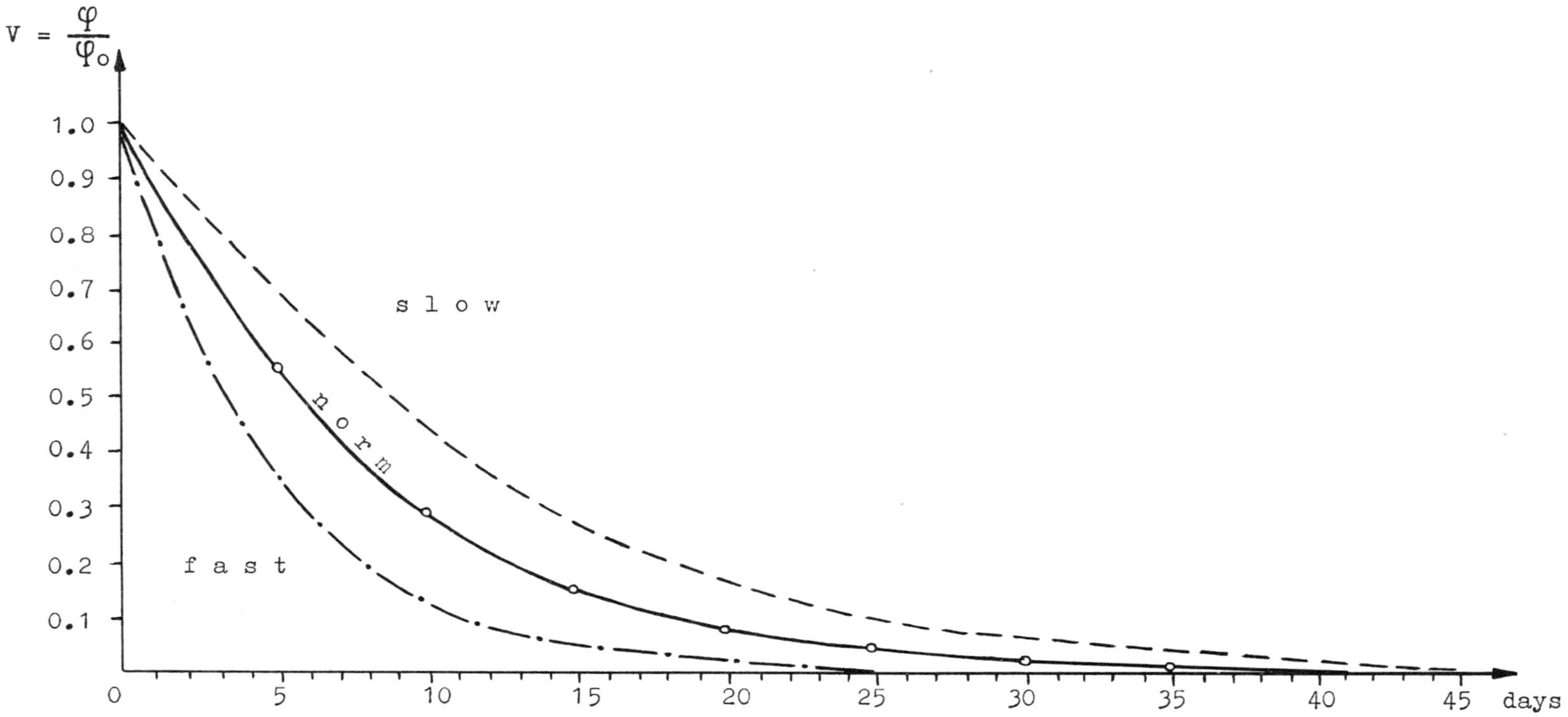

Fig. 1. Universal curve of the liver functional recovery in viral hepatitis smooth course

The patient was hospitalized on the 15th day of illness (on the 5th day of the icteric period) with the medium–grave moderate symptoms of intoxication: flaccidity, 2; appetite, 2; medium ictericity of the skin and sclera, 2. The liver protruded by 1 cm below the costal arch, 1; the spleen by less than 0.5 cm. The urine was dark, the feces discolored. $\varphi_c = 1.75$, $\varphi_b = 1.46$, $\varphi_s = 1.52$. The diagnosis: viral hepatitis A in light form.

The intoxication symptoms disappeared soon; the skin and sclera remained icteric until the 17th day of the icteric period. By the 20th day of the icteric period the liver protruded by 0.5 cm below the costal arch. On the 35th day of the disease (the 25th day of the icteric period) the acute respiratory viral disease (ARVI) developed.

The results of the biochemical blood tests for this patient are the following:

DATE (1975)	9/3	9/10	9/20	9/29	10/8	10/16
ICTERIC PERIOD (days)	5	12	22	31	40	48
INDICES						
Total bilirubin (mg %)	3.75	1.95	1.50	0.38	0.75	0.87
Conjugated bilirubin (mg %)	2.64	0.95	0.75	0.15	0.25	0.13
Free bilirubin (mg %)	1.11	1.00	1.25	0.23	0.50	0.74
Fructose–1–phosphataldolase (units)	6.5	6.0	7.0	9.5	17.0	13.0
Thymol test (units)	49	45	30	22	36	46
β–lipoproteins (units)	43	65	38	41	39	37
Biochemical index	1.46	0.85	0.51	0.33	0.61	0.46
Relative biochemical index	1.00	0.58	0.35	0.22	0.41	0.31

Calculating the values of the relative biochemical index and marking their values on the universal curve (figure 2), we obtained the dynamics of the liver functional recovery in the patient. The table shows the tendency of the liver functional recovery to slow down on the 17th day following t_0 (peak of the disease) while the dynamics of the relative biochemical index goes beyond the upper confidence level. ARVI aggravates the pathological process in the liver due to the intensified cytolytic process in the hepatocyte.

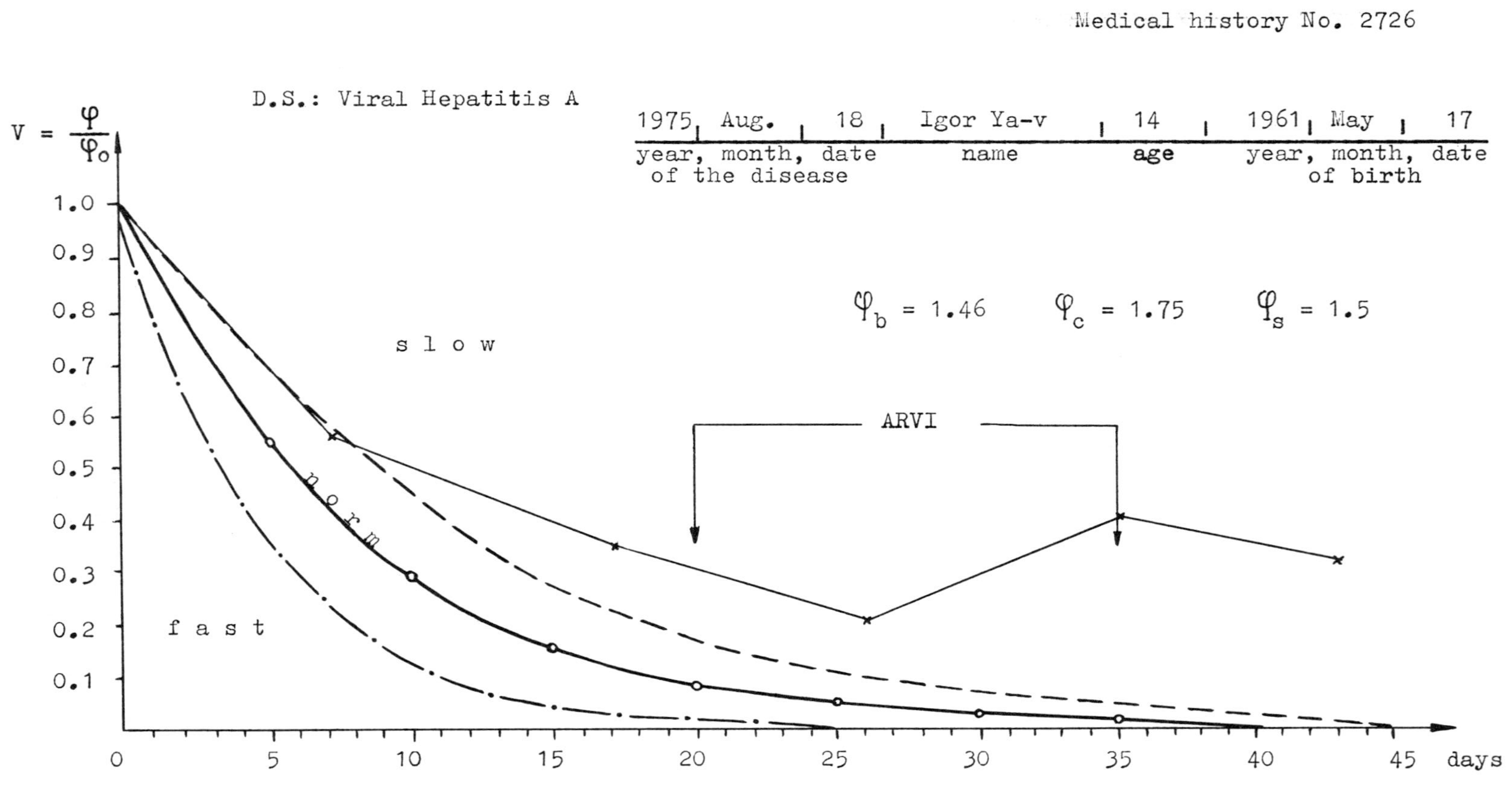

Fig. 2. An example of universal curve application in clinical practice

Using the universal curve to control the dynamics of the liver functional recovery, the clinician will be able to observe the slower recovery well before the biochemical indices reflect the situation and find out the possible causes (the effect of intercurrent diseases, the exacerbation of the previous diseases, etc.), and also determine how the prescribed therapy affects the recovery of the liver functional capacity.

Using a quantitative method for estimating the liver functional capacity—the biochemical index—and the universal curve, which reflects the dynamics of the liver functional recovery, we investigated the problem of estimating the damage to the hepatic functional capacity and the rate of its recovery in acute, protracted and chronic forms of viral hepatitis, in order to obtain the necessary information for diagnosing the disease at the earliest stage. We examined the liver functional damage using the biochemical index in 954 patients with the acute form, 76 patients with protracted form, and 63 patients with chronic form of viral hepatitis. The severity of the liver functional damage during the peak of the illness does not seem to be a factor for the prognosis of the course of disease. However, the majority of patients with the protracted and chronic forms of viral hepatitis showed a smaller damage of the liver during the peak of the illness than those with the acute form. Thus, in patients with the acute and light forms of viral hepatitis the biochemical index was 1.43 during the peak of the illness and in patients with the protracted and chronic viral hepatitis, 1.03 and 0.97, respectively.

Examining the rate of the liver functional recovery for an acute course, we discovered that 8–10 days after the illness peak, the quantitative classification of patients was the following: 78% of patients with normal rate, 16% with slow rate, and 6% with fast rate. At the same time, the slow rate of functional recovery was observed in 50% of the patients with the protracted course and in patients with further chronization. Using the data on the rate of the liver functional recovery in each sample group of patients, we calculated the prognosis probability of the course of viral hepatitis in children, including the liver functional recovery.

With the normal rate of functional capacity, the probability of acute course is equal to 0.93; for protracted course, 0.04, and chronic course, 0.03. Among the patients with a slow rate of functional recovery the probability of chronic form and protracted form increases sharply and is equal to 0.13 and 0.15, respectively. It means that on the average one child out of 8 (with slow rate of functional recovery) may have chronic hepatitis as the outcome of the disease.

The application of the clinical index showed that the rate of clinical recovery in the acute course is approximately equal to the rate of the liver functional recovery, i.e., about 12% a day. The dynamics of the clinical index at the time of the patient's discharge from the hospital slightly slows down compared to the universal curve. This can be caused by the enlarged liver, which is found in 30% of the patients with the light form of the disease and in 50% of the patients with the medium–severe form.

A comparative analysis of the clinical recovery dynamics in patients with acute and chronic forms shows that the clinical recovery is much slower in patients with the chronic viral hepatitis due to a flaccid or no contraction of the liver. Hence, the patients with a slow rate of hepatic functional recovery and with a slow rate of clinical recovery (8–10 days after the peak of the disease) may need additional clinical and laboratory tests, because they may most probably develop a chronic illness. However, we need to take into account the fact that the rate of the liver functional recovery during the peak of the disease in 50% of the patients with potential chronic hepatitis is not different from that given by the universal curve.

Therefore, if the chronic form of viral hepatitis is most probable, the clinician needs to use more than the general biochemical tests; for example, in the persistent splenohepatomegalia, additional tests—such as determination of the isoenzymes LDH and MDH and of the HBs– and HBe–antigens, rheo–hepatography, ultrasonic examination, a puncture biopsy of the liver (if prescribed)—are recommended.

One of the players in the pathogenesis of viral hepatitis is the body's immune system and therefore the immunological indices are of special interest. However, it is difficult to correctly interpret these immunological indices because they are so numerous and ambiguous. Our objective was to devise a generalized immunity index to use in solving particular clinical problems.

To determine such an index, in 179 patients with viral hepatitis of different states of gravity, in addition to a very thorough clinical examination, biochemical tests were made: during the period of illness, 5–7 tests of the blood serum and the tests to determine the concentration of E_t – PFC, E_a – PFC, E_s – PFC, EAC – PFC, and the concentration of G, A, M immunoglobulines. E_t – PFC, E_a – PFC, and E_s – PFC are lymphocytes of the peripheral blood forming rosettes with sheep erythrocytes under different conditions (E_t the total, E_a the active, E_s the stable). The EAC–PFC are lymphocytes forming rosettes with EAC complex (sheep erythrocytes, antierythrocytic rabbit serum, mice complement). The lymphocytes forming rosettes with sheep erythrocytes are T–cells, and the lymphocytes with a EAC–complex are B–cells [2].

To evaluate the dynamics of the pathological process in patients with viral hepatitis, we used a general biochemical index which characterizes the liver functional state.

Certain indices of the cellular and humoral immunity provide some information concerning the immunological condition of the patient. However we, like many other researchers, confronted a difficult problem of appropriately interpreting them in clinical practice—because the changes in the indices are qualitatively and quantitatively inconsistent. Our intention was to generalize the indices containing the largest amount of information on the condition of the body's immune system in order to create a general estimation criterion which characterizes the expressivity of the immune response in children with viral hepatitis, and to see how one can apply this criterion in practice. To this end, we constructed the immunological index Im. Since this index is based on the most informative indices of cellular and humoral immunity, it enables one to estimate the expressivity of an immune response versus normal. The values of this index in healthy children are equal to zero. Thus, the immunological index is defined by the following formula:

$$\mathrm{Im} = A_0 + A_1 \frac{\mathrm{EAC{-}PFC}}{N_{\mathrm{EAC}}} + A_2 \frac{\mathrm{E}_t\mathrm{{-}PFC}}{N_{\mathrm{E}_t}} + A_3 \frac{\mathrm{IgM}/N_{\mathrm{IgM}}}{\mathrm{IgG}/N_{\mathrm{IgG}} + \mathrm{IgA}/N_{\mathrm{IgA}}} + A_4 \frac{\mathrm{IgM}}{N_{\mathrm{IgM}}},$$

where EAC–PFC and E_t–PFC are the indices of cellular subpopulation; IgG, IgM, IgA are the levels of the corresponding fractions of immuno-globulines. N_{EAC}, N_{E_t}, N_{IgA}, N_{IgM}, N_{IgG} are are the corresponding norms. The generalized index is constructed by the methods of multiple linear regression and step regression. The coefficients A_0 – A_4 were obtained using the least squares method; and in our case A_0 = 0.3, A_1 = 1.3, A_2 = −1, A_3 = 0.03, A_4 = 0.04.

The analysis of the values of the immunological index shows that they are not determined by etiology and the degree of gravity of the disease, in other words, there is no obvious difference between the immunological indices Im in patients with viral hepatitis B, viral hepatitis A, and viral hepatitis of unknown etiology, respectively. We have ignored factors of the etiology and severity of the disease. The analysis of the immunological index in patients with an acute course of viral hepatitis (patients with malignant form were studied separately) in the disease dynamics demonstrated that the Im increases during the peak of the illness (0.93 on the average) and gradually decreases by the time of clinical recovery (0.44). It is worth noting that the increasing Im was observed in 100% of patients with viral hepatitis (with variations from 0.2 to 2.3).

We have established that the expressivity of the immune response and the dynamics of the liver functional recovery are closely interrelated (the correlation coefficient for the immunological and the biochemical indices is 0.62). We have also determined that patients in one group (75 people), with the immunological index greater than 0.6 (during the peak) had a higher rate of the liver functional recovery than normal. The patients of the other group (13 people), with the Im smaller than 0.6, had a slower rate. The mean values of Im during the peak of the disease in patients in both groups are presented in table 1. These values are essentially varied ($p \leq 0.005$). For example, the mean Im in patients with normal rate of the liver functional recovery during the peak of the disease is 0.92 ± 0.09; in the case of a slow rate, the mean Im is only 0.44 ± 0.08. These results enable us to hypothesize that the dynamics of the pathological process depends on the expressivity of the immune response: the course will be smooth if Im is high, and slow otherwise.

TABLE 1
The Immunological Index in Patients with Acute and Protracted Forms of Viral Hepatitis During the Peak of the Disease (M ± m)

Disease course	acute		protracted
	rate of the liver functional recovery		
Immunity Index	normal	slow	slow
Im	0.92 ± 0.09	0.44 ± 0.08	0.39 ± 0.09

We have also studied the behavior of the immunological index Im in patients with the protracted course of viral hepatitis. The mean Im in these patients during the peak of disease is 0.39 ± 0.09 (with variations from 0.2 to 0.48). In all of the patients with the protracted course and in 21% of the patients with acute course the Im was less than 0.6. As was noted earlier, patients with an acute course of viral hepatitis (at the peak of the disease Im < 0.6) had a slower rate of the liver functional recovery. Thus, the immunological index lower than 0.6 yields the probability 0.7 of a protracted course of viral hepatitis.

To conclude, mathematical methods for clinical and laboratory data processing helped us quantitatively estimate the degree of the liver functional damage, the patient's clinical condition and the gravity of the hepatic pathological process. The biochemical and clinical indices and the gravity index make it possible to evaluate the gravity of disease and control the dynamics of the pathological process. Furthermore, the clinician can better assess the effectiveness of the prescribed treatment and make a more accurate prognosis for the course of the disease in viral hepatitis patients.

2. Mathematical modelling of the immune process for viral hepatitis B

Mathematical methods for processing the clinical and laboratory data may help clinicians solve concrete problems, but they do not describe the mechanism of the pathological processes. The onset, course and outcome of a particular disease are defined by the dynamics relationship between the pathogenic agent (virus) and the defense system of the organism. Therefore, the model of a viral disease must also describe possible ways of the viral proliferation and the possible reaction of the immune system to the viral antigens.

In 1975, Marchuk [3] developed the simplest mathematical model of a viral disease. This model—a system of four differential equations—accounted for the most characteristic elements of the immune response to an infectious disease and solved problems involving treatment of the chronic form of a disease, simultaneous infection, biinfection, etc. However, the simplest mathematical model did not express many important processes of viral disease. A further step was made when the model of antiviral response was suggested [4].

Let us review the basic notions of the theory, yet incomplete, of antiviral immunity, which, although absent in the simplest mathematical model, constitute the foundation of the antiviral immune–response model:

- the immune response is directed toward a virus freely circulating in the blood and lymph as well as to the infected host cells;
- the recovery process depends on the rate of elimination of the infected cells from the body;
- the ability of cytotoxic lymphocytes of destroying the infected cells determines the organism's defense reaction, but at the same time it causes target–organ and tissue injuries;
- the identification, joint proliferation with effector lymphocytes, and cytotoxic effect of the accumulated T–killers are not initiated by the viral antigen proper, but rather by a complex: virus–transplantation antigen of the general host histocompatibility system;
- the macrophage is a cell which modifies the antigen and forms on its surface a complex consisting of the viral antigens and the antigens of the general host histocompatibility system;
- a double signal is required to stimulate B–lymphocytes and precursors of T–killers: the signals of macrophages stimulated by viruses, and of lymphocyte–helpers.

This model involves ten ordinary differential equations with delay:

1. $$\frac{dV_f}{dt} = n\mathscr{C}_E C_v E + p\mathscr{C}_m C_v - \gamma_f V_f F - \gamma_m M V_f - \kappa\sigma(1-C_v-m)V_f$$

2. $$\frac{dM_v}{dt} = \gamma_M M - \alpha_M M_v - \mathscr{C}_M M_v E$$

3. $$\frac{dH_E}{dt} = \mathscr{C}_H[\zeta(m)\rho_H M_v H_E|_{t-\tau_H} - M_v H_E] - \mathscr{C}_p M_v H_E E + \alpha_H(H_E^* - H_E)$$

4. $$\frac{dH_B}{dt} = \mathscr{C}_H^{(B)}[\zeta(m)\rho_H^{(B)} M_v H_B|_{t-\tau_H^{(B)}} - M_v H_B] - \mathscr{C}_p^{(B)} M_v H_B B + \alpha_H^{(B)}(H_B^* - H_B)$$

5. $$\frac{dE}{dt} = \mathscr{C}_p[\zeta(m)\rho_E M_v H_E E|_{t-\tau_E} - M_v H_E E] - \eta_c \mathscr{C}_E C_v E - \eta_M \mathscr{C}_M E M_v + \alpha_E(E^* - E)$$

6. $$\frac{dB}{dt} = \mathscr{C}_p^{(B)}[\zeta(m)\rho_B M_v H_B B|_{t-\tau_B} - M_v H_B B] + \alpha_B(B^* - B)$$

7. $$\frac{dP}{dt} = \mathscr{C}_p^{(P)}\zeta(m)\rho_p M_v H_B B|_{t-\tau_p} + \alpha_P(P^* - P)$$

8. $$\frac{dF}{dt} = \rho_f P - \eta_f \gamma_f V_f F - \alpha_f F$$

9. $$\frac{dC_v}{dt} = \sigma(1 - C_v - m)V_f - \mathscr{C}_E C_V E - \mathscr{C}_m C_V$$

10. $$\frac{dm}{dt} = \mu \mathscr{C}_E C_V E + \eta \mathscr{C}_m C_V - \lambda ,$$

where $\zeta(m) = 1 - m$.

Here

V_f is the concentration of free virus;

M_v is the concentration of macrophages stimulated by virus;

H_E,H_B are the concentrations of the cells–helpers for the cells–effectors, E– and B–cells, respectively;

E is the concentration of lymphocyte–effectors;

B is the concentration of B–lymphocytes;

P is the concentration of plasma cells;

F is the concentration of antibodies;

C_v is the fraction of target–organ cells infected by virus;

m is the fraction of damaged cells of the target organ.

The initial conditions are given by either the values at the zero moment of time or the values of the delay interval for the variables of the equation with delay. We can regard the above model of antiviral immune response as the prototype of the model of viral hepatitis B. The model describes a phenomenon of great importance: the complete virus elimination from the organism occurs when the cells–effectors have destroyed all the infected cells. Choosing appropriately the values of coefficients qualitatively corresponding to the hepatitis B virus, we obtain numerical solutions. One such solution is shown in figure 3: the behavior of the model variables qualitatively agrees with the available experimental and clinical data. At the same time, the values of some coefficients have been chosen arbitrarily. Those are the coefficients characterizing the processes of interaction between cells of different types. These results agree on the whole with clinical data. According to the latter, the difference between humoral response and cell response to a viral infection imply either chronization of the disease or the unfavorable outcome [5]. The model deals only with the infection with hepatitis B virus. A complete recovery is the most frequent outcome of viral hepatitis. However, chronic hepatitis occurs in approxi–mately 10% of patients. The cases of chronic hepatitis are characterized by various immunological, clinical and morphological factors. Here are two most common variants of viral hepatitis: HB_sAg positive chronic persistent hepatitis (CPH) and HB_sAg positive chronic active hepatitis (CAH). CPH and CAH differ greatly in the disease outcome: CPH often has a favorable course as CAH has frequently an unfavorable outcome.

The investigation of the emergence and of the course of the chronic viral hepatitis B suggests a number of different mechanisms involved. A significant weakened reaction of the T–immune system is observed in patients with CPH as well as in patients with CAH. However, in the CAH patients a considerable immuno–deregulation of T suppressors has been detected [6], [7]. Typical differences between CAH and CPH are repre–sented in table 2. The data of table 2 and the description of mechanisms for chronic hepatitis formation yield the model solutions describing the chronization process in CAH and CPH. We obtained these solutions by de–creasing the values of stimulation coefficients of the T immune system. The corresponding solutions are shown in figures 4 (CPH) and 5 (CAH). It is interesting to note that CAH occupies (in terms of the stimulation coefficients of T system) an intermediate position between the solutions interpreted as an acute form of the disease (figure 3) and as CPH (figure 4). The solution shown in figure 5 has, unlike the solution in figure 4, pronounced fluctuations with a period of about a year. These fluctuations also agree with both clinical data on the stationary CPH course and the alternating remission and aggravation phases in patients with CAH. Let us note that the estimates listed in table 2 are characteristics of the aggrava–tion phase.

In modern immunology there is a general concept of the defensive and destructive action of T–killers with viral infections [5]. The same popula–

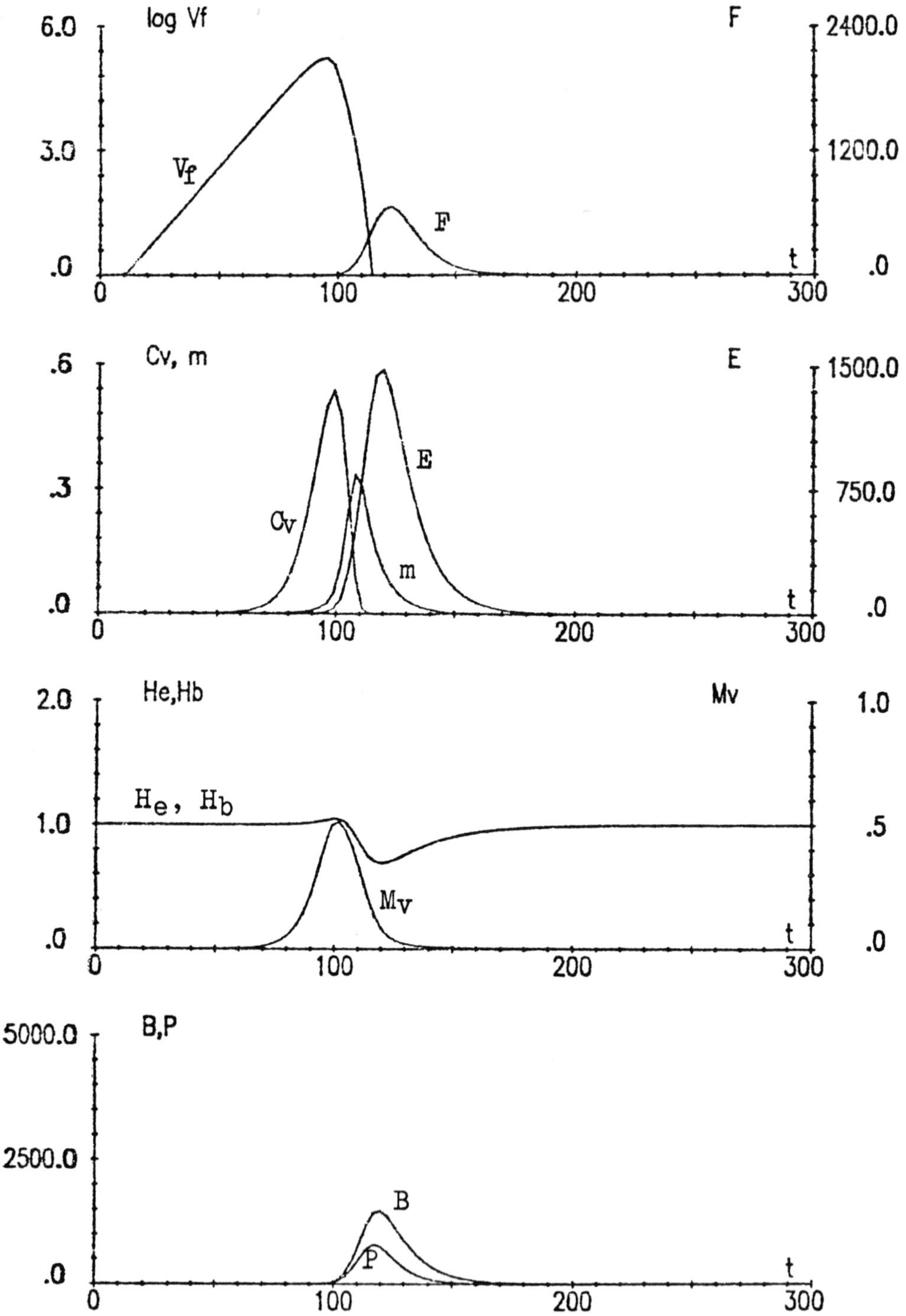

Fig. 3. Antiviral immune–response model solution interpreted as acute form of viral hepatitis B

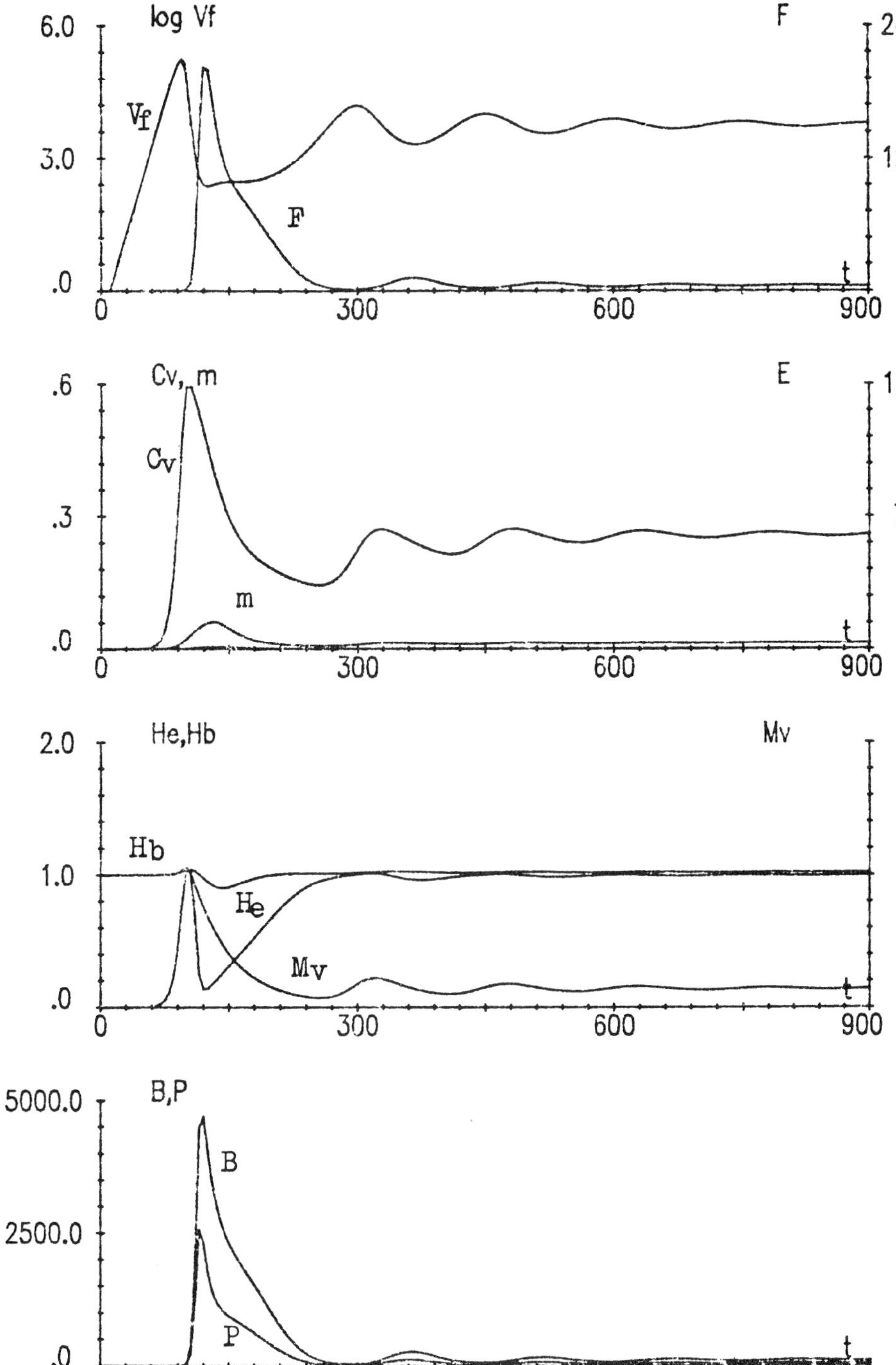

Fig. 4. Antiviral immune–response model solution interpreted as chronic hepatitis

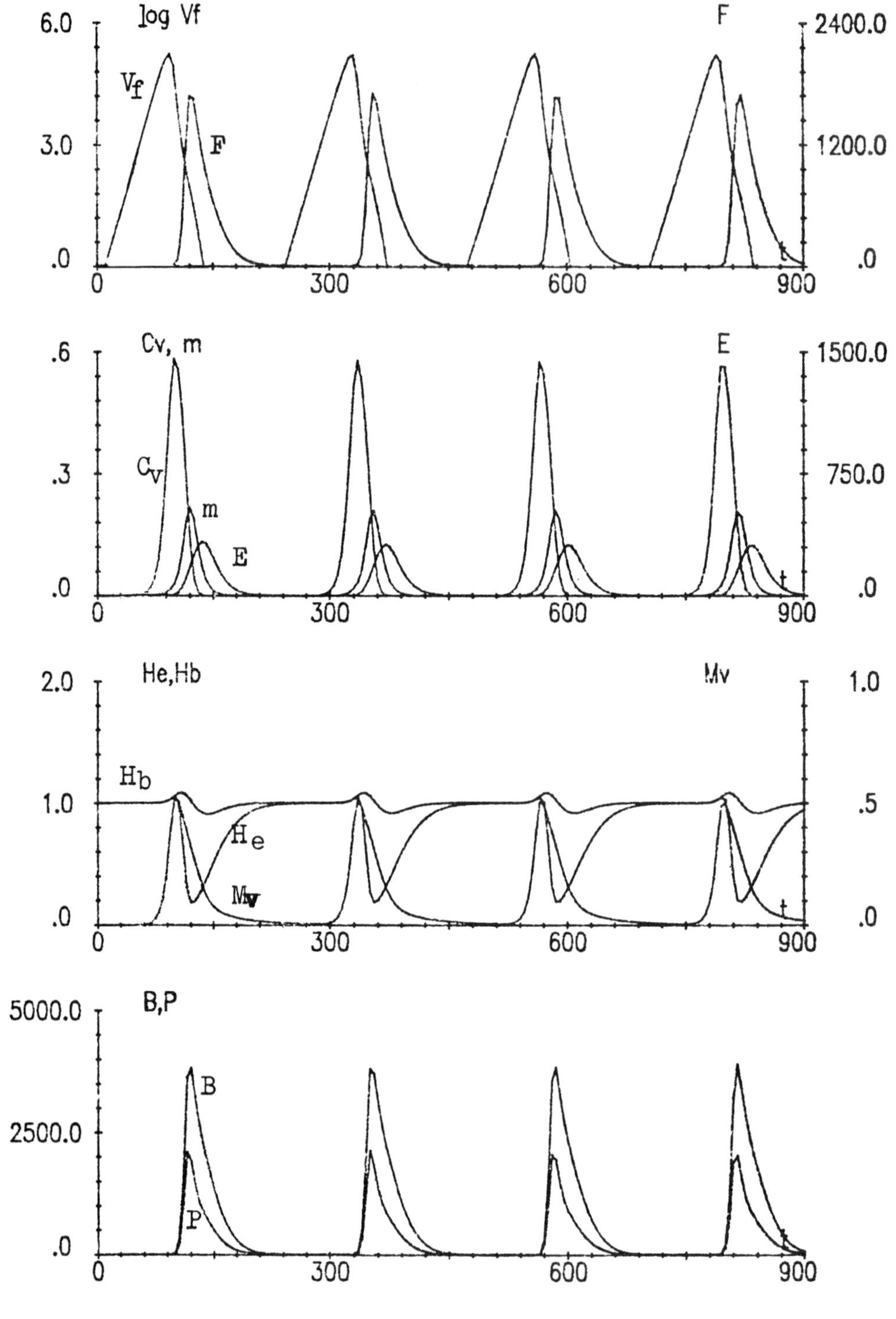

Fig. 5. Antiviral immune–response model solution interpreted as chronic active hepatitis

tion of cytotoxic lymphocytes may cause either recovery or death in animals, as was established in experiments with a viral infection. The researchers came to the conclusion that the earliest development of T cellular immunity reduces the extent of the organ's infection as well as its further damage by T–lymphocyte killers.

The determination of the relation between the gravity of viral disease and the immunity condition of the organism (in particular, T–immune system) is a crucial problem in clinical immunology. The T–immune system can be stimulated before as well as during the illness in a number of ways.

TABLE 2
Typical Values of Model Variables for CAH and CPH

	CPH	CAH	Units
V_f	200	2000	relative concentration
C_v	0.9	0.6	cell fractions
m	0.01	0.1	cell fractions
E	1.5	15	relative units, norm = 1
H	1	1.5	relative units, norm = 1

The model considered was used to examine the dependence of the gravity of viral disease and the process of virus elimination on the reactivity of the T–system and the degree of virus cytopathogenity. Let us explain what exactly (in our model) the characteristics of viral infection are. As the gravity estimate we take $m_{max} = \max_{t \in [0, T]} m(t)$, the model maximum variable on some time interval, which describes the degree of destruction of the target organ. The intensity of the infection–elimination process is given by $V_{f_{min}} = \min_{t \in [0, T]} V_f(t)$, the minimum of V_f, which describes the concentration of free viruses in the organism. The estimates of the immune response associated with rapidly proliferating T– and B–lymphocytes are E_{max} and B_{max}, respectively.

We modelled the process of infecting the organism with one of the three types of virus, which differ in degree of cytotoxicity: viruses of the first type are capable of destroying a cell in 2 days; viruses of the second type destroy a cell in 10 days; viruses of the third type in 100 days. A solution imitating the viral–disease dynamics was obtained and used to determine $m_{\max}$, $V_{f\max}$, $E_{\max}$ and $B_{\max}$. Then, in the equation for T–killers we increased the coefficients $b_p \rho_E$ and $\mathscr{C}_p$ which determine the intensity of proliferation of T–lymphocyte killers. Another solution was obtained for a different reactivity of the immune system. The results are shown in figure 6.

We have established that the protective–destructive action of T–killers having varied virus cytotoxicity is manifested in different ways. With weak cytotoxic viruses, the pathological processes in, say, viral hepatitis B are enhanced (quantitatively) by T–killers, and a greater severity of the disease in patients with a more reactive T–system is the "price" they have to pay for the greater number of viruses ($\mathscr{C}_p$). (See figures 6(a) and 6(b).) We have also determined that there is a rather narrow area of high sensitivity of several characteristics of the disease to a variation of the coefficient $\mathscr{C}_p$, that is the area of T–system reactivity. The use of the model for estimating the effect of a particular drug may lead to a significantly more effective control of the viral process.

The dependence of $B_{\max}$ and $E_{\max}$ on C_p is of interest, too. Figures 6(d) and 6(c) show that the rate of proliferation of B–lymphocytes, after stimulation, diminishes as the concentration of T–killers increases.

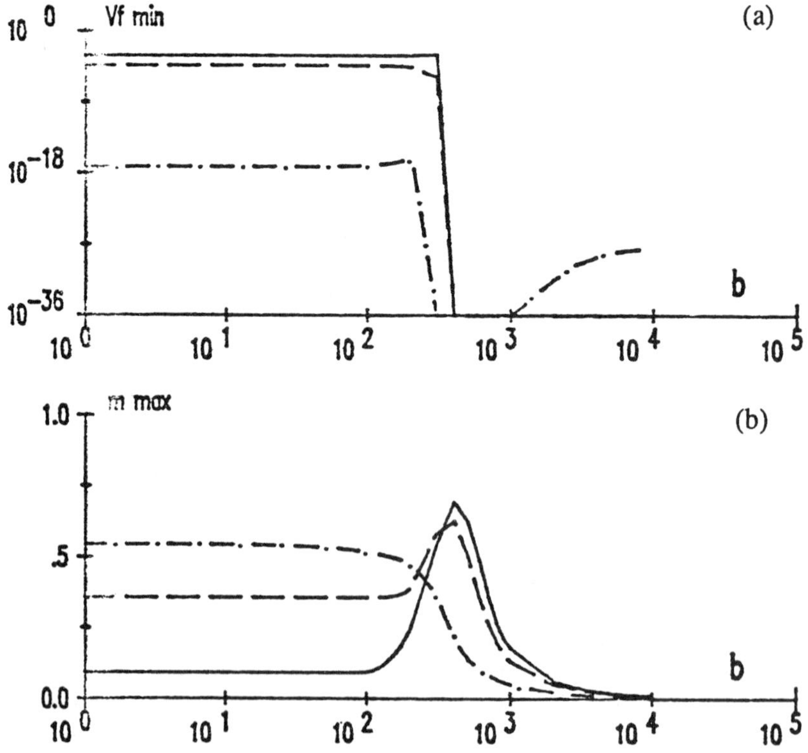

Fig. 6

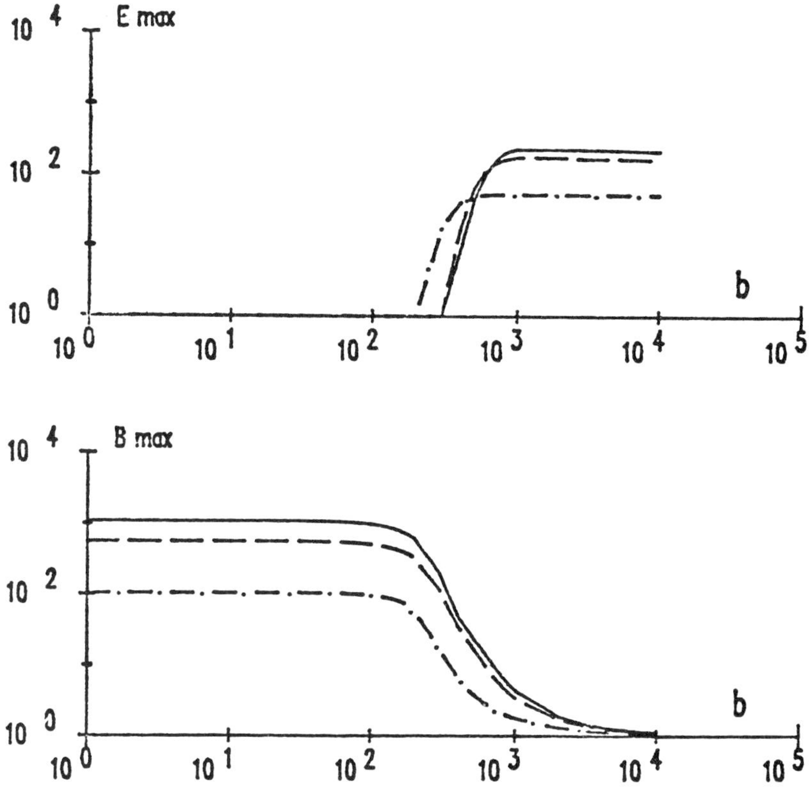

Fig. 6. Dependence of characteristics of antiviral immune response model solution on b–stimulation coefficient of T–killers:

————————	weak cytopathogenic virus
– – – – – -	intermediate cytopathogenic virus
—.—.—.—.	strong cytopathogenic virus

Conclusion

As we have seen, there is still a great gap between the tasks of clinical practice and the capabilities of mathematical models. The reason for this gap is twofold. The first reason is that we still have an inadequate information about quantitative characteristics of the immune processes in viral hepatitis B. The second reason is that mathematical models are yet too abstract and do not account for the whole wealth of clinical data about the virus in particular and the patient in general. For example, we need to include the patient's health background, or the effect of intercurrent illnesses, among other factors. Then mathematical methods will become an efficient and necessary tool in solving urgent clinical, practical problems.

REFERENCES

[1] Nisevich, N.I., Marchuk, G.I., Zubikova, I.I., and Pogozhev, I.B. *Matematicheskoe Modelirovanie Virusnogo Gepatita* (in Russian). Moscow: Nauka, 1981. English translation: Mathematical Modelling of Viral Disease. New York: Optimization Software, Inc., Publications Division. Forthcoming.

[2] Petrov, R.V. *Immunologiya i Immunogenetica* (Immunology and Immunogenetics). Moscow: Izdatel'stvo "Meditsina," 1976.

[3] Marchuk, G.I. *The Simplest Mathematical Model of Viral Disease* (in Russian). Preprint. Computational Center of the USSR Academy of Sciences, Siberian Branch, Novosibirsk, 1975.

[4] Marchuk, G.I., and Petrov, R.V. *Mathematical Model of Antiviral Immune Response* (in Russian). Preprint no. 10, Department of Numerical Mathematics of the USSR Academy of Sciences, Moscow, 1981.

[5] Semenov, B.F., Kaulen, D.R., and Bilandin, I.K. *Kletochnye i Molekulyarnye Printsipy Protivovirusnogo Immuniteta* (Cellular and Molecular Principles of Antiviral Immunity). Moscow: Izdatel'stvo "Meditsina," 1982.

[6] Chisari, F.V., et al. January 1981. Functional properties of lymphocyte subpopulations in hepatitis B virus. *J. of Immunology* 126, no. 1:45–49.

[7] McKay, I.R. 1980. Immunological interactions involving virus and liver: a synthesis. In *Virus and the Liver*, ed. L.W. Bianchi et al., 131–35. Lancaster, England: Publisher.

THE MECHANISM OF IMMUNE RESPONSE AMPLIFICATION BY STIMULATOR OF ANTIBODY PRODUCTION (SAP) (STUDIES BY MEANS OF A MATHEMATICAL MODEL)

R.V. Petrov, R.N. Stepanenko, and Yu.I Skalko

Department of Immunology
Second Moscow State Medical Institute
Moscow, USSR

Cytokinins play an important role in the control of proliferation and differentiation of B–cells [1–4]. Our laboratory has investigated the soluble factor involved in the differentiation of B–cells into mature antibody–forming cells [5–7]. This humoral factor is released by bone marrow cells in the absence of antigenic stimulation, and it increases the number of plasma cells in the effector phase of immune response. It was isolated from supernatants of murine bone marrow cultures, and was active both in vitro and in vivo [8]. This factor is heat stable, and it has a molecular mass of about 1000–3000 daltons. It is assumed that SAP performs the regulatory function of bone marrow cells at the level of maturation and differentiation of the cells of B type. However, the mechanism of SAP action is still unknown. It can be assumed that SAP promotes the drawing of an additional number of cells in antibody synthesis which cannot participate in antibody production without these stimulants. It is also possible that the factor released by bone marrow cells regulates the duration of antibody synthesis by plasma cells in the effector phase of immune response.

To study the mechanism of the SAP action, a computer simulation was initiated, using the simple mathematical model of immune response suggested by Gurij Ivanovich Marchuk in 1975 [9] .

The statement of the problem

Figure 1 shows the antibody response process according to the theory of immune–cell cooperation. The antigen is absorbed by microphages and then recognized by T–lymphocyte helpers and B–lymphocytes. The T–cell helpers deliver different signals (F_1, F_2, F_3, etc.) triggering differentiation of B–lymphocytes into antibody producers. F_1 (antigen–specific signal) is a soluble factor which has an antigen–binding area and Ia antigens deriving from the I region of the major histocompatability complex. Other signals (F_2 and F_3) are antigen–nonspecific. They were generally designated as factors replacing T–cells or interleukins 2 and 3 [10–12]. Interleukin 2 exerts a stimulating influence over proliferation of antibody–producer precursors, and interleukin 3 influences the differentiation of immature plasma cells. This factor is necessary for differentiation of the immediate precursors of plasma cells into antibody–forming cells. The population of antibody producers is formed as a result of such cooperation of immune cells. Subsequently the antibodies synthesized by plasma cells bind the antigen and form immune complexes which activate the negative feedback control of antibody production. The mechanisms of this control are still not properly understood, and we shall not discuss them in this paper.

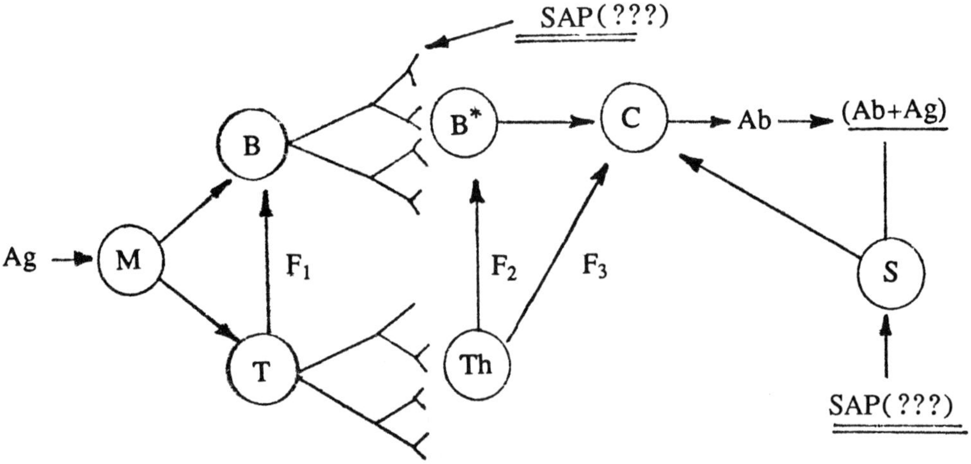

Fig. 1. Scheme of the immune cells' cooperation during the antibody response

Ag – antigen
M – macrophage
T – T–lymphocyte
B – B–lymphocyte
B* -- immediate precursors of plasma cells
Th – helper T–lymphocyte
C – plasma cells
Ab – antibodies
(Ab+Ag) – immune complex
S – system of control over the duration of Ab synthesis by plasma cells
F_1, F_2, F_3 – soluble factors released by T–lymphocytes

According to the theory briefly sketched above, the mechanism of SAP action can be one of the following two possible versions. It is known that in the production phase of antibody response there is a number of plasma cells (the so–called "silent" cells) which do not produce antibodies, although they have an apparatus that is necessary for synthesis of antibodies of given specificity [13]. By the first hypothesis, the SAP involves these "silent" cells which do not introduce antibodies into antibody production, thus increasing the number of antibody producers. The second hypothesis states that the SAP suppresses the cells controlling the duration of the antibody synthesis. An increase in the duration of the antibody synthesis of some plasma cells can result in a greater total sum of antibody producers in the effector phase of antibody response. Hence, by the first hypothesis, the SAP acts on B^*; by the second hypothesis, it acts on S (fig. 1).

In order to determine which of the two hypotheses is correct, we have constructed mathematical models of SAP action in the effector phase of the antibody response.

Description of the models

We have constructed three models:

M_0 – the model of immune response without SAP action (normal immune response, control);

M_1 – the model based on the hypothesis that SAP action leads to an increase of mature antibody–producer lifetime;

M_2 – the model based on the hypothesis that SAP action involves "silent" precursors into antibody production

These models were tested by computer simulation. If the models M_1 and M_2 lead to qualitatively different results, we could determine (by comparison with the results of laboratory experiments) which of the hypotheses is correct.

The simple mathematical model of immune response (M_0), suggested by G.I. Marchuk in 1975, was taken as a mathematical model of antibody response without SAP action [9]. The equations of this model have the following form:

$$\frac{dV}{dt} = -\gamma FV ,$$

$$\frac{dF}{dt} = \rho C - \eta\gamma FV - \mu_f F , \qquad (M_0)$$

$$\frac{dC}{dt} = \alpha FV|_{t-\tau} - \mu_c(C-C^*) ,$$

$$V(0) = V_0, \quad C(0) = C^*, \quad F(0) = F^* = \frac{\rho C^*}{\mu_f} .$$

Three variables in these equations respectively denote the concentration of a nonreproducing antigen ($V(t)$), the concentration of antibodies ($F(t)$), and the concentration of plasma cells producing antibodies ($C(t)$). It is assumed that the rate of antigen inactivation is proportional to the antibodies' concentration. The first term on the right side of the equation for plasma cells denotes the increase of plasma cells due to stimulation of the lymphocytes by the bound antigens. It is known that in the formation of plasma–cell clones from lymphocytes, their proliferation and differentiation takes some time. In the models this period of time is expressed by a time-delay term τ, which is the time interval from the beginning of lymphocyte stimulation up to the plasma cells' clone formation. The second term represents the aging of plasma cells with constant μ_c, which is the inverse value of their mean lifetime. Here C^* is the constant characterizing the level of plasma cells in an organism.

The first term on the right side of the equation for antibodies denotes the production of antibodies by plasma cells with rate ρ; the second term describes the decrease of antibodies due to neutralization of antigens; the third, the natural decay of antibodies with constant rate μ_f equal to the inverse of the antibodies' half–life. We have used these model parameters to simulate the antibody response to lymph nodes, induced by a subcutaneous injection of sheep red blood cells in foot [14]. In this experiment, the peak of concentration of plasma cells in the effector phase of immune response is 10^3 higher than before antigen injection. The progression of the number of plasma–cells in time is the following: plasma cells appear on the second and third day after the antigen injection, and on the fourth day their number reaches its peak, followed by a decrease.

The model M_1 is constructed in the following way: before SAP is injected the immune response develops according to the model M_0. By the first hypothesis, SAP injection will cause an increase of the lifespan of C–cells; therefore after SAP injection on the 4th day, the parameter μ_c decreases so that the new parameter $\mu_c' < \mu_c$.

The model M_1:

$$\frac{dV}{dt} = -\gamma FV ,$$

$$\frac{dF}{dt} = \rho C - \eta\gamma FV - \mu_f F , \qquad (M_1)$$

$$\frac{dC}{dt} = \alpha FV|_{t-\tau} - \mu_c'(C-C^*) .$$

All parameters of the model M_1 are the same as in the model M_0 with the exception of the parameter μ_c'. The parameter μ_c' is chosen according to the following experimental data: SAP injection on the 4th day after the antigen injection causes an increase in the number of plasma cells to be three times as large.

The following model is taken as M_2. According to this model, in the production phase of antibody response there is a number of plasma cells (B) which do not produce antibodies (so–called "silent cells"). In the model M_2 the first three equations are the same as in the model M_1. The fourth equation is added to describe the accumulation of "silent" plasma cells. We consider two populations: mature plasma cells (C–cells) and "silent" plasma cells (B–cells). It is assumed that B–cells after SAP injection mature in plasma cells. The parameter μ_B approximately corresponds to the inverse lifespan of precursors turning to mature antibody–producers. In this case the development of the immune response can be described by the following system of differential equations (the model M_2):

$$\frac{dV}{dt} = -\gamma FV ,$$

$$\frac{dF}{dt} = \rho C - \eta\gamma FV - \mu_f F ,$$

$$\frac{dC}{dt} = \alpha FV|_{t-\tau} - \mu_c(C - C^*) + \delta_B B , \qquad (M_2)$$

$$\frac{dB}{dt} = \alpha_2 FV|_{t-\tau} - \mu_B B - \delta_B B .$$

The parameters in the model M_2 are taken the same as in the model M_0. It was assumed that the parameter μ_B is very small (i.e., precursors live for a long time); in what follows we assume it to be zero. In the third and fourth equations we added the terms $+\delta_B B$, $-\delta_B B$ describing the change of pre–cursors into plasma cells. The parameters α_2 and δ_B are chosen according to the experimental data, i.e., SAP injection must lead to the threefold increase in the number of plasma cells. In both M_1 and M_2 a limited time during which the factor is acting was taken into account. It is supposed that the factor has been removed from the organism 1.5 days after injection and thereafter the immune response developed in accordance with the model M_0.

The models M_0, M_1 and M_2 are reduced to the dimensionless form as in [17]. All further experiments are carried out with dimensionless models and the results are given for dimensionless values.

Computer simulation

Using the appropriate values of model parameters, the development of antibody response after SAP action was simulated and compared with the experimental data. Some findings are shown below.

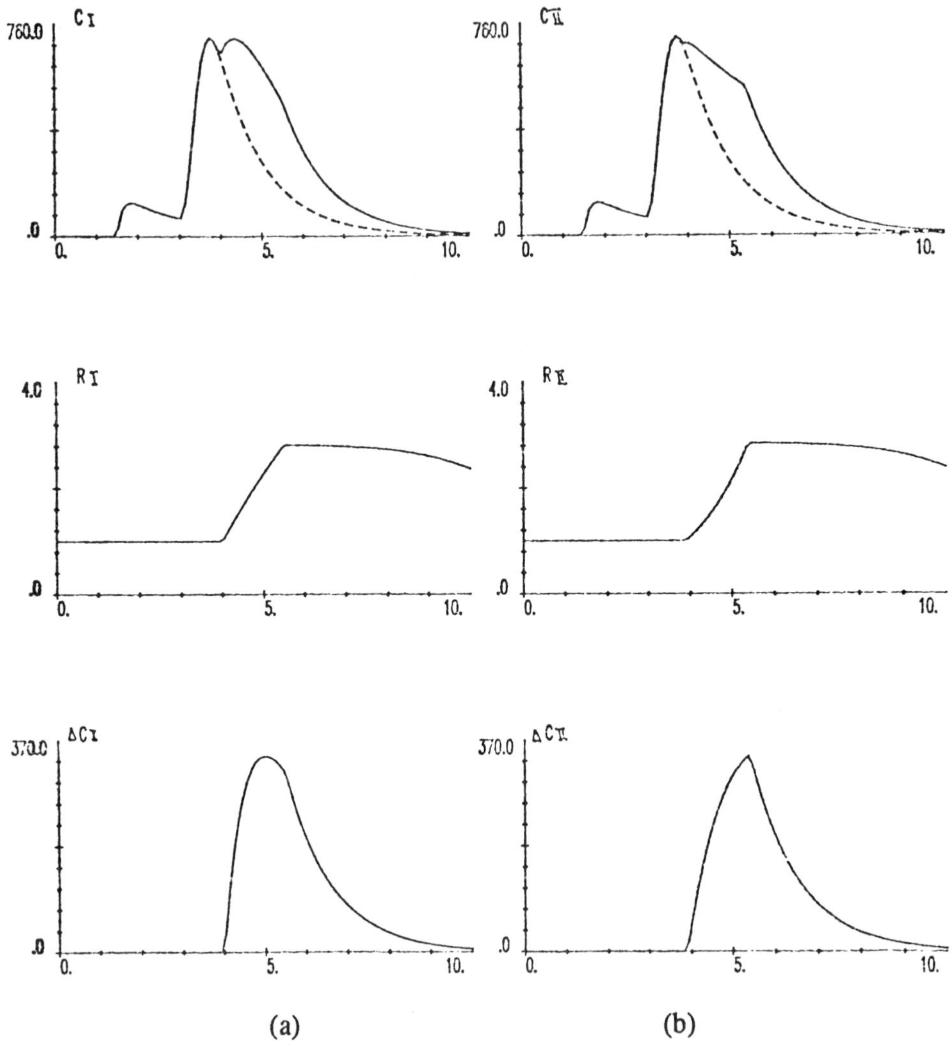

Fig. 2. Injection of SAP factor at the peak of the immune response

a. results on the model M_2;

b. results on the model M_1.

Control experiment (model M_0) shown by dotted line

EXPERIMENT 1

SAP injection at the peak of the immune response, i.e., on the fourth day after immunization, was simulated. The computer results are shown in fig. 2. In the right part of fig. 2, computed curves referring to the model M_1 are given. Computed curves referring to the model M_2 are introduced in the left part. The dynamics of C–cells in the experiment without SAP action (the model M_0) is depicted by the dotted line in fig. 2. In addition, fig. 2 shows the dynamics of the so–called coefficient of immune response amplification $R(t)$, which is equal to the ratio of the number of C–cells (the models M_1 and M_2 describing SAP action) to their number in the control version (the model M_0);

— the dynamics of the value ΔC which is equal to the difference between the number of C–cells of the model describing SAP action (M_1 and M_2) and their number in the control version. The cited results show that the models M_1 and M_2 in this experiment lead to qualitatively equal dynamics of the number of mature antibody–producers $C(t)$, coefficient of amplification $R(t)$, and value $\Delta C(t)$. Therefore from this immunological experiment we cannot infer the correctness of either hypothesis.

EXPERIMENT 2

The dependence between the SAP action and the moment of injection was investigated. In this experiment, the factor injection on the first, second and third day after the peak of immune response was simulated. The results represented in fig. 3 show that the models M_1 and M_2 predict qualitatively different dynamics of the process development. In accordance with the model M_2, one more peak is observed in the dynamics of mature antibody producers. This peak gets higher and more expressive than in the case of the later SAP injection. For $C(t)$ the model M_1 yields the dynamics qualitatively equivalent to those in the previous experiment. The dynamics of the amplification coefficient $R(t)$ is worth of interest. In accordance with the model M_1, if SAP is injected on the fifth, sixth or seventh day after immunization, the peak of $R(t)$ moves to the right on the time axis and its magnitude remains invariable. According to the model M_2, the later SAP injection also makes the peak of $R(t)$ shift; in this case the values of $R(t)$ increase substantially.

For the ΔC value, the model M_1 predicts that the later injection of the factor results in the situation where the ΔC value reaches its maximum much later. In this case the magnitude of the ΔC value decreases substantially. According to the model M_2, the magnitude of the ΔC value does not depend significantly on the time of factor injection.

We have thus drawn the conclusion: a comparison of the simulation results using the models M_1 and M_2 with the results of the immunologic experiments involving the SAP injection on the 5th, 6th and 7th day after the antibody immune response induction enables us to establish which of the two hypotheses is correct. The corresponding experiments were then carried out. The agreement

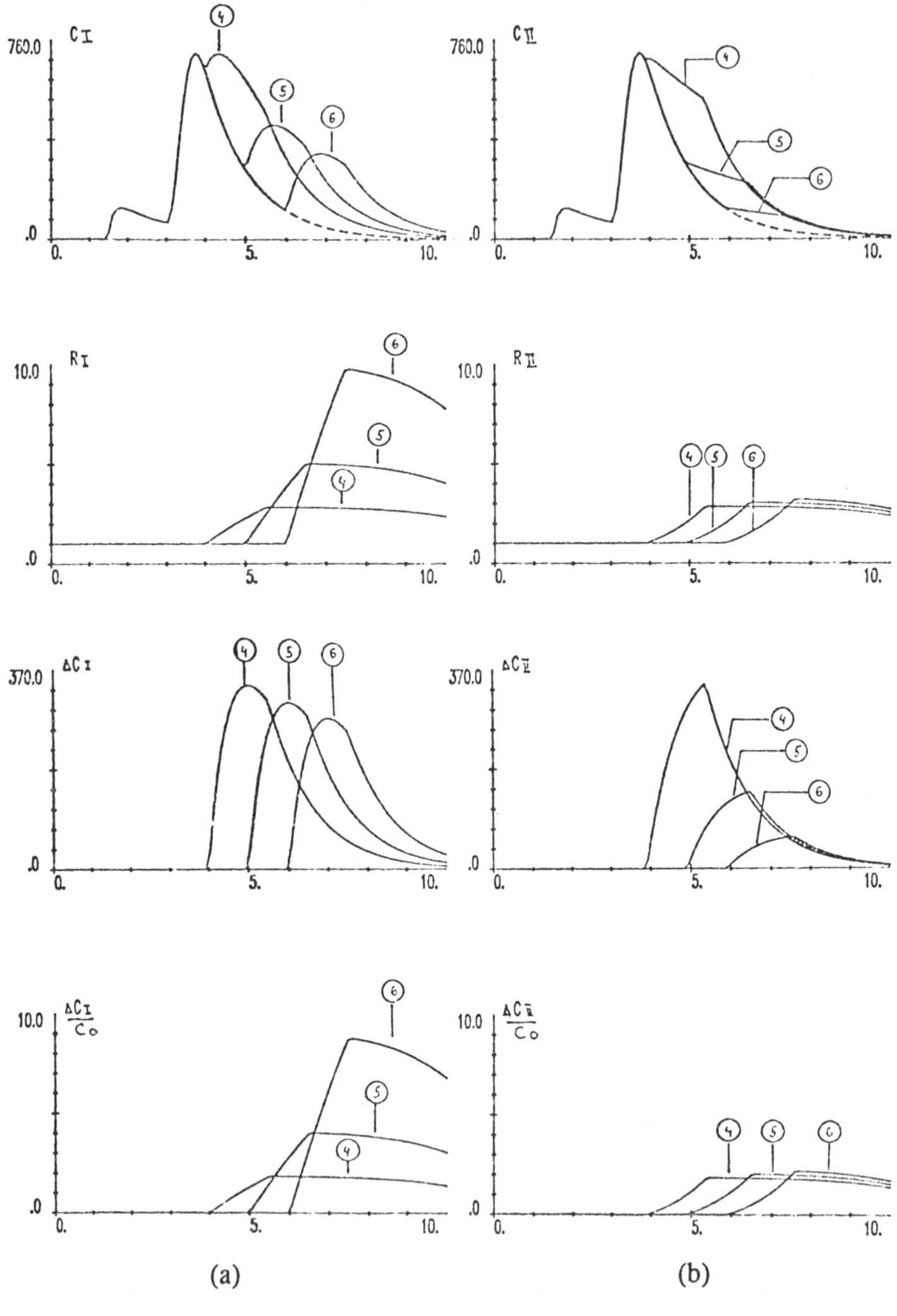

(a) (b)

Fig. 3. Injection of SAP factor on the fourth (curve 4), fifth (curve 5), sixth (curve 6) day after immunization

a. results on the model M_2;

b. results on the model M_1.

Control experiment (model M_0) shown by dotted line

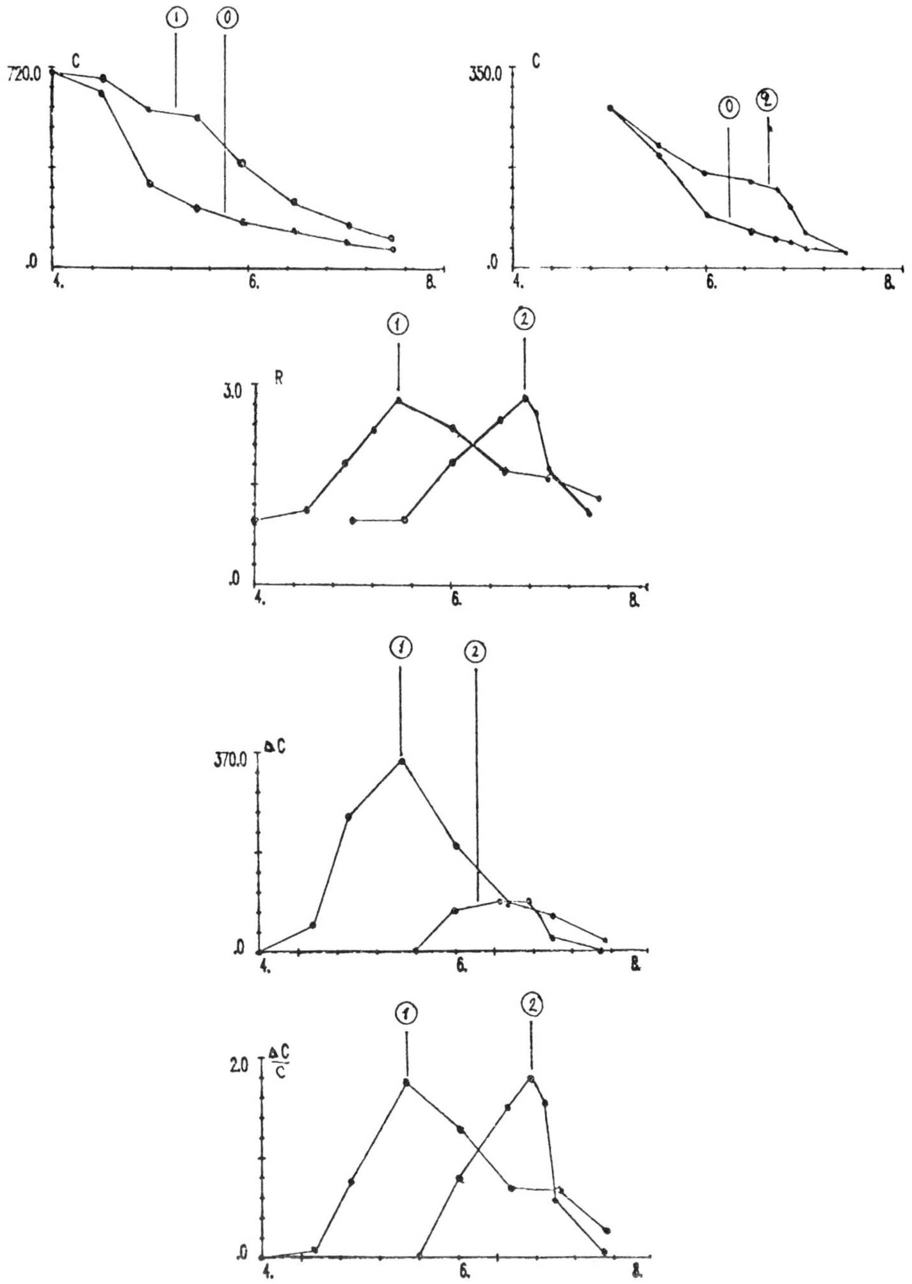

Fig. 4. Results of experiments on animals

0 – experiment without SAP factor (control);

1 – injection of SAP at the peak of the immune response, on the fourth day

2 – injection of SAP on the fifth day after immunization

between the simulated curves and the development of antibody response after the SAP injection in the experiments is the evidence that the model M_2 describes the kinetics of C–cells more accurately than the model M_1 (fig. 4).

Therefore we can conclude that SAP injection causes an increase in the lifespan of C–cells. However, we can see that the compound curves are somewhat different from the experimental curves. Therefore, the model M_2 needs to be more precise.

One more remark is in order. Computer simulation does make it possible to determine which particular experiments are required. To carry out an experiment one has to make adjustments, which requires a more precise model and new computer simulation. And this will in turn lead to a new experiment, and so on. It is obvious that mathematical modelling is of great help in stimulating and guiding experimental work. We are confident that the mathematical analysis will bring us to a better understanding of the immune processes and in consequence of that to more effective therapeutic methods.

REFERENCES

[1] Dutton, R.W., Falkoff, R., and Hirst, J.A. 1971. Is there evidence for an non-antigen-specific chemical mediator from the thymus-derived cell in the initiation of immune response? *Prog. Immunology* 1:3-55.

[2] Harwell, L.,Kappler, J., and Marrack, P. 1976. Antigen-specific and nonspecific mediators of T-cell/B-cell cooperation. III. Characterization of the nonspecific mediator(s) from different sources. *J. Immunology* 116:13-79.

[3] Kishimoto, T., Miyake, T., Nishizawa, Y., Watanabe, T., and Yamamura, Y. 1975. Triggering mechanism of B-lymphocytes I. Effect of antiimmunoglobulin and enhancing soluble factor on differentiation and proliferation of B-cells. *J. Immunology* 115:11-79.

[4] Parker, D.C. 1982. Separable helper factors support B-cell proliferation and maturation to Ig secretion. *J. Immunology* 129:4-69.

[5] Petrov, R.V., Mikhajlova, A.A., Stepanenko, R.N., and Zakharova, L.A. 1975. Cell interactions in the immune response: effect of humoral factor released from bone marrow cells on the quantity of mature antibody producers in the culture of immune lymph node cells (in Russian). *Kletochnaya Immunologiya* 17:342-50.

[6] Petrov, R.V., et al. (in Russian). *Bull. Eksper. Biol.*, vol. 4 (1978): 563-66.

[7] Petrov, R.V., Stepanenko, R.N., Saipbaev, B.S., and Golenkov, A.K. 1984. A stimulator of antibody producers isolated from human bone marrow cell cultures in healthy body and with different diseases (in Russian). *Bull. Eksper. Biol.* 8 :129-256.

[8] Petrov, R.V., Mikhajlova, A.A., and Zakharova, L.A. 1980. Cell interaction at the level of mature antibody producers; the properties of the bone marrow humoral factor stimulating antibody production. *Ann. Immunology* 131D:161-71.

[9] Marchuk, G.I. 1979. Mathematical models in immunology and their interpretation. In *Modelling and Optimization of Complex Systems*. Proceedings of the IFIP TC-7 Working Conference, Novosibirsk, July 1978, 114-29. Berlin New York Heidelberg Tokyo: Springer-Verlag.
[10] Leibson, H., Marrack, P., and Kappler, J. 1981. B-cell helper factors. Requirement for both IL-2 and another 40000 M factor. *J. Exper. Med.* 154:1681.
[11] Swain, S., Dennert, G., Warner, J., and Dutton, R. 1981. Culture supernatants of a stimulated T-cell line have helper activity that synergizes with IL-2 in the response of B-cells to antigen. *Proc. Natl. Acad. Sci. USA* 78:2517.
[12] Agadzhanyan, N.G., Gurvich, A.E., and Grigor'eva, O.S. (in Russian). *Doklady Akademii Nauk* 242, no. 4 (1978): 968-70.
[13] Marchuk, G.I. *Mathematical Models in Immunology*. New York: Optimization Software, Inc., Publications Division, 1983.

DETERMINATION OF THE DISEASE MODEL PARAMETERS BASED ON OBSERVATIONAL DATA

Sergej M. Zuev

Department of Numerical Mathematics
The USSR Academy of Sciences
Moscow, USSR

Introduction

This paper deals with some probabilistic approaches to the determination of parameters in mathematical models of disease processes, based on observed data.

Wide application of mathematical models in this area is determined primarily by the need to consolidate all the results obtained by different researchers with respect to varied aspects of disease. It allows one to analyze the development of a disease in its totality and test them using the model before they are used in clinical practice.

For various purposes of modelling, stochastic differential equations are frequently used. This paper deals with models represented by systems of ordinary differential equations which describe the change in the number of cell populations participating in the immune–response process [1]. The characteristic feature of these models is that they are constructed to investigate the mechanisms of some "abstract" disease caused by a particular initial dose of antigen. By antigen we mean viruses, bacteria, or malignant tumor cells. That is why modelling and simulation are essential in investigating various diseases. The progress made in immunological studies allows us now to describe systematically the mechanisms of various diseases in terms of the interaction between the antigen and the immune system.

The general mathematical descriptions of various diseases permit us to solve problems of processing and interpreting clinical and laboratory data, which can be analyzed using theoretical results of a mathematical model. Therefore, most practical problems can be reduced to determining the model parameters using the observational data (clinical observations or results of experiments on animals). This can be done because the model parameters calculated on the basis of real data are in fact estimates of the parameters of a living organism—real system, which we try to control by using drugs in order to bring about a desirable dynamics of the disease process. With a mathematical model, choosing appropriately the parameters, one can always obtain a solution, simulating the transition from pathological state to healthy state of the organism. To implement such transitions in the real system under investigation, it is necessary to know the quantitative characteristic effect of a given drug on real parameters. This can be established, for example, by determining the model parameters using the observations made in groups of patients treated with drugs of various doses. The data can be used to make a comparative analysis of the efficiency of various therapeutic methods. Let us also note that the quantitative data on the effect of drugs on the organism's parameters (the model) allow us to envisage the optimal control of the treatment process, which is obviously one of the goals of the application of mathematical models in medicine.

Thus in drawing inferences from experimental data on the basis of mathematical models, determination of unknown parameters using the results of observations plays a key role.

We can clearly distinguish in the modern literature in immunology two directions in solving this problem, depending on the model chosen. If the model is a system of ordinary differential equations, then we are led to an inverse problem. The methods of solution of such a problem are examined in [2]. If the model is stochastic, the solution is based on filtering theory [3], [4], [5]. The observation models we need to treat would appear to be substantially different from these, however.

1. Mathematical models and experimental data

First, let us describe the models and the experimental data under consideration.

The literature on the mathematical modelling of diseases (see, for example, the *Proceedings of the International Conference on Mathematical Modelling in Immunology and Medicine* [6]) shows wide application of ordinary differential equations systems such as the following:

$$\begin{gathered} \dot{x}^i = \sum_k a_k^i x^k + \sum_{k,j} b_{kj}^i x^k x^j + \sum_{k,j,l} c_{kjl}^i x^k x^j x^l + \cdots , \\ x^i(0) = x_0^i, \quad t \in [0,T], \quad i = 1,2,\ldots,n , \end{gathered} \tag{1}$$

$x(t) = (x^1(t), x^2(t), \ldots, x^n(t))$ is the vector of state variables, components of which are both the concentration of cells taking part in immune response and concentration of various substances which influence the disease dynamics. Products on the right side of the system (1) take into account the interaction between state variables. The coefficients a_k^i, b_{kj}^i, $c_{kjl}^i, \ldots$ are assumed to be constant.

Since the immune reaction is the process of interaction between the antigen and cell populations of an organism, the mathematical models describing this process can be represented generally by the system (1). An extensive application of such models is well explained by this fact. It should be noted that (1) might be interpreted as an appropriate feedback control of bilinear systems, which have been extensively studied, e.g., in [7].

Thus, let us suppose the model to be a system of ordinary differential equations:

$$\dot{x}_t = f(x_t,\alpha), \quad x_t\big|_{t=0} = x_0, \quad t \in [0,T] \,, \qquad x_t = (x_t^1, x_t^2, \ldots, x_t^n) \,, \tag{2}$$

where $x_t \in \mathbf{R}^n$ is the vector of state variables, $\alpha \in \mathbf{R}^\ell$ is a vector of coefficients or parameters. Unless otherwise specified, we shall view the vector as a matrix $(m\times 1)$. The peculiarity of the model (2) is that it is *linear* with respect to α. Let us denote the solution of the problem (2) by $x_t(\alpha)$, $t \in [0,T]$.

Let the trajectory of the model variables be obtained by experiments on animals or from clinical observations. This means that there is a set of times

$$\theta = \{t_0, t_1, \ldots, t_N\}, \quad 0 \le t_0 < t_1 < \cdots < t_N \le T \,,$$

and the values of the variables measured at these times are $X = \{x_{t_0}, x_{t_1}, \ldots, x_{t_N}\}$. If the experiment is carried out in a group of m animals, there is a group of trajectories $X_m = \{X^i, \ i = 1,2,\ldots,m\}$, in which the trajectory $X^i = \{x^i_{t_0}, x^i_{t_1}, \ldots, x^i_{t_N}\}$ corresponds to the observation of the ith animal. The experiments are carried out of course with animals of a same strain, and therefore the set of trajectories X_m is the result of an m-times-repeated experiment with one organism.

With animals of varied strain, the result is not a set of trajectories but m_t independent observations for $t \in \theta$, i.e., $X' = \{X^i_t, \ i = 1,2,\ldots,m_t, \ t \in \theta\}$. This case takes place while performing the experiment in the following way. At time $t = 0$, a group of $m = \sum_{t\in\theta} m_t$ animals receive the same quantity of antigen. At $t = t_0 > 0$ the model state variables on m_{t_0} animals are measured. These animals are sacrificed as a result, and a group of $m - m_{t_0}$ survives. Then the measurements are repeated at the instants of time $t_1, t_2, \ldots, t_N$.

We shall discuss the choice of model variables, which are to be measured and the choice of the set θ for the determination of parameter vector α. We deal with these problems in the final part of the paper. In this section we shall only indicate the special features of the problem. The mathematical model, parameters of which we wish to estimate, is deterministic, whereas the real trajectories of state variables are random; thus they cannot be realized in the frame of model (2) with one constant value $\alpha = \overline{\alpha}$.

It should be noted that the random character of the real values of the model state variables can be stipulated not only to account for the measurement error, but also for the influence of various factors not taken into account in the model.

The mathematical model (2), in fact, takes into consideration only those factors which define the dynamics of the process and allow us to explain the mechanism of the phenomenon. That is why in constructing the model a great number of inessential details are discarded, and the model under study becomes "isolated" from the system in which it takes place. If our knowledge about the mechanisms of the phenomenon in hand corresponds to reality, then the factors that do not influence the process would be thrown aside, and the model might qualitatively describe the main features of the process. The influence of these factors is such that real trajectories of the observed variables have short–term random deviations from some general regularity $x_t(\overline{\alpha})$, which we would like to investigate by the model (2). Naturally, we study stationary trajectories, i.e., those which we can regard as the result of m experiments on one organism. Therefore, on the basis of qualitative analysis of the model and the type of the experimental trajectories, it is possible to indicate approximately a set D containing the unknown value $\overline{\alpha}$. For example, D is a set of parameter values corresponding to aperiodic solutions if the observed trajectories are aperiodic, etc.

It is natural to suppose that the model (2) for some $\alpha = \overline{\alpha}$ describes the real trajectories on the average. That is, if we denote the real process by $\{x_t,\ t \in [0,T]\}$ and take X_m as a set of realizations of the process given on θ, we assume that there exists an $\overline{\alpha} \in D$ such that

$$\overline{x}_t = \mathrm{E}(x_t) = x_t(\overline{\alpha}) ,$$

where E is the mathematical expectation operator.

This assumption is the basis for the solution of the problem we are interested in. The methods for the solution of this problem can be divided into deterministic and statistical ones. In the first case we mean the methods of the solution of the inverse problem for equation (2) using observational data $\{\overline{x}_t,\ t \in [0,T]\}$ [2]; in the second, the methods of statistical estimation of the model parameters, based on the use of stochastic models of state [3], [4], [5]. Let us examine the main notions of both methods.

2. Solution of inverse problems by variational methods

Let us assume that the results of the experiment X_m or X' are processed using statistical methods, and we estimate the trajectory $\{\overline{x}_t,\ t \in \theta\}$. For example, the estimates

$$\tilde{x}_t = \frac{1}{m_t} \sum_{i=1}^{m_t} x_t^i, \quad t \in \theta$$

are taken in the capacity of $\bar{x}_t$, $t \in \theta$. These estimates are calculated with the required estimated confidence level. Then α can be estimated by minimizing the mean square deviation:

$$J(\alpha) = \sum_{t \in \theta} (\tilde{x}_t - x_t(\alpha))^2 \tag{3}$$

Note that if we use not the averaged trajectory $\bar{x}_t$ but the sample ensemble X_m, then to obtain the parameter estimate, which is the best in the sense of statistical criteria, we should construct, according to [8], the sum of the variances:

$$J(\alpha) = \sum_{t \in \theta} \frac{1}{m_t} \sum_{i=1}^{m_t} (x_t^i - x_t(\alpha))^{\mathrm{T}} K_t^{-1} (x_t^i - x_t(\alpha)) , \tag{4}$$

where K_t is the covariance matrix which is a priori unknown.

An alternate approach more consistent with immunological physiology is suggested in [2].

According to [2], let us assume the solution $x_t(\alpha^0)$ to correspond to some standard undisturbed state of the system. Let us assume the solution $x_t(\alpha^0)$ to be known.

Furthermore, assume that the observed state $\bar{x}_t$ (called the *disturbed state*) is described by the model (2) with

$$\alpha = \bar{\alpha} = \alpha^0 + \delta\alpha ,$$

where $\delta\alpha$ is assumed to be small as compared to α^0.

Using the assumption $\bar{x}_t = x_t(\alpha^0) + \delta x_t$, we obtain

$$\dot{x}_t(\alpha^0) + \frac{d}{dt}\delta x_t = f(x_t(\alpha^0)+\delta x_t, \alpha^0+\delta\alpha) . \tag{5}$$

Assuming enough smoothness of the right side in (2) and supposing the δx_t to be much smaller than $x_t(\alpha^0)$, let us examine the expansion

$$f(x_t(\alpha^0)+\delta x_t, \alpha^0+\delta\alpha) = f(x_t(\alpha^0),\alpha^0)$$
$$+ A(x_t(\alpha^0),\alpha^0)\delta x_t + F(x_t(\alpha^0),\alpha^0)\delta\alpha + \cdots ,$$

where $A(x,y) = (\partial f_i(x,y)/\partial x_j)$, $F(x,y) = (\partial f_i(x,y)/\partial y_j)$. Substituting this expression into (5) and limiting ourselves to the first-order terms, we obtain

$$\begin{aligned} \frac{d}{dt}\delta x_t - A(x_t^0,\alpha^0)\delta x_t &= F(x_t^0,\alpha^0)\delta\alpha , \\ x_t^0 &= x_t(\alpha^0), \quad \delta x_0 = 0, \quad t \in [0,T] . \end{aligned} \tag{6}$$

Equation (6) describes small deviations of the solution from an undisturbed state. For simplicity of notation, let us introduce the operator

$$L = \frac{d}{dt} - A(x_t^0, \alpha^0)$$

and denote

$$\delta F = F(x_t^0, \alpha^0)\delta\alpha \, . \tag{7}$$

Then (6) assumes the following form:

$$L\delta x = \delta F \, . \tag{8}$$

Let us examine the adjoint equation

$$L^*\varphi^* = p \, , \tag{9}$$

where L and L^* are adjoint operators:

$$(Lg,h) = (g,L^*h) \, , \tag{10}$$

where the inner product $(g,h) = \int_0^T g_t h_t \, dt$, g and h are the elements of a Hilbert space on which the operators L and L^* are defined. The function p will be determined later.

Taking (8), (9) and (10) into account yields

$$(\varphi^*, \delta F) = (\delta x, p) \, . \tag{11}$$

Let us choose $p_i = \delta(t-t_i)$, where $t_i \in \theta$, and $\delta(t-t_0)$ is a delta function. Then from (11) we obtain

$$(\varphi_i^*, \delta F) = \delta_\Sigma x_{t_i}, \quad \delta_\Sigma x_{t_i} = \sum_{k=1}^{n} (\bar{x}_{t_i}^k - x_{t_i}^k(\alpha^0)), \quad i = 1,\dots,N \, .$$

If δF depends linearly on $\delta\alpha$, then for $N = \ell$ ($\delta\alpha \in \mathrm{R}^\ell$) we obtain a system of linear algebraic equations to define the vector $\delta\alpha$.

Thus, after calculating $\delta\alpha$ we can easily define the vector of parameters $\bar{\alpha} = \alpha^0 + \delta\alpha$ corresponding to the observed regime in the system.

It should be noted that this solution depends on the choice of the initial value of parameter vector α^0, i.e., how close the latter is to $\bar{\alpha}$. According to [2], for a more accurate definition of $\bar{\alpha}$, it is possible to construct an iterative process in which the estimates $\bar{\alpha}$ are used as initial data, and the algorithm repeats.

Such an approach seems to be effective in the cases when the experimental data have small variances and the trajectory $\bar{x}_t$ can be estimated with a high confidence level by a small quantity of real trajectories. However, there are examples [9] when such averaging requires a great number of experimental curves. In immunological experiments and clinical observations this involves substantial costs. Moreover, if we speak of the determination of parameters of a single individual, then we should discard averaging. In this case on the right side of the algebraic equation system with respect to $\delta\alpha$

$$(\varphi_i^*, F(x_t^0, \alpha^0)\delta\alpha) = \delta_\Sigma x_{t_i}, \quad i = 1, \ldots, N,$$

$\delta_\Sigma x_{t_i}$ are random. Therefore we can try to solve the problem of filtering of a random component [3], [8] which occurs in real trajectories.

Thus we have examined the statistical approach to the determination of the model parameters.

3. The stochastic model for the description of disturbed motion

Following the idea proposed in section 2, we assume the undisturbed state to correspond to $x_t(\overline{\alpha})$, while the observed or disturbed one is realized in the model (2) with $\alpha = \overline{\alpha} + \delta\alpha_t$, where $\delta\alpha_t \in \mathbf{R}^\ell$ is a function of time. With respect to thei^{th} real trajectory, we assume that

$$x_t^i = x_t(\overline{\alpha} + \delta\alpha_t^i), \quad t \in [0,T], \; x_t^i \in \mathbf{R}^n ,$$

where $x_t(\overline{\alpha}+\delta\alpha_t^i)$ is the solution of problem (2) at $\alpha = \overline{\alpha}+\delta\alpha_t^i$. Since $X^i = \{x_t^i, \; t \in \theta\}$ is the realization of a random process given on the set θ, then the function set

$$\{\delta\alpha_t^i, \; t \in [0,T], \; i = 1,2,\ldots,m\}$$

is also a set of realizations of some random process $\delta\alpha$.

Thus we come to the following stochastic model for the description of the disturbed state of the system:

$$\dot{x}_t = f(x_t, \overline{\alpha}+\delta\alpha_t), \; t \in [0,T] . \tag{12}$$

To proceed, let us assume, like in section 2, the disturbances to be small. To emphasize this fact we should denote the disturbed motion by x_t^ε and rewrite the model (12) as follows:

$$\dot{x}_t^\varepsilon = f(x_t^\varepsilon, \overline{\alpha}+\delta\alpha_t) = \varphi(\varepsilon, x_t^\varepsilon, \overline{\alpha}, \omega) , \tag{13}$$

where x_0^ε is fixed, $\varepsilon > 0$ is a small parameter, $\omega \in \Omega$, and Ω is a sample space of the random process

$$\{x_t^\varepsilon(\omega), \; t \in [0,T], \; \omega \in \Omega\} .$$

We say that random disturbances on the right side of (13) are small if for small $\varepsilon > 0$, x_t is close to $x_t(\overline{\alpha})$ with a high confidence level:

$$\lim_{\varepsilon \to 0} p\{ \sup_{0 \le t \le T} |x_t^\varepsilon - x_t(\overline{\alpha})| > \delta\} = 0$$

for any $\delta > 0$.

This equality means that with small random disturbances, the process realizations (13) lie in the vicinity of the undisturbed trajectory $x_t(\overline{\alpha})$ with probability close to one. The equality can be interpreted as a formalized assumption that the observed trajectories have a common law $x_t(\overline{\alpha})$. To construct the model (13), let us take into consideration the fact that the random deviations $x_t - x_t(\overline{\alpha})$ are short–lived; this means that they are caused by a fast random variable. Therefore in equation (12) we assume

$$\delta\alpha_t = \xi_{t/\varepsilon} ,$$

where ξ_t is a random process with values in $\mathbf{R}^\ell$, $\varepsilon > 0$ is a small parameter. In this case

$$\dot{x}_t^\varepsilon = f(x_t^\varepsilon, \overline{\alpha} + \xi_{t/\varepsilon}), \quad t \in [0,T] , \tag{14}$$

The parameter ε on the right side of the model takes into account the division of variables into fast and slow. In fact, introduce a new variable

$$y_{t/\varepsilon}^e = x_t^\varepsilon$$

to pass to a new time $S = t/\varepsilon$. Then from (14) we find that

$$\dot{y}_S^\varepsilon = \varepsilon f(y_t^\varepsilon, \overline{\alpha} + \xi_s), \quad s \in [0, T/\varepsilon] .$$

The multiplier ε on the right side of this system shows that the state variables are slow. The observed trajectories were assumed earlier to be homogenous. The model (14) implies that the disturbances are of unsystematic nature, i.e., $E\xi_t = 0$ for all t. Moreover, since the random process is fast, let us assume that for arbitrary $S > 0$ and $\delta > 0$, $x \in \mathbf{R}^n$ and for any $t \in [0,T]$,

$$\lim_{\varepsilon \to 0} p\{ |\int_t^{t+S} f(x, \overline{\alpha} + \xi_{S/\varepsilon}) ds - Sf(x, \overline{\alpha})| > \delta\} = 0 . \tag{15}$$

In this case, according to (10), we can show that with $\sup_t E|f(x,\xi_t)^2 < \infty$ for any $T > 0$, $\delta > 0$

$$\lim_{\varepsilon \to 0} p\{ \sup_{0 \le t \le T} |x_t^\varepsilon - x_t(\overline{\alpha})| > \delta\} = 0 .$$

Thus, the model (14) describes small random deviations of the disturbed state from the undisturbed $x_t(\alpha)$.

Condition (15) is satisfied, e.g., if, as $\tau \to \infty$,

$$\mathrm{cov}(\xi_t, \xi_{t+\tau}) \to 0 .$$

Such an assumption is natural, and it agrees with the fact that ξ_t is the fast variable. So, $\mathrm{cov}(\xi_t, \xi_{t+\tau})$ decreases fast enough provided $\tau < T$, where T is the characteristic time of a slow variable change. Strictly speaking, we can assume that the process ξ_t satisfies the strong mixing condition [10] with a mixing coefficient $\gamma(\tau)$, which decreases fast with the growth of τ.

Then taking into account the assumptions concerning the right side of the model (2) and following the lines of [10], we can prove the following theorem.

Theorem. *Let components of a vector function $f(x,y)$ have continuously bounded, through the whole space, first and second partial derivatives. Assume that the random process ξ_t with values in $\mathbf{R}^\ell$ has, with probability 1, piecewise–continuous trajectories and fulfills the strong mixing condition with a coefficient $\gamma(t)$ such that*

$$\int_0^\infty \tau[\gamma(\tau)]^{1/5}\, d\tau < \infty$$

and

$$\sup_{x,\,t} \mathrm{E}|f(x,\xi_t)|^3 < M < \infty .$$

Then the process

$$\zeta_t^\varepsilon = (x_t^\varepsilon - x_t(\overline{\alpha}))/\sqrt{\varepsilon} ,$$

as $\varepsilon \to 0$, converges weakly on the interval $[0,T]$ to the Gauss–Markov process ζ_t^0, which satisfies the system of linear differential equations

$$\dot{\zeta}_t^0 = A(x_t(\overline{\alpha}),\overline{\alpha})\zeta_t^0 + \dot{w}_t^0, \quad \zeta_t^0 = 0 , \tag{16}$$

where w_t^0 is a Gaussian process with independent increments, zero mean and covariance matrix K_t,

$$K_t^{ij} = \mathrm{E}w_t^i w_t^j = \int_0^t Q^{ij}(x_s(\overline{\alpha}))ds , \tag{17}$$

$$Q^{ij}(x) = \lim_{T\to\infty} \frac{1}{T}\int_0^T \int_0^T Q_1^{ij}(x,s,t)\, ds\, dt ,$$

$$Q_1^{ij}(x,s,t) = \mathrm{E}f^i(x,\xi_t)f^j(x,\xi_s), \quad i,j = 1,2,\ldots,n ,$$

$A(x,\alpha)$ is a square matrix,

$$A(x,\alpha) = (\partial f^i(x,\alpha)/\partial x^j) ,$$

where $f^i(x,\alpha)$ and x^j are the elements of vectors $f(x,\alpha)$ and x, respectively.

Thus, assuming only a division of variables in the system into fast and slow components, we have shown that, with essential difference of characteristic times of variable changes, the deviation process $x_t^\varepsilon - x_t(\alpha)$ is approximately Gaussian–Markov and satisfies the equation

$$\frac{d}{dt}(x_t^\varepsilon - x_t(\overline{\alpha})) = A(x_t(\overline{\alpha}),\overline{\alpha})(x_t^\varepsilon - x_t(\overline{\alpha})) + \sqrt{\varepsilon} w_t^0 . \quad (18)$$

Equation (18) determines the correspondence between the set of real (random) trajectories of the model variables and the solution $x_t(\overline{\alpha})$. We can now proceed to solve the problem of filtering the fast random variable ξ_t and estimate the model parameters.

4. Estimation of the model parameters by the maximum–likelihood method

Using our results let us examine the statistical estimation of the model parameters based on the principle of maximum likelihood, as for example in [11].

Thus we have the model as a system of ordinary differential equations

$$x_t = f(x_t,\alpha), \quad x_0 = q, \quad t \in [0,T] , \quad (19)$$

where $x_t(\alpha)$ is a solution of the problem (19), $\alpha \in \mathbf{R}^\ell$ is a vector of unknown parameters. The vector function $f(x,\alpha)$ is linear with respect to α, and its elements have bounded continuous first and second partial derivatives in $x \in \mathbf{R}^n$.

As a result of experimental or clinical observations, the ensemble X_m of real trajectories of the model state variables has been obtained. We assume that the ensemble X_m is given on θ by the set of realizations of the random process $\{x_t^\varepsilon,\ t \in [0,T]\}$. It is assumed that there exists a vector $\overline{\alpha}$ such that

$$x_t(\overline{\alpha}) = \mathrm{E}x_t^\varepsilon, \quad t \in [0,T] .$$

The solution $x_t(\overline{\alpha})$ is regarded as undisturbed motion, and the observed trajectories as the result of small random disturbances of the system (19), i.e.,

$$\dot{x}_t^\varepsilon = f(x_t^\varepsilon, \overline{\alpha} + \xi_{t/\varepsilon}), \quad x_0^\varepsilon = x_0, \quad t \in [0,T] ,$$

where ξ_t is a random process with the values in $\mathbf{R}^\ell$ such that $\mathrm{E}\xi_t = 0$,

$$\lim_{T\to\infty} \frac{1}{T} \int_0^T \int_0^T \mathrm{E}\xi_t^i \xi_s^j \, ds \, dt = g^{ij} ,$$

where ξ_t^i is the ith component of vector ξ_t, and $G = g^{ij}$, $i, j = 1,2,\ldots,\ell$ is its matrix of intensiveness.

Taking into account the results cited above, we have the system of linear differential equations for the deviation $\delta x_t = x_t^\varepsilon - x_t(\overline{\alpha})$:

$$\frac{d}{dt}\delta x_t = A(x_t(\overline{\alpha}),\overline{\alpha})\delta x_t + \dot{w}_t^0 \sqrt{\varepsilon} . \tag{20}$$

To simplify, let us assume G to be diagonal. Then, taking into account linearity of the right side with respect to coefficients and the expression (19), we can rewrite the model for the deviations (20) as follows:

$$\frac{d}{dt}\delta x_t = A(x_t(\overline{\alpha}),\overline{\alpha})\delta x_t + B(x_t(\overline{\alpha})\Gamma_1 \dot{w}_t , \tag{21}$$

where Γ_1 is a matrix with elements $(\varepsilon g^{ij})^{1/2}$; $B(x)$ is such that

$$f(x,\alpha) = B(x)\alpha ;$$

w_t is the standard Wiener process.

Denote $M_t = \mathrm{E}\delta x_t$, $R_t = \mathrm{cov}(\delta x_t, \delta x_t)$. Then using the technique cited in [13], we find that M_t and R_t satisfy the equations

$$\begin{aligned} \dot{M}_t &= A(x_t(\overline{\alpha},\overline{\alpha})M_t , \\ \dot{R}_t &= A(x_t(\overline{\alpha}),\overline{\alpha})R_t + R_t A^{\mathrm{T}}(x_t(\overline{\alpha}),\overline{\alpha}) + C(\overline{\alpha},\Gamma,t) , \end{aligned} \tag{22}$$

where the elements of matrix $C(\overline{\alpha},\Gamma,t)$ have the forms

$$C^{ij}(\overline{\alpha},\Gamma,t) = b^i(x_i(\alpha))\Gamma(b^i(x_t(\alpha)))^{\mathrm{T}}, \quad \Gamma = \Gamma_1\Gamma_1 .$$

Here $b^i(x)$ is the ith row of the matrix $B(x)$. To estimate the vector α and the matrix diagonal Γ for the set X_m =, we write the density function

$$p(X_m|\alpha,\Gamma) .$$

Since the process δx_t is Markov, for a single trajectory we have

$$p(X|\alpha,\Gamma) = \prod_{i=1}^{N} p(\delta x_{t_i}|\delta x_{t_{i-1}}; \alpha,\Gamma) .$$

And since we assume the trajectories to be independent,

$$p(X|\alpha,\Gamma) = \prod_{i=1}^{N} \prod_{j=1}^{N} p(\delta x_{t_i} | \delta x_{t_{i-1}}; \alpha,\Gamma) ,$$

where δx_t^i is a deviation vector of the ith trajectory at time t. It follows from (21) that the conditional densities under the product sign are Gaussian:

$$p(\delta x_{t_i} | \delta x_{t_{i-1}}; \alpha,\Gamma) \tag{23}$$
$$= ((2\pi)^n \det(R_{t_j}))^{1/2} \exp\{-\tfrac{1}{2}(\delta x_{t_j}^i - M_{t_j}^i)^{\mathsf{T}} R_{t_j}^{-1} (\delta x_{t_j}^i - M_{t_j}^i)\} ,$$

where $M_{t_j}^i$ and R_{t_j} are determined by equations (22) on the interval $[t_{j-1}, t_j]$ satisfying the initial conditions:

$$M_{t_{j-1}}^i = \delta x_{t_{j-1}}^i = x_{t_{j-1}}^i - x_{t_{j-1}}^i(\alpha), \; R_{t_{j-1}}^i = 0 .$$

Parameter estimates can be obtained from the condition of the function minimum [8]:

$$\phi(\alpha,\Gamma) = -\ln p(X_m | \alpha,\Gamma) .$$

If instead of X_m we are given a set of independent values X', then the problem becomes simple for $t \in \theta$. M_t, R_t can be found from equations (22) on the interval $[0,T]$ with initial conditions $M_0 = 0$, $R_0 = 0$. This means that $M_t = 0$ for all $t \in [0,T]$. In this case the estimates of parameters α,Γ minimize the following function:

$$\tilde{\phi}(\alpha,\Gamma) = \sum_{t \in \theta} \sum_{i=1}^{m_t} [\ln \det R_t + (x_t^i - x_i(\alpha))^{\mathsf{T}} R_t^{-1} (x_t^i - x_i(\alpha))] . \tag{24}$$

Estimating the parameters in this way, we should take into account two specific features of the experimental data: (1) not all state variables of the model are measured in practical situations and (2) the real trajectories are given not on the whole interval $[0,T]$ but on the discrete set $\theta = \{t_0, t_1, \ldots, t_N\}$.

To define which of the model state variables should be measured during the experiment for the further estimation of parameters, let us note that according to model (20), vector α is chosen in such a way that

$$\mathrm{E}\delta x_t = \mathrm{E}(x_t^e - x_t(\alpha)) = 0 \tag{25}$$

for all $t \in [0,T]$. If this value of the vector α is found, the problem is solved.

Among n variables of the model $x_t = (x_t^1, \ldots, x_t^n)$ let the first k be observed: $x_t^1, x_t^2, \ldots, x_t^k$, $k < n$. With these observations, we can choose a α such that for $i = 1,2,\ldots,k$

$$\mathrm{E}\delta x_t^i = \mathrm{E}(x_t^{\epsilon i} - x_t^i(\alpha)) = 0, \ t \in [0,T] ,$$

i.e., $M_t^i = \dot{M}_t^i = 0$.

But we have a system of equations for the vector M_t

$$\dot{M}_t = A(x_t(\overline{\alpha}),\overline{\alpha})M_t .$$

Therefore, if for all $t \in [0,T]$, substituting into it $M_t^i = \dot{M}_t^i = 0$, $i = 1,2,\ldots,k$, it follows that for all $t \in [0,T]$

$$M_t^i = 0, \ i = k{+}1, k{+}2,\ldots,n .$$

Thus to estimate the model parameters, the data on the dynamics of the first k variables are sufficient.

The second peculiarity of real data leads to equality (25) at the points $t \in \theta$ with various values of the coefficient vector α. Indeed, if for example two solutions $x_t(\alpha_1)$ and $x_t(\alpha_2)$, $\alpha_1 \neq \alpha_2$ intersect at the points $t \in \theta$ in such a way that

$$x_t(\alpha_1) = x_t(\alpha_2) = \mathrm{E}x_t^\epsilon, \ t \in \theta , \tag{26}$$

then the estimation problem does not have a unique solution, since both α_1 and α_2 can be chosen as $\overline{\alpha}$.

In practical problems, the qualitative analysis of the model (19) and the observed trajectories make it possible, as a rule, to define the feasible area D of the coefficients α. For example, we can find the values corresponding to "subclinical" form, "acute form with recovery," and "chronic" form [1].

In this case for fixed D the set θ should be such that for any $\alpha_1 \neq \alpha_2$, $\alpha_1 \in D$, $\alpha_2 \in D$

$$x_{t_k}(\alpha_1) \neq x_{t_k}(\alpha_2)$$

for some t_k. This condition excludes equality (26) and guarantees that the estimates α_m, $m = 1,2,\ldots$, with probability 1 have only one limit point $\overline{\alpha}$. In simple cases we can determine for any set D the possible number of intersections of two solutions belonging to the set

$$\{x_t(\alpha), t \in [0,T], \alpha \in D\} .$$

In these cases $\theta = \{t_0,t_1,\ldots,t_N\}$ should be constructed in such a way that the inequality $N > r$ holds.

We have thus examined a typical situation that one encounters in determining disease model parameters using observational data. Or, what is more precise, we have taken into consideration some special features of this problem, that is the fact that the model is deterministic, whereas the observed trajectories of state variables are of random nature. We can estimate the coefficients of the deterministic model without averaging the real trajectories, so that in particular we can calculate the parameters from a single trajectory. This is significant in determining the characteristics of the immune system of an individual organism. It is worth mentioning that if we try also to take into account the random measurement error, in the real data X_m, we can use the technique presented in [12].

REFERENCES

[1] Marchuk, G.I. *Mathematical Models in Immunology*. New York: Optimization Software, Inc., Publications Division, 1983.

[2] ——————. *Methods of Computational Mathematics*. New York Berlin Heidelberg Tokyo: Springer–Verlag, 1981.

[3] Liptser, R.S., and Shiryaev, A.N. *Statistics of Random Processes*. Vols. 1 and 2. New York Berlin Heidelberg Tokyo: Springer–Verlag, 1977–78.

[4] Balakrishnan, A.V. *Stochastic Differential Systems*. Lecture Notes in Economics and Mathematical Systems, vol. 84. Berlin New York Heidelberg Tokyo: Springer–Verlag, 1978.

[5] Sage, A.P., and Melsa, J.L. *Estimation Theory with Applications to Communications and Control*. New York: McGraw–Hill Publ. Co., 1971.

[6] Marchuk, G.I., and Belykh, L.N., eds. *Mathematical Modeling in Immuno–logy and Medicine*. Proceedings of the IFIP TC–7 Working Conference on Mathematical Modeling in Immunology and Medicine, Moscow, 5–11 July, 1982. Amsterdam New York Oxford: North–Holland Publ. Co., 1983.

[7] Mohler, R.R., and Kolodziej, W.J. 1975. *Modelling and Control in Biochemical Science*. Lecture Notes in Biomathematics, vol. 6. Berlin New York Heidelberg Tokyo: Springer–Verlag.

[8] Balakrishnan, A.V. *Kalman Filtering Theory*. New York: Optimization Software, Inc., Publications Division, 1984.

[9] Zuev, S.M. 1982. Statistical estimation of dynamics parameters of a functional recovery process. In *Matematicheskoe Modelirovanie v Immunologii i Meditsine*, ed. Marchuk, G.I., 93–100. Moscow: Nauka.

[10] Vetsel, A.O., and Frejdlin, M.I. *Fluctuations in Dynamic Systems Caused by Small Random Disturbances* (in Russian). Moscow: Nauka, 1979.

[11] Zuev, S.M. 1983. Statistical estimation of immune response mathematical models coefficients. In *Mathematical Modeling in Immunology and Medicine*, ed. Marchuk G.I. and Belykh, L.N., 255–64. Proceedings of the IFIP TC–7 Working Conference on Mathematical Modeling and Medicine, Moscow, 5–11 July 1982. Amsterdam New York Oxford: North–Holland Publ. Co.

[12] Balakrishnan, A.V. In this volume. A note on the Marchuk–Zuev identification problem.

[13] Evlanov, L.G., and Konstantinov, V.M. *Sistemy so Sluchajnymi Parametrami* (Systems with Random Parameters). Moscow: Nauka, 1976.

V.F. Dem'yanov, and L.V. Vasil'ev
Nondifferentiable Optimization
1985, xvii + 455 pp.
ISBN 0-911575-09-X Optimization Software, Inc.
ISBN 0-387-90951-6 Springer-Verlag New York Berlin Heidelberg Tokyo
ISBN 3-540-90951-6 Springer-Verlag Berlin Heidelberg New York Tokyo

A.A. Borovkov, Ed.
Advances in Probability Theory: Limit Theorems For Sums of Random Variables
1985, XII + 301 pp.
ISBN 0-911575-17-0 Optimization Software, Inc.
ISBN 0-387-96100-3 Springer-Verlag New York Berlin Heidelberg Tokyo
ISBN 3-540-96100-3 Springer-Verlag Berlin Heidelberg New York Tokyo

V.F. Kolchin
Random Mappings
1986, approx. 250 pp.
ISBN 0-911575-16-2 Optimization Software, Inc.

B.T. Polyak
Introduction to Optimization
1986, approx. 450 pp.
ISBN 0-911575-14-6 Optimization Software, Inc.

V.P. Chistyakov, B.A. Sevast'yanov, and V.K. Zakharov
Probability Theory For Engineers
1986, approx. 200 pp.
ISBN 0-911575-13-8 Optimization Software, Inc.

V.F. Dem'yanov, and A.M. Rubinov
Quasidifferential Calculus
1986, approx. 300 pp.
ISBN 0-911575-35-9 Optimization Software, Inc.

N.I. Nisevich, G.I. Marchuk, I.I. Zubikova, and I.B. Pogozhev
Mathematical Modeling of Viral Diseases
1986, approx. 400 pp.
ISBN 0-911575-06-5 Optimization Software, Inc.

Continued on page 382

L. Telksnys, Ed.
Change Detection in Random Processes
1986, approx. 250 pp.
ISBN 0-911575-20-0 Optimization Software, Inc.

V.A. Vasilenko
Spline Functions: Theory, Algorithms, Programs
1986, approx. 280 pp.
ISBN 0-911575-12-X Optimization Software, Inc.

I.A. Boguslavskij
Filtering and Control
1986, approx. 400 pp.
ISBN 0-911575-21-9 Optimization Software, Inc.

R.F. Gabasov, and F.M. Kirillova
Methods of Optimization
1986, approx. 350 pp.
ISBN 0-911575-02-2 Optimization Software, Inc.

V.V. Ivanishchev, and A.D. Krasnoshchekov
Control of Variable Structure Networks
1986, approx. 200 pp.
ISBN 0-911575-05-7 Optimization Software, Inc.

V.G. Lazarev, Ed.
Processes and Systems in Communication Networks
1986, approx. 250 pp.
ISBN 0-911575-08-1 Optimization Software, Inc.

A.N. Tikhonov, Ed.
Problems in Mathematical Physics and Computational Mathematics
1986, approx. 500 pp.
ISBN 0-911575-10-3 Optimization Software, Inc.

G.I. Marchuk, Ed.
Computational Processes and Systems
1986, approx. 350 pp.
ISBN 0-911575-19-7 Optimization Software, Inc.

Continued on page 384

TRANSLITERATION TABLE

R	E	R	E
а А	a	р Р	r
б Б	b	с С	s
в В	v	т Т	t
г Г	g	у У	u
д Д	d	ф Ф	f
е Е	e	х Х	kh
ё Ё	e	ц Ц	ts
ж Ж	zh	ч Ч	ch
з З	z	ш Ш	sh
и И	i	щ Щ	shch
й Й	j	ъ Ъ	"
к К	k	ы Ы	y
л Л	l	ь Ь	'
м М	m	э Э	eh
н Н	n	ю Ю	yu
о О	o	я Я	ya
п П	p		

I.E. Kazakov, and S.V. Mal'chikov
State Space Theory
1986, approx. 350 pp.
ISBN 0-911575-15-4 Optimization Software, Inc.

B.A. Berezovskij, et al.
Multicriteria Optimization: Theory and Applications
1986, approx. 200 pp.
ISBN 0-911575-11-1 Optimization Software, Inc.

Yu.I. Merzlyakov, Ed.
Advances in Probability Theory: Groups and Algebraic Systems With Endpoint Constraints
1986, approx. 300 pp.
ISBN 0-911575-33-2 Optimization Software, Inc.

V.M. Glushkov, V.V. Ivanov, and V.M. Yanenko
Modelling of Evolution Systems
1986, approx. 400 pp.
ISBN 0-911575-32-4 Optimization Software, Inc.